12·14·11   56996   36.68

EDISON COMMUNITY COLLEGE
LIBRARY
1973 EDISON DRIVE
PIQUA, OHI 45356
937-778-8600

COLLEGE

OXFORD MEDICAL PUBLICATIONS

Emergencies in Children's and Young People's Nursing

Published and forthcoming titles in the Emergencies in ... series:

Emergencies in Anaesthesia, Second Edition
Edited by Keith Allman, Andrew McIndoe, and Iain H. Wilson

Emergencies in Cardiology, Second Edition
Edited by Saul G. Myerson, Robin P. Choudhury, and Andrew Mitchell

Emergencies in Children's and Young People's Nursing
Edited by Edward Alan Glasper, Gillian McEwing, and Jim Richardson

Emergencies in Clinical Radiology
Edited by Richard Graham and Ferdia Gallagher

Emergencies in Clinical Surgery
Edited by Chris Callaghan, J. Andrew Bradley, and Christopher Watson

Emergencies in Critical Care
Edited by Martin Beed, Richard Sherman, and Ravi Mahajan

Emergencies in Nursing
Edited by Philip Downing

Emergencies in Obstetrics and Gynaecology
Edited by S. Arulkumaran

Emergencies in Oncology
Edited by Martin Scott-Brown, Roy A.J. Spence, and Patrick G. Johnston

Emergencies in Paediatrics and Neonatology
Edited by Stuart Crisp and Jo Rainbow

Emergencies in Palliative and Supportive Care
Edited by David Currow and Katherine Clark

Emergencies in Primary Care
Chantal Simon, Karen O'Reilly, John Buckmaster, and Robin Proctor

Emergencies in Psychiatry
Basant K. Puri and Ian H. Treasaden

Emergencies in Respiratory Medicine
Edited by Robert Parker, Catherine Thomas, and Lesley Bennett

Emergencies in Trauma
Aneel Bhangu, Caroline Lee, and Keith Porter

Head, Neck and Dental Emergencies
Edited by Mike Perry

Medical Emergencies in Dentistry
Nigel Robb and Jason Leitch

Emergencies in Children's and Young People's Nursing

Edited by

Edward Alan Glasper

Professor of Children's and Young People's Nursing
Faculty of Health Sciences
University of Southampton
Southampton, UK

Gillian McEwing

Lecturer in Nursing (Child)
School of Nursing and Midwifery
Faculty of Health
University of Plymouth
Plymouth, UK

Jim Richardson

Pennaeth Adran (Gofal Teulu)
Head of Division (Family Care)
Cyfadran Iechyd, Chwaraeon
a Gwyddoniaeth/Faculty of Health, Sport & Science
Prifysgol Morgannwg/University of Glamorgan
Glyntaf, Pontypridd, UK

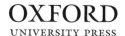

OXFORD
UNIVERSITY PRESS

OXFORD

UNIVERSITY PRESS

Great Clarendon Street, Oxford OX2 6DP

Oxford University Press is a department of the University of Oxford.
It furthers the University's objective of excellence in research, scholarship,
and education by publishing worldwide in

Oxford New York

Auckland Cape Town Dar es Salaam Hong Kong Karachi
Kuala Lumpur Madrid Melbourne Mexico City Nairobi
New Delhi Shanghai Taipei Toronto

With offices in

Argentina Austria Brazil Chile Czech Republic France Greece
Guatemala Hungary Italy Japan Poland Portugal Singapore
South Korea Switzerland Thailand Turkey Ukraine Vietnam

Oxford is a registered trade mark of Oxford University Press
in the UK and in certain other countries

Published in the United States
by Oxford University Press Inc., New York

© Oxford University Press, 2011

The moral rights of the author have been asserted
Database right Oxford University Press (maker)

First published 2011

All rights reserved. No part of this publication may be reproduced,
stored in a retrieval system, or transmitted, in any form or by any means,
without the prior permission in writing of Oxford University Press,
or as expressly permitted by law, or under terms agreed with the appropriate
reprographics rights organization. Enquiries concerning reproduction
outside the scope of the above should be sent to the Rights Department,
Oxford University Press, at the address above

You must not circulate this book in any other binding or cover
and you must impose this same condition on any acquirer

British Library Cataloguing in Publication Data
Data available

Library of Congress Cataloging in Publication Data
Data available

Typeset by Glyph International, Bangalore, India
Printed in China
on acid-free paper through
Asia Pacific Offset

ISBN 978-0-19-954719-7

10 9 8 7 6 5 4 3 2 1

Oxford University Press makes no representation, express or implied, that the
drug dosages in this book are correct. Readers must therefore always check the
product information and clinical procedures with the most up-to-date published
product information and data sheets provided by the manufacturers and the most
recent codes of conduct and safety regulations. The authors and publishers do not
accept responsibility or legal liability for any errors in the text or for the misuse or
misapplication of material in this work. Except where otherwise stated, drug dosages
and recommendations are for the non-pregnant adult who is not breastfeeding.

Foreword

For many children, young people, and their families, their first contact with hospital services will be via the Emergency Department of their local hospital. Most hospitals have now established specific expertise within their Emergency services for children and young people, often through the appointment of children's nurses; however these staff will be operating within the wider Emergency service.

When a child or a young person is sick it is a very worrying and frightening time for them and their families, and their experience will have a long-lasting impact. It is therefore essential that staff are able to quickly and confidently establish a positive rapport to put everyone at their ease and to instil confidence in all those involved.

The children's nurse in an Emergency Department is likely to be the most experienced nurse and it is their responsibility to take the lead in ensuring a positive experience for children, young people, and their families. They do this by working with the whole multi-professional team to develop their knowledge and skills so that they can establish that rapport, communicate well with the child and family, recognise and respect the needs and rights of children and their families, and develop exemplary standards for the observation, assessment, management and delivery of care to children and young people, in an environment tailored for their needs.

In addition the children's emergency nurse requires an extensive range of knowledge and skill in the identification of illness, recognition of signs and symptoms, history taking, potential differential diagnosis, examination and treatment of common children's problems likely to present in an Emergency Department, Walk-in Centre or Acute Admissions Unit, so that he/she is able to advocate in the best interests of the child or young person.

This book has efficiently summarized this range of knowledge into a handy and very readable text, signposting additional sources of information and further reading. It effectively addresses the whole patient journey built on best practice principles of care using a systematic physiological approach, but also grounded in well-established and evidenced philosophies of patient care. I am sure all those working in this field of children's nursing will find this book a useful and easily accessible source of knowledge and point of reference.

Liz Morgan
Chief Nurse and Director of Education
Great Ormond Street Hospital for Children NHS Trust

Acknowledgements

We would like to thank Hayley Coates, Ophthalmic Photographer, for taking the photographs used in chapter 9.

We thank Patsy Bedford, Ophthalmic Nurse Practitioner at Southampton Eye Casualty, and Mr Narman Puvanchandra MB BChir, MA, FRCOphth, Ophthalmology Spr Southampton Eye Unit, for their input of knowledge, experience, and advice.

With thanks for her advice to Faith Constantine, Senior Paediatric Radiographer, Derriford Hospital, Plymouth.

Contents

Detailed contents

List of Contributors

Victoria Abbott
Senior Paediatric A&E Sister
Emergency Department
East Surrey Hospital
Redhill, UK

Louise Adams
Paediatric Staff Nurse
Emergency Department
Southampton General Hospital
Southampton, UK

Sarah Barton
Lead Paediatric Nurse
Accident and Emergency
  Department
Basildon and Thurrock University
  Hospital Foundation Trust
Essex, UK

Karen Blair
Lecturer, Child Nursing
Department of Health, Wellbeing
  and Family
Canterbury Christ Church
  University
Canterbury, UK

Jill Bleiker
Teaching Fellow in Radiology
Centre for Medical Imaging
University of Exeter
Exeter, UK

Neil Bloxham
Charge Nurse and Clinical
  Educator
Children's High Dependency Unit
Derriford Hospital
Plymouth, UK

Eileen Brennan
Nurse Consultant Paediatric
  Nephrology
Great Ormond Street Hospital
  for Children
London, UK

Maria Brenner
Head of Children's Nursing
School of Nursing, Midwifery and
  Health Systems
University College Dublin
Dublin, ROI

Keith Bromwich
Nurse Practitioner
Rugby Urgent Care/Walk in
  Centre
Hospital of St Cross/UHCW
  NHS Trust
Rugby, UK

Mark Broom
Senior Lecturer
Cyfadran Iechyd, Chwaraeon a
  Gwyddoniaeth/
Faculty of Health,
  Sport & Science
Prifysgol Morgannwg/University
  of Glamorgan
Glyntaf, Pontypridd, UK

Pauline Cardwell
Teaching Fellow, Children's
  Nursing
School of Nursing and Midwifery
Medical Biology Centre
Queens University Belfast
Belfast, UK

Pauline Carson
Teaching Fellow, Children's
  Nursing
School of Nursing and Midwifery
Medical Biology Centre
Queens University Belfast
Belfast, UK

Stefan Cash
Senior Lecturer Clinical Skills/
  Child Health
Birmingham City University
Birmingham, UK

Margaret Chambers
Lecturer in Nursing
Faculty of Health
University of Plymouth
Plymouth, UK

Carol Chamley
Senior Lecturer and Course
  Director
Children and Young People's
  Nursing
Coventry University
Coventry, UK

Alan Charters
Queen Alexander Hospital
Portsmouth Hospitals Trust
Portsmouth, UK

Karen Currell
Senior Lecturer in Child
  Nursing
University of Huddersfield
Huddersfield, UK

Mary Donnelly
Senior Lecturer in Children's
  Nursing
University of Hertfordshire
Hatfield, UK

Amy Dopson
Child Health Tutor
University of Surrey
Guildford, UK

Sarah Doyle
Urology Advanced Paediatric
  Nurse Practitioner
Alder Hey NHS Foundation
  Trust
Liverpool, UK

Amanda Driffield
Lecturer Children's Nursing
Child Health Studies
School of Healthcare
University of Leeds
Leeds, UK

Judith Ellis
Executive Dean
Faculty of Health and Social Care
London Southbank University
London, UK

Andrew Fitzell
Paediatric Nurse Lead
Family Breaks Devon, Action For
  Children
Devon, UK

Helen Frizell
Lead Educator in Maternal and
  Child Health
Basingstoke and
  Northamptonshire NHS
  Foundation Trust
Basingstoke, UK

Chris Gale
Lecturer-Practitioner in Child
  and Adolescent Mental
  Health and Brookvale Youth
  Mental Health Team
University of Southampton
Southampton, UK

Laura Gilbert
Senior Lecturer in Child Nursing
Department of Health,
  Wellbeing and the Family
Faculty of Health and Social Care
Canterbury Christ Church
  University
Canterbury, UK

Stephen Gill
Paediatric Dermatology Nurse
Dunedin Hospital
Dunedin, New Zealand

Edward Alan Glasper
Professor of Children's and Young
  People's Nursing
Faculty of Health Sciences
University of Southampton
Southampton, UK

Elizabeth Gormley-Fleming
Senior Lecturer in Children's
  Nursing
University of Hertfordshire
Hatfield, UK

Laura Hall
Paediatric Staff Nurse
Emergency Department
Southampton General
  Hospital
Southampton, UK

Jan Heath
Skills for Practice Lead
Southampton University
  Hospitals Trust
Southampton General Hospital
Southampton, UK

Kevin Humphreys
Lecturer
School of Health Sciences
University of Southampton
Southampton, UK

Sian Ireland
Consultant in Emergency
  Medicine
Department Lead for
  Paediatric Emergency
  Medicine
Royal Cornwall Hospital
Truro, UK

Emma Jasper
Whitehorse Assessment Unit
Derriford Hospital
Plymouth, UK

Melanie Kelly
Ward Manager
Royal Cornwall Hospital Trust
Truro, UK

Kate Khair
Nurse Consultant in
  Haemophilia
Great Ormond Street Hospital
  for Children
London, UK

Suzanne Knight
Emergency Nurse Practitioner/
  Senior Sister, Emergency
  Department
Southampton University Hospitals
  NHS Trust
Southampton, UK

Gillian W. Langmack
Lecturer - Child Branch
School of Nursing
University of Nottingham, and
  Lincoln County Hospital
Lincoln, UK

Gillian M. Lewis
Child Health Nurse Lecturer
Capital and Coast Health District
  Health Board
Wellington Hospital
Wellington South, New Zealand

Lorraine Major
Paediatric Nurse Practitioner in
  Maternal and Child Health
Basingstoke & Northamptonshire
  NHS Foundation Trust
Basingstoke, UK

Lindy May
Nurse Consultant, Paediatric
  Neurosurgery
Parrot Ward
Great Ormond Street Hospital
  for Children
London, UK

Gillian McEwing
Lecturer in Nursing (Child)
School of Nursing and Midwifery
Faculty of Health
University of Plymouth
Plymouth, UK

Brian McGowan
Lecturer
School of Nursing
Faculty of Life and
  Health Sciences
University of Ulster
Jordanstown, UK

Amanda Miller
Lecturer
University of Salford
Salford, UK

Simon Minford
Course Leader, Paediatric
  Clinical Examination
Liverpool John Moores
  University
Liverpool, UK

Philomena Morrow
Nurse Lecturer
Medical Biology Centre
Queens University Belfast
Belfast, UK

Gary Mountain
Senior Child Health Lecturer
School of Healthcare
University of Leeds
Leeds, UK

Iain Neely
Clinical Nurse Educator
Children's Emergency
  Nottingham University
  Hospital
Nottingham, UK

Jody Neville
Staff Nurse, Paediatric
  Assessment Unit/HDU
Royal Cornwall Hospital
Truro, UK

Annie Noble
Paediatric Resuscitation
  Officer
University Hospitals Bristol
  NHS Foundation Trust
Bristol, UK

Sharon Nurse
Senior Teaching Fellow
School of Nursing and
  Midwifery
Queens University Belfast
Belfast, UK

Michele O'Grady
Senior Sister
Children's Emergency Department
Watford General Hospital
West Hertfordshire Hospitals
  NHS Trust
Watford, UK

Helen Pearson
Staff Nurse
Paediatric Oncology
The Royal Marsden Hospital NHS
  Foundation Trust
Surrey, UK

Jenny Pinfield
Senior Lecturer in Child Health
Institute of Health and Society
University of Worcester
Worcester, UK

Rebecca Platt
Senior Sister & ENP
Children's Emergency Department
Watford General Hospital
West Hertfordshire Hospitals
  NHS Trust
Watford, UK

Emma Powditch
Sister
Eye Casualty
Southampton Eye Unit
Southampton University Hospitals
  NHS Trust
Southampton, UK

Sarah Price
Nurse Practitioner
Eye Casualty
Southampton General Hospital
Southampton University Hospitals
  NHS Trust
Southampton, UK

Jennie Quiddington
Lecturer
School of Nursing and Midwifery
University of Southampton
Southampton, UK

Christine Rhodes
Senior Lecturer Child Nursing/
  Principal Lecturer
Lead for Service User Involvement
School of Human & Health
  Sciences
University of Huddersfield
Huddersfield, UK

Jim Richardson
Pennaeth Adran (Gofal Teulu)
  Head of Division (Family Care)
Cyfadran Iechyd, Chwaraeon
  a Gwyddoniaeth/Faculty of
  Health, Sport & Science
Prifysgol Morgannwg/University of
  Glamorgan
Glyntaf, Pontypridd, UK

Dawn Ritchie
Lecturer (Child Health)
School of Nursing
University of Nottingham
Queen's Medical Centre
Nottingham, UK

Giovanni Riva
Senior Paramedic
Welsh Ambulance Services
  NHS Trust
Wales, UK

Sheila Roberts
Senior Lecturer
Children's Nursing Team
University of Hertfordshire
Hatfield, UK

Jennie Robertson
Sister, Emergency Department
Southampton University Hospitals
  NHS Trust
Southampton, UK

Sarah Shelley
Named Nurse for Safeguarding
  Children
Safeguarding Children Team
Plymouth Hospital
Plymouth, UK

Mary Smith
Senior Lecturer and SCPHN
  Award Leader
Cyfadran Iechyd, Chwaraeon a
  Gwyddoniaeth/
Faculty of Health, Sport & Science
Prifysgol Morgannwg/University
  of Glamorgan
Glyntaf, Pontypridd, UK

Sue Smith
Principal Lecturer in Children's
  Public Health
University of Huddersfield
Huddersfield, UK

Hannah Solomon
Staff Nurse
Royal Cornwall Hospital Trust
  Treliske
Truro, UK

Magi Sque
Senior Lecturer
School of Health Sciences
University of Southampton
Southampton, UK

Kathryn Summers
Canterbury Christchurch
  University
Canterbury, UK

John Thain
Senior Lecturer in Children's
  Nursing
School of Health and Wellbeing
University of Wolverhampton
Walsall, UK

Shelley Thomas
Matron
University of Bristol Dental
  Hospital and Bristol Eye
  Hospital
Bristol, UK

Denise Toplis
Senior Staff Nurse
Royal Devon and Exeter NHS
    Foundation Trust
Exeter, UK

Ruth Trengove
Clinical Development Nurse
Paediatric High Dependency Unit
Louisa Cary Ward
Torbay Hospital
Torquay, UK

Jacqueline Vasey
Senior Lecturer, Child Nursing
University of Huddersfield
Queensgate, UK

Jacki Wain
Staff Nurse
Paediatric Assessment Unit
Royal Berkshire NHS
    Foundation Trust
UK

Sandra Walters
Sister
Emergency Department
Southampton General Hospital
Southampton, UK

Andy Watson
Charge Nurse
Children's Emergency
Nottingham University Hospital
Nottingham, UK

Katy Weaver
Brighton Children's Hospital
Brighton, UK

Caroline Williams
Practice Development Nurse
    Emergency Unit
West Wales General Hospital
Carmarthen, UK

Jo Williams
Advanced Nurse Practitioner
    ENT
Birmingham Children's Hospital
Birmingham, UK

James Wilson
Lecturer in Mental Health
School of Health Sciences
University of Southampton
Southampton, UK

Jane Wilson
Senior Sister
Paediatric Accident and
    Emergency
St George's Hospital
London, UK

Maureen Wiltshire
Paediatric Lead/Senior Nurse
Southampton NHS Walk In
    Centres
Southampton, UK

Janet Youd
Nurse Consultant
Emergency Care
Calderdale & Huddersfield NHS
    Foundation Trust
Huddersfield, UK

Principles of care

⑦ **Children's rights**

Introduction
- A convention is an agreement between countries to obey the same law.
- Once a country has ratified a convention it agrees to obey the rules that are set out in the convention.

The United Nation's Convention on the Rights of the Child (UNCRC)
- The UNCRC (United Nations General Assembly 1989) applies to all children until their eighteenth birthday.
- Ratified by the government of the United Kingdom (UK) on 16 December 1991.
- The government of the UK must ensure that all children enjoy the rights set out in the convention, except in those areas where the government has entered a specific reservation.
- Separated into 54 'articles' —most give children social, economic, cultural or civil and political rights; some describe how governments must publicize or implement the convention.
- Some children and young people, e.g. disabled children, have additional rights to ensure that their needs are met.

What the UNCRC means
- The convention came into force in the UK on 15 January 1992.
- All children in the UK have specific rights which include the following which are important for health and social care professionals to be aware of and respect:
  - The right to life and normal growth and development
  - The right to a family name and nationality
  - The right, wherever possible, to be cared for by their own parents
  - The right to have their views respected and their best interests to be taken into consideration
  - The right to health, healthcare, and social security
  - The right to access information held about them
  - The right to education, leisure, culture, and the arts
  - The right to think freely and to practise their religion
  - The right to privacy and confidentiality.

The Committee for the Rights of the Child
- The Committee for the Rights of the Child is responsible for ensuring that each of the countries signed up to the UNCRC follows its rules.
- The Committee is made up of an international body of experts in children's rights.

The Children's Commissioners
- Children's Commissioners are responsible for promoting children's views and the rights enshrined in the UNCRC.

Further reading

UK Department for Education and Skills (2003). Every child matters (Green Paper). London: The Stationery Office

Franklin B (2001). The new handbook of children's rights (2nd edition). London: Taylor and Francis Ltd

United Nations General Assembly (1989). United Nations Convention on the Rights of the Child. UN Treaty collection. http://treaties.un.org/Pages/ViewDetails.aspx?src=TREATYandmtdsg_no=1V-11andchapter=4andlang=en

⑦ Consent to treatment in children and young people

Definition
- Informed consent is a legal state whereby persons are said to have given their consent based on a full understanding of the facts, implications and consequences of a given action.
- In order to give informed consent a person must first be competent to do so.

Age of consent
- In the United Kingdom, a young person is considered to be a minor until he/she reaches their eighteenth birthday.
- This means that all young people over the age of eighteen years who are competent to consent have the right in law to give consent to treatment and to refuse treatment.
- This consent or refusal cannot be overridden by anyone else, including those with parental responsibility for the young person.

Parental responsibility
- Parents or guardians may have the right to give consent to medical, surgical and dental treatment on behalf of a minor for whom they have parental responsibility.
- Mothers automatically have parental responsibility for their children.
- Fathers have parental responsibility for their children if they were married to the mother at the time of conception or birth, or if they got married to her later.
- Unmarried fathers have parental responsibility if they have acquired legal responsibility for their child through one of these three routes: (after 1 December 2003 stated in The Adoption and Children Act 2002) by being named on the birth certificate with the mother, by a parental responsibility agreement with the mother, by a parental responsibility order, made by a court (Department of Health 2001).

Consent and young persons aged 16 and 17 years
- Persons aged 16 and 17 have a statutory right to give consent.
- However, they are not considered to be adults in law, so those who make decisions on their behalf must be able to justify such decisions and document them.
- Where a young person aged 16 or 17 years is unable to give consent, parents or guardians may consent on their behalf.
- A health professional may act in the 'best interests' of a young person when they are unable to do so, and where a parent or guardian is also unable to give consent on their behalf.
- While young persons have a right to give consent to medical, surgical and dental treatment, they do not have the right to refuse treatment

that may be life saving, and any such refusal can be overridden by the parents, guardians or the court.
- Where the treatment required by the young person is judged to be not in their best interests, the parents or guardians could seek to make them a ward of court or ask for the matter to be brought before the court.

Children aged under the age of 16 years
- Do not automatically have the right to consent to treatment. The validity of the child's consent depends upon whether or not he or she is deemed to be competent to give consent.
- Gillick competence is a term used in medical law to decide whether a child of 16 years or under is able to consent to his or her own medical treatment, without the need for parental permission or knowledge.
- The decision as to whether a child is Gillick competent or not relies on the judgement of the individual clinician.
- The Fraser Guidelines relate specifically to a child's right to consent to contraceptive treatment while under the age of 16 years.

For young people over 18 years the Mental Capacity Act needs to be considered
- The NMC (2002) states that you should presume that every adult patient is legally competent unless otherwise assessed by a suitably qualified practitioner.
- A patient is legally competent if they have the capacity to understand and retain information regarding the treatment or procedure, and can use this to make an informed choice.
- If a person is sectioned under the Mental Health Act 1983 they may have their rights to consent restricted (www.dh.gov.uk).

Capacity is defined by the Mental Capacity Act (2005) as 'the everyday ability to make decisions or take actions that influence their life'.
It has 5 key principles:
- A presumption of capacity
- An individual is supported to make their own decisions
- Unwise decisions do not indicate that a person does not have the capacity to consent
- All actions (decisions) must be performed with the intention of best interest for the individual at all times
- Everything done for or on behalf of the person must be the least restrictive option, with minimal impact on their basic rights and freedoms.

The Mental Capacity Act (2005) also defines what is considered to be incapacity. This is when a person is unable to make or communicate decisions because of an impairment or disturbance in the function of their mind or brain at the time a decision has to be made. An assessment process should be used, and the Act gives some suggestions of criteria:
- Failing to demonstrate relevant understanding of the information given to them when making a decision
- Being unable to retain information relevant to the decision

- Being unable to demonstrate that they can consider the pros and cons of information given to them
- Being unable to communicate their decision by any means.

Following an assessment, a decision will be made on the patient's behalf if this is considered to be in their best interests. This will be considered a duty of care.

Further reading

Dimond B. (2001a) Legal aspects of consent 7: young people aged 16–17 years. *British Journal of Nursing* 10:732–33
Dimond B. (2001b) Legal aspects of consent 8: children under the age of 16 years. *British Journal of Nursing* Department of Health (2001) Consent – what you have a right to expect, a guide for parents. London: DH 10:797–99

⑦ Communicating with a child in preparation for an emergency procedure

The hospital environment can be very frightening both for children and for their parents/carers, especially if it is the child's first experience of hospital. When a child is bought to the accident and emergency department they may be feeling unwell and experiencing some pain or discomfort. They also find themselves in a strange environment where they may experience things that are frightening, unfamiliar, and often invasive and painful. Combined with panic, this fear and unfamiliarity can make it difficult for the child and their family to make sense of the situation, and may affect their behaviour and responses.

Some children will cope with their experience of an emergency department (ED) or an emergency procedure with minimal distress or anxiety, especially when in a parent's presence. It is the parents who largely facilitate clinical access to a child and enhance their cooperation.

Preparation

Preparation uses play to help the child to understand his or her illness and treatment/procedures, share information, and discuss options and to provide the opportunity to correct any misconceptions. Preparation helps to:

- Educate and help them to understand their illness, injury or the required procedure
- Aid compliance, and the promotion of choice aids co-operation
- Correct any misconceptions or fantasies
- Reduce short/long term effects of a hospital admission/visit
- Increase the child's ability to cope with treatment and procedures
- Give the child an opportunity to express feelings (i.e. anxiety, fear)
- Encourage them to trust hospital staff
- Return the element of control
- Enable informed consent
- Speed recovery.

In emergency situations the opportunity to prepare a child for a procedure is very limited. However, preparation does not need to be extensive or elaborate. Simply sharing information sensitively at the appropriate level can be very beneficial, and can help to reduce distress and anxieties in patients and carers considerably. If you do not have time to prepare the child, you may be able to involve them during the procedure: you could give them simple choices, such as whether they would like to sit or lie down, or whether they would like to watch or look away, in an effort to return the element of control.

You must always be honest to build and maintain trust, which will influence the relationship made with the child. Also, you should never make promises that you are unable to keep.

Some techniques you could use to prepare a child and family for a procedure are:
• Role play/modelling, to act out the procedure
• Doll play
• Discussion/explaining the procedure
• Photo books showing a collection of photos put together to show the child what happens during the required procedure (DH, 2003)
• Story books of hospital experiences
• Look at real equipment if appropriate and safe
• Discuss any available choices and make a plan of how the patient would like the procedure to be performed.

Your choice of technique for any form of therapeutic play should always be based on the child's age and stage of development, and should take into account any special needs/requirements to ensure it is suitable and beneficial.

Further reading

Chambers M. (2008) Therapeutic play in hospital. In: Kelsey J., McEwing G. (eds). Clinical Skills in Child Health Practice. Edinburgh: Elsevier. Pp. 18–26
Cleaver K, Webb J (eds). (2007) Emergency Care of Children and Young People. Oxford: Blackwell Publishing

⑦ Preserving autonomy and respect

The Universal Declaration of Human Rights (www.un.org) states in Article 1 that, 'All human beings are born free and equal in dignity and rights'. This includes children and young people under the age of 18, who may have particular need to have their dignity respected because of their developmental stage and relative immaturity.

Article 3 of the UN Convention on the Rights of the Child (www.unicef. org) states that, 'In all actions concerning children the best interests of the child shall be a primary concern'.

In order to ensure a respectful and humane relationship, children's and young people's nurses will have to be mindful of children's rights in all aspects of their work. These will include:

- The right to be treated in a kind and respectful manner
- The right to be heard and involved in discussions
- The right to be treated fairly
- The right to be treated in the same way as others, i.e. equity and freedom from discrimination
- The right to be given information and told the truth
- The right to be protected from harm
- The overall right to have their fundamental dignity protected.

All of these rights will also apply to the child's family and carers, since the child may be immature in their development and understanding and therefore dependent on their primary carers and wider family.

It is particularly important that the child and their family are protected from being judged or treated negatively on the basis of perceived or assumed attributes. Such prejudice can be highly damaging and distressing, and might potentially be based on such factors as:

- Ethnicity and nationality
- Skin colour
- Age
- Gender
- Belief and religion (or lack of this)
- Social origin and class
- Language, dialect and accent
- Disability
- Political viewpoint.

Respecting rights and treating children and their families respectfully and with humanity promotes their ability to act autonomously. This might be achieved by:

- Taking time to listen and hear
- Trying to understand the child and family's perception and experience of the situation they find themselves in
- Trying to gauge the child and family's understanding of the situation and identifying learning and information needs to underpin coping and autonomy
- Being open in communication which is pitched for understanding without being patronising

- Respecting cultural beliefs and needs based on these, e.g. health beliefs, modesty requirements, etc.
- Being aware of yourself and the impression you give others
- Being committed to antidiscriminatory practice
- Being committed to protecting and promoting child and family autonomy

Further reading

Alderson, P. (2008) Young Children's Rights: exploring beliefs, principles and practice. Second edition. London: Jessica Kingsley.
Invernizzi, A, Williams, J. (2008) Children and Citizenship. London: Sage.
Universal Declaration of Human Rights (www.un.org)

⑦ **Health care policy standards for children's emergency care**

The Direction of Travel Consultation published by the Department of Health (2006) highlights the necessity of integrating urgent and emergency services in such a way that people get the right care at the right time as close to their homes as is clinically safe. With the reduction of out-of-hours general practitioner services, such policy recommendations are crucial in the care of sick children requiring urgent, unscheduled, and emergency care. The primary problems that families find frustrating are delays and a disjointed health care journey. Parents want an appropriate response to an urgent need, such as how to care for their sick child, through advice from an agency such as NHS Direct or a Walk-in Centre. In addition, they require a rapid response in an emergency situation, either from an emergency department or from a paediatric emergency assessment unit. Importantly, families want their children assessed and cared for at the point of first contact by a skilled workforce. This has important ramifications for emergency departments and walk-in centres that may have insufficient trained children's nurses as part of the caring team. It should be stressed that some nurses, especially those who have registered after undertaking an adult field of practice course, may be practising outside the boundaries of their NMC registerable qualification.

As safety is of paramount importance, aspects of the 'Direction of Travel' policy document, such as the workforce and skill mix, must be resolved.

The 'Direction of Travel' is one of many policies that are pertinent to the emergency department and emergency care. Crucially, standard 7 of the National Service Framework (NSF) for Children, Young People and Maternity Services has set a bench mark which states that children and young people should be cared for in a separate paediatric emergency area/department where a lead adolescent professional role has been established. Importantly nurses should ascertain:

- Where children and young people are triaged, to avoid children experiencing hostile sights and sounds
- That privacy, dignity and safety are assured
- That the ambience and facilities where children are cared for are appropriate
- That there are facilities for breast-feeding, nappy changing, etc.
- That facilities for disabled children are available
- That the ratio of paediatric staff including staff with adolescent mental health experience is appropriate
- That there is a lead adolescent role established within the emergency department
- That there are links to social workers for young person admissions (e.g. self harmers)
- The quality of play areas
- The availability of play specialist
- The quality of waiting accommodation.

The presence of appropriately trained children's nurses in all areas where children and young people are seen as emergencies is of prime importance.

Further reading

Department of Health (2006) Direction of travel for urgent care: A discussion document. Crown Copyright
Department of Health (2004) The National Service Framework for Children, Young People and Maternity Services. www.dh.gov.uk

⑦ Communication through play

Good communication skills are essential when interacting with children in any situation but in a hospital setting there are other things to be considered. The child may not absorb information so easily due to distress, fear or pain and there will be lots of sounds and distraction.

Points to consider:
- Assess the child's needs. A distressed child will be much more receptive if calmed and reassured before attempting any discussion. They may have hearing/visual impairment or special needs. English may be their second language, which will need to be fully reflected. Additionally, children with special needs may use specific communication techniques such as makaton.
- Be aware of body language – remember children see the world very differently to us and may spend a lot of time seeing things from an adult's knee/waist height for example. Always get down to their level.
- Eye contact and facial expression can have a huge effect on the way children perceive and respond.
- Tone of voice – children can pick up on anxieties and emotions projected in our voices.
- Language – this should always be age and stage appropriate. Try to keep words simple and consistent (don't use different words to describe the same thing).
- Involve the parents/carers (and siblings if appropriate) wherever possible, as the child may respond better to information from carers. It will also help them to feel involved when they are often feeling worried and helpless and hopefully allay some of their concerns. Also, carers usually know their child best and can help to explain things in a way their child will understand.
- Repeat information if necessary to allow the child and family to absorb it.
- Allow and encourage the family to ask questions. They may be feeling unsure but scared to ask questions, through fear of getting in the way, delaying necessary procedures or just sounding 'silly'.
- Some children may have debilitating fears such as 'needle phobia' where special techniques such as guided imagery may need to be used.

Distraction

Although opportunities to prepare children are limited, you can still make use of other therapeutic play techniques, such as distraction, wherever possible, which will help to reduce levels of stress, anxiety and procedural pain in some cases.

Distraction is a therapeutic play technique that involves using simple activities/toys or games to distract the child and act as a temporary barrier between the child's mind and the actual procedure for the duration of the procedure. It helps to reduce anxiety, aid compliance, encourage the child to be more relaxed and in turn reduce perceptions of pain.

Some distraction techniques include:
- Simple two way conversation on their choice of topic
- Books, preferably interactive, e.g. musical, find the object or optical illusion books

- Puzzles
- Music/videos/DVDs
- Telling jokes
- Simple games like 'I spy' and 'snap'
- Counting games ('how many butterflies can you see on the wall?')
- Finger puppets and story telling
- Singing/musical toys
- Interactive toys like pop-up toys and wind up animals
- Bubbles.

It sometimes helps to let the child choose the activity they would like to do during the procedure and to be adaptable. It is important to constantly assess the child's involvement and responses throughout, and to adopt an alternative technique when the child loses interest or if the original plan isn't as successful as hoped.

Nonpharmacologic interventions, such as the therapeutic play techniques mentioned, are not designed to replace other methods of pain control, but can be powerful adjuncts in reducing anxiety and pain in children and young people.

Further reading

Weaver K, Groves J (2007). Fundamental aspects of play in hospital. In: Glasper A, Aylott M, Prudhoe G, eds. Fundamental Aspects of Children's Nursing Procedures. Quay Books: London
Sinha M, Christopher NC, Fenn R, Reeves L (2006). Evaluation of Nonpharmacologic Methods of Pain and Anxiety Management for Laceration Repair in the Pediatric Emergency Department. *Pediatrics* 117:1162–8
Weaver K, Battrick C, Glasper EA (2007). Developing a Hospital Play Guideline and Protocol for Sick Children with Debilitating Fears. *Journal of Children's and Young People's Nursing* 1:143–9

① Breaking significant news during an emergency

Giving significant news is a task which most professionals have little experience of and find incredibly difficult. How this news is given will affect the adjustment and future coping mechanisms of the recipients.

Significant news is any information which adversely and seriously affects an individual's view of their future.

- Its impact depends on the gap between the patient's expectations and the reality of the situation.
- Religion, race, culture, and previous experiences of both patient and staff will affect how the information is given and received.
- Usually the most senior clinician gives the information; this should be someone who will have ongoing involvement in the patient's care.
- The primary nurse should attend the interview; this enables them to support the family after the event and feedback to colleagues as they will have knowledge of what information was given and the terminology used.
- Rarely will the recipient remember all the information given, so things may have to be repeated.
- Parents should be told together so they receive the same information and can support each other.
- Failure to provide sensitivity, support, honesty and realism can lead to the recipients experiencing fear, anxiety and despair.
- Participate in the recipient's decision-making if expert knowledge is required.
- Be willing to discuss the possibility of death if this could be an outcome.

Several steps are suggested for professionals to progress through when breaking significant news.

Although there are guidelines on how to break significant news, the approach used will need to be adapted on an individual basis.

Further reading

Dias L, Chabner BA, Lynch T, Penson R (2003). Breaking Bad News: A Patient's Perspective. *The Oncologist* 8:587–96

Gavaghan S, Carroll D (2002). Families of critically ill patients and the effect of nursing interventions. *Dimensions of Critical Care Nursing* 21:64–71.

http://www.breakingbadnews.co.uk/guidelines.asp

Price J, McNeilly P (2008). Breaking bad news to parents. In Kelsey J, McEwing G (eds) (2008). Clinical Skills in Child Health Practice. Elsevier: Edinburgh, pp. 388–394

⑦ Writing patient information leaflets for families discharged from emergency environments

Standard 7 of the National Service Framework (NSF) for Children, Young People and Maternity Services has set a benchmark stating that written child- and young person-focused information for ongoing care must be available for all appropriate conditions when children are discharged from emergency care environments.

- Information leaflets should be available and used in emergency care areas.
- Where appropriate such leaflets, for ongoing care and so on, should be translated into other languages.
- There should be a lead professional within the emergency care areas who has the responsibility for developing policies/protocols for children, young people and their families.

Key points when designing discharge information material include making it:
- Comprehensible – ensure the reader will be able to understand the text
- Written for a child, a young person or a family carer as appropriate
- Usable/readable – can the reader apply the information?
- Accessible – can the reader find the information easily, or is it lost in a sea of ambiguous text?

Before rushing to your computer to produce your information leaflet

- Know your purpose. What is it you want to achieve for this child on discharge from an emergency situation?
- Know your subject. Do you have the knowledge to write the material?
- Know your audience – involve children, young people or carers at the design stage.
- Know the setting under which your family member will read the leaflet.

When writing information leaflets ensure that they contain

- 'Awareness information' which allows the reader to relate to the contents of the information leaflet.
- 'How-to information' which allows your reader to optimise the purpose of the leaflet. (For individuals with poor literacy consider comic style embellishments as in Jones et al 2000.)
- 'Principles' information which gives easy to understand focused information, e.g. on why certain drugs actually work. This is important for medication compliance.

It is important to stress that health care professionals such as nurses may not possess the necessary skills to write information leaflets. Seeking help, e.g. from a librarian, may help in the production of a leaflet that contains up-to-date evidence-based information, and importantly is usable for the child, young person or adult carer.

Designing the style of information leaflets for emergency care environments

Remember that time is critical in emergency care areas where sick children and young people may have very short stays.

- Use informative not descriptive headings, e.g 'MP3 player Disease' is not very inspiring, 'What is MP3 player Disease? is better, and 'Living with MP3 player Disease' is the best of all.
- Try to personalise the leaflet by using personal pronouns (I, we, us or you).
- Use decisive language which is clear and unambiguous.
- Describe actions positively, e.g. 'do not administer unless the client is developing a fever' is bad; 'give only when the patient has a temperature above 38 degrees Centigrade' is much clearer.
- Use familiar words. For instance 'your child has broken his lower arm' is better than 'your child has fractured his radius'. Medical jargon is poorly understood by the general public.
- Use short paragraphs with strong topic sentences.
- Use simple visual images.
- Use at least 12 point type, and larger text for younger and older readers.

Consider placing emergency care leaflets clearly signposted on the Trust web pages. Advise families to seek additional information from the children first website on http://www.childrenfirst.nhs.uk/.

Further reading

Lang TA (1999). Developing Patient Education Handouts. Department of Scientific Publications: The Cleveland Clinic Foundation. Available at http://www.tomlangcommunications.com/ Expanded_Patient_Ed_chapter.pdf

Jones R, Finlay F, Crouch V, Anderson S (2000) Drug information leaflets: adolescent and professional perspectives. *Child: Care, Health and Development*, 26:41–48

⑦ **Family-centred care**

Family-centred care (FCC) is now considered a central tenet of the care of children and young people. At its core is the recognition that the family is a central part of a child or young person's life, and that therefore they should be cared for within the context of their family. It is a multi-faceted concept that has evolved throughout the past 50 years, and terms such as parental involvement and parent participation are often used to describe its application in practice. Family-centred care can be defined as:

'The professional support of the child and family through a process of involvement, participation, and partnership underpinned by empowerment and negotiation' (Smith et al 2002)

This wider definition suggests that family-centred care is more than just involvement and participation by parents, instead being a process brought about through negotiation with, and empowerment of, the child and their family. Family-centred care is therefore about nurses and other health care professionals empowering families and negotiating their involvement, participation, and partnership. It is a partnership between the family and the professionals, whereby parents are supported in their central caring role and actively involved in the care to the extent that they wish. The level and extent to which this takes place will vary, and will depend upon factors such as individual family needs and circumstances, and where they find themselves on their child's illness journey. The family-centred care practice continuum has been developed to illustrate this, and suggests that parental input can occur anywhere on the continuum, varying from entirely nurse-led to sharing equal status and being parent-led. The suggestion is that this enables nurses to facilitate family-centred care according to individual family needs rather than applying a blanket approach that may not always be achievable. This is particularly important in the emergency department, where the family's needs and circumstances are likely to be very different to those in a ward setting. The care here is more likely to be towards the nurse-led end of the continuum; however, this does not mean that family-centred care cannot be implemented and achieved.

Essential requirements for family-centred care
- Acknowledgement that the family is a central part of the child/young person's life
- Good communication skills
- Good assessment skills
- Empowering families
  - Building relationships: acknowledge that there may be times when parents do not want to actively participate in their child's care.
  - Information giving: a planned approach should be used to provide and share information verbally, through the use of literature or other media or teaching skills. Information for children and young people should be age appropriate and for younger children facilitated through the use of play.

- Facilitating participatory experiences:
  - Discussions with members of the multi-disciplinary team
  - Parenting tasks and nursing tasks.
- Negotiating care:
  - Awareness of individual family members' needs
  - Utilize appropriate and effective communication skills
  - Plan care in partnership with the family.

Which policies reflect FCC?

- Every Child Matters (2003)
- National Service Framework (2003)
- Standards for Better Health (2006)
- Aiming High for Disabled Children: Better Support for Families (Shields et al 2007).

The main conclusion from this review is that more research, using measurable outcome factors, is needed to assess whether FCC really works to improve a child's experience of hospitalization.

Further reading

Smith L, Coleman V, Bradshaw M (2002). Family-centred care concept theory and practice. London: Palgrave

http://www.familycenteredcare.org. American based institute providing a resource for health professionals through training, information dissemination, policy and research initiatives.

Shields L, Pratt J, Davis L, Hunter J (2007). Family-centred care for children in hospital. Cochrane Database of Systematic Reviews, Issue 1, Art. no . CD004811

⑦ Emergency care of children: abiding by the NMC Code

There are elements of your practice that you must think about before you undertake any emergency procedure. These procedural elements of the care you deliver are supported by all aspects of the Nursing and Midwifery Council (NMC) Code which constitutes standards of conduct, performance and ethics for nurses and midwives (see Table 1.1, NMC 2008).

Table 1.1 The NMC Code

1: Make the care of people (i.e. children and young people and their families/carers) your first concern, treating them as individuals and respecting their dignity
2: Work with others to protect and promote the health and wellbeing of those in your care, their families and carers, and the wider community
3: Provide a high standard of practice and care at all times
4: Be open and honest, act with integrity and uphold the reputation of your profession

There are some aspects of the Code which directly pertain to the carrying out of procedures on children and young people.

1 Make the care of people (i.e. children and young people and their families carers) your first concern, treating them as individuals and respecting their dignity

The NMC Code instructs all nurses to treat people as individuals. It is therefore crucial that you treat all children, young people and their families or carers as individuals and respect their dignity. To achieve this, a children's nurse must always consider aspects of dignity, which are sometimes difficult to achieve in some emergency care environments. For example, in order to maintain child patient dignity, consider the provision of toileting and bathroom facilities. The health care professionals who deliver care to children and young people in emergency health care environments need to act in such a way that they respect the privacy and dignity of the child throughout their health care journey.

The NMC Code also asks that nurses treat all people kindly and considerately, act as advocates for those families in their care, and help families to access relevant information and support. Helping families to navigate the labyrinth of information in the real and virtual world is a skill all children's nurses must harness.

The NMC Code asks each children's nurse to respect children's, young people's and families' right to confidentiality. It states that you must ensure that people are informed about how and why information is shared by those who will be providing their care. Only in safeguarding situations can a children's nurse not promise confidentiality. In these situations, the NMC Code states that you must disclose information if you believe a child may be at risk of harm.

Importantly for nurses working in emergency environments, the NMC Code specifically asks (children's) nurses to support families in self-caring activities to improve and maintain their health. This aspect of the Code is of paramount importance when discharging families from emergency care areas. Additionally the NMC Code emphasizes the need for nurses to make arrangements to meet families' language and communication needs, highly pertinent in contemporary emergency care settings. Therefore, the NMC Code states that you must share with children and their families in a way that they can understand the information they want or need to know about their health.

The NMC Code asks each nurse to ensure that consent is gained before any treatment or procedure is commenced.

Of crucial importance to any children's nurse are the criteria which are utilized when ascertaining if an individual child achieves Gillick competence.

In this context the child or young person should be able to demonstrate that they:
- Understand simple terms, and the nature, purpose and necessity of the proposed treatment
- Believe the information applies to them
- Retain the information long enough to make a choice
- Make a choice free from pressure

Having to make children and young people accept procedures or treatments against their will may perpetuate psychological trauma, and exacerbate any future encounter or procedure in the future. However, remember that the NMC Code states that you must be able to demonstrate that you have acted in someone's (i.e. a child's) best interests if you have provide care in an emergency.

The NMC Code states that you must refuse any gifts, favours or hospitality that might be interpreted as an attempt to gain preferential treatment. Likewise the NMC Code clearly indicates that you must establish and actively maintain clear sexual boundaries at all times with children and young people in your care, their families and carers.

2 Work with others to protect and promote the health and wellbeing of those in your care, their families and carers and the wider community

The NMC Code asks each nurse to work with colleagues to monitor the quality of their work and to maintain the safety of those in their care. Additionally, the NMC Code asks nurses to consult with and take advice from colleagues when appropriate. The NMC Code clearly states that you must make a referral to another practitioner when it is in the best interest of someone in your care. This is particularly pertinent to novice practitioners who may still be developing their skills. Secitons of the Code apply to the delegation of tasks or specific procedures to students and untrained members of staff. It is your responsibility under the NMC Code to confirm the outcome of any delegated task, and to ensure that the required standards are met.

The NMC Code is emphatic that nurses should manage risk and therefore child patient safety. The NMC Code therefore asks each nurse to act without delay if they believe that they or a colleague or anyone else has put someone at risk. Therefore, the NMC Code states that you must inform someone in authority if you experience problems that prevent you working with the Code or other nationally agreed standards.

The NMC Code explicitly states that you must report your concerns in writing if problems in the environment of care are putting your children and their families at risk. Prior to undertaking any procedure a nurse must always ensure that health and safety, infection control and local and, if applicable, national policies and procedures are adhered to.

3 Provide a high standard of practice and care at all times

To do this the NMC Code insists that nurses use the best available evidence. Furthermore the NMC Code states that you must keep secure, clear and accurate records.

4 Be open and honest, act with integrity and uphold the reputation of your profession

This NMC Code element states that you must inform any employers you work for if your fitness to practice is called into question.

Further reading

Larcher V (2005). Consent, Competence and Confidentiality. *British Medical Journal* 330:353–56
Nursing and Midwifery Council (2008). The Code: Standards of conduct, performance and ethics for nurses and midwives. NMC, London.

⑦ Record keeping

Record keeping is an integral part of nursing practice, and part of the duty of care owed to the child patient by the nurse. It facilitates the care process, and should reflect consultation and discussion between members of the multiprofessional team and the patient. The principles of good record keeping are well established, and are equally applicable to paper and computerized records. Records provide the outward evidence of communication. Failure to maintain accurate records can lead to professional misconduct. From a medico-legal aspect, the emergency department (ED) record is a prime source of evidence.

Health records

A health record is any electronic or paper information recorded about a person for the purpose of managing their healthcare. These include doctor's records, nursing records, all primary care records, X-rays, pathology reports, allied health professional reports, and pharmacy records.

Importance of record keeping

Owing to the important nature of health care, nurses and healthcare practitioners must ensure that the quality of their interventions is substantiated in the patient's written records.

The primary purpose of record keeping is to provide an accurate account of the care and treatment given to the patient. This facilitates the monitoring of the care given and allows a clinical history to be developed. Continuity of care is enabled by the maintenance of accurate health records. A high standard of record keeping by nurses is essential, as it may be used to inform the multidisciplinary team who are subsequently involved in the care of the child and young person. Healthcare records also have an important legal function.

Legal and professional aspects of record keeping

The healthcare record may be used by employers, defence lawyers, and litigant patient counsel as evidence. Any material document that records any aspect of the care of the child or young person may be used as evidence – including notes on scraps of paper, which if relevant could be subpoenaed by the court. In most situations, the patient record is the first source of enquiry when any investigation into care is initiated. The courts take the view that if it is not written down then it did not happen.

The Data Protection Act (1998) provides a legal right of access to all health records to living people. For the deceased patient, there is a limited statutory right of access to records under the Access to Health Records Act (1990). There should be no surprises for the child and family in their records, as good practice dictates that their opinions are sought, considered, and documented, along with being informed and consulted at all stages of the treatment process. When access to a child's health record is requested, any person with parental responsibility may apply independently. If the child's parents live apart and share parental responsibility they may individually apply. If the competent child requires access, they may apply and they must give their consent if their parents seek to obtain access to their records, as they must be afforded the same duty of confidentiality as an adult. Records must be retained until the child's 21st birthday.

Regardless of occupational role of the nurse or clinical setting, they are expected to maintain contemporaneous records of the individual's care in a factual and logical manner. This is the mark of a skilled and safe practitioner.

Record keeping in the ED environment

Resuscitation room

It is essential to delegate the role of 'scribe' to a competent team member who will keep a record of all procedures, medication, investigations, and care given during the resuscitation procedure. As soon as possible, the staff directly involved should document in the health record information on the care they gave and the condition of the child/young person.

General ED attendance

Presenting complaint

Make sure records address in detail why the child is presenting at ED, onset of condition or time of injury. Note who is presenting the information and their relationship to the child, and what others have observed, e.g. paramedics.

Previous relevant history

This should include any prior ED attendance, a comprehensive past medical history, and in the case of an infant their birth history. Child protection registers should be cross-checked.

Current medication

Current medication including any complementary therapies should be documented.

Triage/exam findings

Details of assessment undertaken at triage and any physical examination should be documented.

Investigations ordered

A list of investigations ordered should be recorded and notes made as they are completed.

Treatment

Any treatment given must be documented, noting the patient's response to that treatment. A contemporaneous approach to this must be taken. Evidence that consent has been obtained, where intimate procedures are required, must also be documented in patient's records. The journey through the ED should be recorded. How is the child? Have they improved drastically or deteriorated?

Discharge advice should be documented as should discharge location.

Child and family involvement

The child and family should be viewed as equal partners in the care process and should contribute to the written record.

Best practice in record keeping
- Records must be clear, factual and accurate.
- They must be completed as soon as possible after an event has occurred.
- Records must not be tampered with or altered in any way.
- If alterations or additions are justified, then they must be dated and signed, with the original entry still legible.
- Records must be recorded in terms that the child and family can understand.
- Abbreviations, jargon, speculation, subjectivity and meaningless phrases should not be included.
- All entries should be dated, timed and signed to ensure that your role in care is documented.
- Records must be kept secure.
- If delegating the task of record keeping to a pre-registration student of nursing or to a health care support worker, the registered nurse must ensure they have the knowledge and skills to undertake this role and are adequately supervised. Counter-signing is required if they are not deemed competent.
- Professional judgement and local standards will determine frequency of entries.

The future
The implementation of a new integrated information technology system should assist with the standardization of health records, improve communication and enable information to be shared.

Further reading
Tingle J (1998). Nurses must improve their record keeping skills. *British Journal of Nursing* 7:245.
The Data Protection Act (1998) http://www.opsi.gov.uk
The Access to Health Records Act (1990) http://www.opsi.gov.uk
The Freedom of Information Act (2000) http://www.opsi.gov.uk
The Caldicott Report (1997) http://www.opsi.gov.uk
Nursing and Midwifery Council (2007). Record Keeping. NMC, London.
Nursing and Midwifery Council (2008). The Code: Standards for conduct, performance and ethics for nurses and midwives. NMC, London.
Department of Health (1998). Information for Health: An Information Strategy for the Modern NHS. DH, London.
http://www.dh.gov.uk/en/Publicationsandstatistics/Publications/PublicationsPolicyAndGuidance/DH_4007832

⑦ Interprofessional working

Children and families who require emergency care are exposed to more than one professional. The number of professionals involved and the importance of their ability to work collaboratively increases with the complexity of the child's needs. New initiatives to improve management of disease processes invariably point out the need for interprofessional collaboration. UK government policy, in an effort to address patients' safety, reduce clinical errors, and improve organizational performance, is encouraging health care staff to blur traditional roles, in a drive to increase joint working between practitioners. There is currently a lack of clarity regarding the impact that changes to traditional working practices might have on staff delivering the services, or on patient care. However, the expectation is that team-based models of care will avoid gaps, which are seen as important risk factors for patient safety (Bion and Heffner 2004).

Elements that contribute to skilful and effective team work

- Effective administrative structures and leadership
- An organizational culture that fosters the importance of teamwork
- Encouragement of new ways of working together
- Development of common goals
- Clear lines of communication
- Cooperation and co-ordination, and active participation of all members
- Clear guidelines, protocols and procedures
- Effective mechanisms to resolve conflict
- Mechanisms to overcome resistance to change
- Educational structures that encourage interprofessional learning and understanding of the professional roles/responsibilities of each member

Successful teams

- Recognize the professional and personal contributions of all members
- Promote individual development and team interdependence
- Recognize the benefits of working together
- See accountability as a collective responsibility
- Implement team interventions embedded in initiatives working to improve quality of care

Barriers to interprofessional collaboration

- Differences in history and culture
- Differences in language and jargon
- Varying levels of preparation, qualifications, and status
- Limited understanding of how to work together
- Poor leadership
- Differences in requirements, regulations, and norms of professional education
- Fears of diluted professional identity
- Differences in accountability, payment, and rewards
- Concerns regarding clinical accountability

Irrespective of barriers that are present, most health professionals have at least one characteristic in common, a personal desire to learn, and they have at least one shared value, to meet the needs of their patients or clients.

Improved health outcomes usually lie outside the scope or control of any single practitioner.

Real improvements are likely to occur only if the range of professionals responsible for providing a particular service are brought together to:
- share their different knowledge and experiences
- agree what improvements they would like to see
- test these in practice
- jointly learn from their results.

A powerful incentive for greater teamwork among professionals is created by directing attention to the areas where changes are likely to result in measurable improvements for the patients they serve together, rather than concentrating on what, on the surface, seem to be irreconcilable differences. Gains in child and family outcomes can be realized if staff regularly interact to negotiate and agree on their working practices.

The role of education in encouraging interprofessional working is considered to make a positive contribution to collaborative working, and findings from systematic reviews are now beginning to substantiate these claims (Barr et al 2005). These reviews have indicated that interprofessional education can make a positive contribution to collaborative knowledge and skills, and also contribute to improvements in delivery of care.

Further reading

Barr H, Koppel I, Reeves S (2005). Effective interprofessional education. Assumption, argument and evidence. London: Blackwell
Bion JF, Heffner MD (2004). Challenges in the care of the acutely ill. *The Lancet* 363:970–977

ⓘ **Safeguarding children: information sharing**

Introduction

Nurses should:
- Know when information can be shared and when it is inappropriate to do so.
- Remember that the welfare of the child is paramount!

Sharing information: guiding principles
  www.everychildmatters.gov.uk/informationsharing

- Explain openly and honestly to children, young people and their families.
- Seek agreement on what information will, or could, be shared and why and how, UNLESS to do so:
  - would put the child, young person or others at increased risk of significant harm
  - would undermine the prevention, detection or prosecution of a serious crime
  - would interfere with a potential investigation.
- Ensure the child's safety and welfare are their overriding consideration.
- Share information given without consent if there is sufficient need to override the lack of consent (see consent and confidentiality below).
- If in doubt, seek advice especially regarding possible significant harm to a child or serious harm to others.
- Ensure information is:
  - accurate
  - up-to-date
  - relevant
  - shared only with those people who need to see it
  - shared securely.
- Always record the reasons for their decision – whether it is to share information or not.

Consent and confidentiality

- Information is NOT confidential when it is:
  - already lawfully in the public domain
  - available from a public source
  - shared by someone in the knowledge that it will be shared with others.
- Information IS confidential when it is:
  - sensitive information and not any of the above.
- Consent must be informed.
- Explicit consent given verbally or in writing is good practice.
- Written consent is often preferable.
- Consent may be required from the person with parental responsibility – it is important to know who has parental responsibility.

- A young person may give or refuse consent to sharing information if aged 16 or 17, or if a child under 16 who has the capacity to understand.
- You can lawfully share confidential information without consent IF it can be justified in the public or child's interest; for example:
  - evidence that the child is suffering or is at risk of suffering significant harm
  - reasonable cause to believe that a child may be suffering or at risk of significant harm
  - the prevention of significant harm to children including the prevention and detection of serious crime (i.e. any crime which causes or is likely to cause significant harm)
  - a Court Order is made for release of records.

Information sharing checklist

- Is there a legitimate purpose for you or your agency to share the information?
- Does the information enable a person to be identified?
- Is the information confidential?
- If the information is confidential, do you have consent to share?
- Is there a statutory duty or court order to share the information?
- If consent is refused, or there are good reasons not to seek consent to share confidential information, is there a sufficient public interest to share information?
- If the decision is to share, are you sharing the right information in the right way?
- If in doubt seek advice from the named or designated nurse or doctor in child protection/safeguarding children.
- Have you properly recorded:
  - what decision is reached, i.e. whether to share or not to share information?
  - reasons and justification for the decision?
- Who has access to records?
- How securely are they kept?

Remember: where nurses have reasonable cause to suspect that a child may be suffering or at risk of suffering significant harm, they should refer their concerns to children's social care. In general, nurses should seek to discuss concerns with the family, and if possible seek agreement to sharing information BUT NOT if such a discussion places a child at increased risk of significant harm OR interferes with any potential investigation.

- The child's interest must be given overriding consideration.

Further reading:

Department for Education and Skills (2006) Information sharing: Further guidance on legal issues. DfES available online at: www.everychildmatters.gov.uk/informationsharing

Information Commissioner's Office (2007) Framework code of practice for sharing personal information. Wilmslow. ICO

ⓘ **Identifying abuse and mistreatment in emergency care**

Introduction

This section will consider the importance of the recognition of abuse in children. It is the duty of professionals to report concerns regarding the possibility that a child is the victim of neglect or physical, emotional, or sexual abuse. Recognizing signs and responding appropriately can save a child's life.

Definitions of abuse

- Physical abuse: the causing of physical harm to a child.
- Emotional abuse: the persistent emotional maltreatment of a child to cause severe and persistent adverse effects on the child's emotional development.
- Sexual abuse: the forcing or enticing of a child to take part in sexual activities, whether or not they are aware of what is happening.
- Neglect: the failure to meet a child's basic physical and/or psychological needs.

Signs of abuse

Table 1.2 highlights some common signs of abuse to be vigilant for.

Procedures for an abused child

The key role of a nurse is to:
- Recognize injuries and presentations that may not be accidental and recognize children who are neglected or about whom you have concerns.
- Treat the injury or presentation.
- Refer the child appropriately.

Every child that attends the emergency department should be assessed appropriately. The assessment process has been divided into three phases.

Initial assessment
- Is the child subject to a child protection plan?

This is essential information to every child that attends the ED. If the child is subject to a child protection plan social services need to be informed; however, it does not mean that their presentation is a result of abuse. Likewise, if the child is not known to social services it is not conclusive that they have not been abused.

- How many attendances has the child had to the ED?

This can be an important factor for recognising abuse especially if the child has had multiple attendances for limb problems, overdoses or poisoning, head injuries, and many more. However, remember some children have a number of attendances for genuine reasons so be careful not to jump to conclusions.

- Are the child's details documented correctly?

Table 1.2 Common signs of abuse

Types of abuse	Signs of abuse
Physical	Bruises, especially finger sized marks
	Burns and scalds
	Bites
	Suspicious fractures
	Head injuries
	Poisoning
Emotional	Self-deprecation
	Expressionless face
	Abnormally affectionate to strangers
	Neurotic behaviour, e.g. rocking and self-harming
Sexual	Anogenital bruising and tears
	Sexually transmitted infections
	Pregnancy
	Genital itching and/or pain
	Usually there are no physical signs
Neglect	Unkempt dirty appearance
	Faltering growth
	Severe nappy rash
	Sores
	Hunger
	Poor relationship between child and parent/carer

Documentation is both highly important and a legal requirement. Make sure that the child's name, address, date of birth, next of kin, doctor's practice and school attended are documented correctly. These are essential to look for previous admissions, find medical notes and to check whether the child is subject to the child protection plan.

Taking a history
• Where is the injury?
• Does it look suspicious?
• How did the injury occur?
• When did the injury occur?

All these questions help to determine whether the injury is consistent with the story given, or if there has been a delay in presentation to the ED.

Physical examination

Every nurse when doing an initial assessment should be vigilant of the following:

• Does the child look unkempt?

This observation can help determine that the child may have been neglected.

• Is the child underweight?

This can be determined against a growth chart; many abused and neglected children are often seen to have faltering growth.

• What are the injuries like? Are there any other marks on the child?

It is important to look at the injuries and to determine whether there are other marks, e.g. bruises, burns or bites. Make sure a description of injuries and a clear diagram of the injuries are documented by either a nurse or a doctor.

Once the assessment stage has been completed and if there are any concerns it is important that the senior emergency doctor and nurse in charge are informed immediately. The senior doctor will then inform and refer the child to a paediatric specialist registrar. If a child is suspected to be a victim of abuse, a thorough physical examination and investigations will then be carried out by the senior doctor or paediatric specialist registrar. These include:

• X-rays and skeletal surveys to find old or other fractures.

• Photographs, useful for evidence in court.

• Pregnancy testing and cultures, to assess for/rule out sexually transmitted infections and pregnancy in sexually abused patients.

• Blood tests, to assess for/rule out haematological causes of excessive bruising.

It is important that any child about whom there are concerns is admitted to hospital and not discharged by anyone except a specialist registrar or consultant.

A flowchart has been adapted as a guideline for the recognition and treatment of children at risk, following the recommendations that came out of the Laming Report concerning Victoria Climbie (see Fig. 1.1).

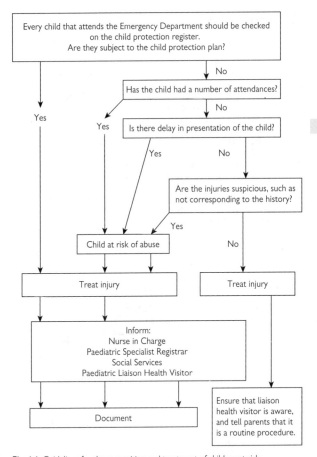

Fig. 1.1 Guidelines for the recognition and treatment of children at risk

Further reading

National Collaborating Centre for Women's and Children's Health (2009) When to suspect child maltreatment. NCCWCH, London.

Flanagan, N (2002). The child protection register: A tool in the accident and emergency department? *Emergency Medical Journal* 19:229–30.

ⓘ Sexual abuse

Sexual abuse (the law and policy relating to sexual abuse and criminality are different across the four countries of the UK, and therefore readers are advised to consult their local procedures) refers to situations where a child (for brevity, child refers to those under 18 years of age) has been forced, enticed, or subjugated to take part in sexual activities be these physical (penetrative or non-penetrative) or non-physical (e.g. being forced to watch pornographic materials). Such victims could include those who have been abused by parents or siblings, involved in prostitution, trafficked for sex slavery purposes, raped, or assaulted through non-consensual acts with peers. It can happen to children of all ages, including babies, as well as those with complex disabilities or conditions where they are not able to articulate the abuse. In rare cases, a child who is critically ill resulting from sexual assault may die en route, and so the team will be dealing with a child who may have been murdered as well as abused. Each of these situations raises differing challenges for dealing with the victims in emergency situations. It is also important to consider that most acts of sexual abuse will be perpetrated alongside other forms of abuse, including physical and emotional abuse, as well as neglect. Exacerbating this will be the effects on the child of being in a strange environment, the involvement of different professionals, and the potential for separation from parent(s)/others if they are suspected of being perpetrators.

In the emergency situation specific concerns need to be addressed to ensure that the child is both treated and protected.

Provision of emergency medical and nursing care

The level of emergency care required for the child will depend on the nature and extent of the sexual abuse or assault as well as their age. The younger the child the more likely there are to be physical injuries; the risk of, e.g., haemorrhage, fractures, or internal injury from penetration is higher. As with any other emergency scenario, triage, life support, and follow-on management will be implemented depending on the child's status and the injuries found.

Documentation

Documentation of the child's status and any interventions is important in every case, but in these cases it is especially important to consider that records may be used in child protection procedures and for criminal proceedings. If the child dies, then a Child Death Review may be undertaken to investigate the events surrounding the death, and contemporaneous documentation is crucial.

Preservation of forensic evidence

Sexual activity with a child is a criminal offence, and in order for prosecution to take place the police may need to collect forensic evidence. This is undertaken using local protocols and in collaboration with the health team, although in some areas forensic nurse practitioners will provide this service. Nonetheless, the nursing team need to be cognizant of the need to preserve items for future forensic examination.

Immediate referral and protection of the child

Each local authority will have specific protocols for both referring children at risk of harm and the sharing of information where sexual abuse may have taken place. The status of the child will initially determine the level of immediate protection required, for example if resuscitation is necessary. However, it is not the health team's responsibility to identify the perpetrator; rather it is to ensure that those accompanying a child are not placing the child at risk. Normal safeguarding procedures require a member of the emergency team (and this may be anyone so long as that person is clearly identified) to make a referral to social services and/or the police. Clearly, where the child appears to be at immediate risk from an accompanying person the police must be informed; they then have the power to intervene. Any referral must be followed up in writing, and therefore contemporaneous and comprehensive documentation is crucial.

Emotional support

Any child who has undergone a sexual assault may have endured a range of abuses often over a period of time and therefore requires sensitivity in how they are cared for both generally and during any necessary interventions. Similarly, parents and carers may equally be emotionally traumatized if the event has been perpetrated by others, and will naturally be angry as well as upset. The nurse needs to be aware of these possible emotions and be responsive to them.

Further reading

Department for Education and Skills (2006). What to do if you are worried a child is being abused. Nottingham: DfES

HM Government (2006). Working Together to Safeguard Children. A guide to inter-agency working to safeguard and promote the welfare of children. London: TSO.

Nursing and Midwifery Council (2008). The Code: Standards of conduct, performance and ethics for nurses and midwives. London: NMC. Available at http://www.nmc-uk.org/aArticle. aspx?ArticleID=3057

Powell C (2007). Safeguarding Children and Young People. A Guide for Nurses and Midwives. Maidenhead: Oxford University Press

Thain J (2007) Sexual Assault. In Glasper EA, McEwing G, Richardson J (eds). Oxford Handbook of Children's and Young People's Nursing. Oxford: Oxford University Press

① Transport and transfer of the sick or injured child

Indications
- To move from the ED for definitive care or treatment (e.g. to the ward or operating theatre)
- To move for diagnostic investigations (e.g. CT scan or X-ray)
- To move to a tertiary hospital for specialized care or treatment (e.g. burns centre or paediatric intensive care)

Principles of transfer
As a general rule, only children whose condition has been assessed and stabilized should be moved from the emergency department. Thus, transfer of the child, whether into or out of a hospital, should be a carefully planned event. This will minimize the risk of any unexpected complications either en route or at the destination. Only in very exceptional circumstances should an unstable child be moved from the ED (e.g. the need for immediate life-saving surgery).

Planning for any transfer should include
- Ensuring optimum preparation and stabilization of the child
- Communication with the destination
- Identification of transfer personnel
- Identification of transport means
- Identification of equipment to take
- Appropriate documentation
- Communication with the child and family

Ensuring optimum preparation and stabilization of the child (reference APLS)
- Ensure full assessment and primary interventions are completed.
- Ensure airway, breathing and circulation are assessed and any interventions completed. In particular ensure any airway or venous access devices are properly secured.
- Complete diagnostic imaging where appropriate.
- Ensure adequate analgesia.

Communication with the destination
Allocate one member of staff to communicate with the destination. Ensure communication of the following parameters:
- Name of the child
- Age
- Weight
- Allergies
- History
- Treatment received
- Current condition including equipment/drugs in use
- Obtain name of receiving staff (medical and nursing) and record in notes
- Name/relationship of accompanying family
- Clarify who will arrange the transportation

- Estimated time of arrival
- Record any treatment requested by the receiving destination (e.g. drug/ fluid administration for burned patients)

Identification of transfer personnel

The transfer staff should include at least one nurse with training in pae- diatric life support and transportation of the sick child. This nurse should ideally have first-hand knowledge of the child and any treatment he/she has received in the emergency department.

If medical intervention en route is predictable (e.g. if the patient is semi-conscious or likely to need drugs or resuscitative measures) then an appropriately trained doctor should also accompany. If any airway manoeuvres are likely, the doctor should be an anaesthetist with appropriate paediatric training.

The transfer of a sick child can be a good learning opportunity for junior medical and nursing staff. Consideration should be given to taking junior staff if the space is available and departmental circumstances will allow.

Identification of transport means

For intra-hospital transfer, consideration should be given as to whether the child needs to be on a trolley or would be safe and psychologically better sitting on a parent's knee in a wheelchair.

For inter-hospital transfer, land ambulance is the usual mode of transport. Communication should occur with the ambulance service to establish:

- time for collection
- specifics of destination
- clinical condition of the child
- personnel accompanying
- equipment to be taken.

Some specialist units have retrieval teams. These units often have specially equipped vehicles and specially trained staff for transfer of the critically sick or injured child.

Identification of equipment to take

Most departments have a 'transfer bag' of equipment pre-prepared for use in the transfer of children. All staff who may be involved in a transfer should be familiar with the contents of the bag. It should include any size-appropriate equipment needed for the resuscitation of the child. In addi-tion, any specific drugs (including oxygen) or specific equipment needed for the child (e.g. syringe drivers or IV pumps) should be taken. For long journeys take spares, as batteries quickly fail. Keep a checklist of equip-ment taken to ensure it is all brought back.

Always ensure any pre-prepared equipment bags are checked regularly to ensure equipment is in working order and within expiry date.

Appropriate documentation

- Ensure copies of all documentation are taken with the child to the destination.
- Ensure copies of diagnostic images are also taken if they are not available in electronic format by the receiving unit.
- Ensure there is documentation for recording events/vital sign monitoring en route.

Communication with the child and family

- If clinically and developmentally appropriate, ensure the child is aware of his/her condition and the need for transfer.
- Ensure a senior member of the team caring for the child liaises with the parents/legal guardian of the child to ensure they are clear about the need for transfer.
- Decide whether it is appropriate for a parent to accompany the child.
- Ensure they know exactly where they are going (provide a map if necessary).
- Stress the importance of NOT following behind the ambulance.
- Ensure they know who will be caring for their child at the destination, and thus who to ask for.
- Provide transport if necessary.

On return

- Ensure all equipment is appropriately cleaned or disposed of, and that any pre-prepared bags are checked and restocked.

Further reading

Children's Acute Transport Service: www.cats.nhs.uk

⚠ Safe discharge of children from the emergency department

Safe discharge of children from the ED requires consideration of the following aspects:
- Holistic assessment of the infant, child or young person
- Assessment of the family's ability to provide care
- Coordinated multi-professional approach
- Ongoing support and services

Immediate management
- Assessment of the child's presenting condition
- Assessment of any existing condition the child may have, such as long-term illness
- Examination of the child, including current clinical observations
- Ascertain parent(s) perceptions of their child's health status
- Documentation of care delivery and discussions

Nursing management
Referral for ongoing care and support
- Identify services needed and their availability, e.g. health visitor, community children's nurse or social services.
- Discharge summary to their general practitioner (GP).
- Assess the needs of the family in caring for the child following ED attendance.

Provision of supplies, medications or equipment
- The nurse must ensure that resources such as equipment and medicines are supplied or available to the child and family.

Education and information needs of child and family
- The child's safety and wellbeing must be the first priority of the nurse.
- Parental education, providing information to the parents, and assessing their ability to deliver care required.
- Additional support services may be needed to support the child's care provision following discharge information, and they should also be supported by written guidelines to aid the continuity of care.
- Documentation of care delivered.

Follow-up appointments
- Review appointments should be arranged prior to the child leaving the department.
- Referral to community services with consent from the child's family.

Review or unplanned reattendance
- Educate the child and family regarding indicators of improvement or deterioration.
- Contact details for the department.
- Advice about accessing GP services or other support during the child's illness.

Risk assessment/management
- Accurate assessment and documentation of the child's condition, prior to discharge.
- Parents advised to return or seek help if concerned about child's condition.

Discharge protocol
- Local/trust policy adhered to regarding discharge process.
- Multi-professional process: joint decision with parents, nurse and medical staff involved.
- Care delivery clearly documented.

Further reading

Department of Health (2004) 4-Hour Checklist: reducing delays for A and E patients. DH, London.
Department of Health (2003) Discharge from hospital: pathway, process and practice. DH, London.
Royal College of Nursing (2004) Discharge planning. RCN, London.

① Observational assessment

Assessing children (for brevity children refers to all age groups from 0–18 years) is a fundamental role of the nurse and one which requires the utilization of many skills and tools. Within the emergency situation nurses routinely use a variety of technological tools to assess different physiological states of children, including the measurement of temperature, oxygen saturations, pulse and blood pressure, cardiac monitoring, and invasive assessments, e.g. that of blood glucose levels. Similarly, assessments may be undertaken using specific tools including ABC, AVPU, and the Glasgow Coma Scale (GCS), and those for pain such as FACES and FLACC.

Despite all these methods, the nurse has an equally powerful set of readily available measurement tools, which are often underestimated in preference to the use of technology. These tools are the senses of sight, hearing, touch, and to an extent smell, all of which can provide valuable information about the status, changes, and responses of a child (and family) to a specific situation or condition.

Sight

Sight is one of the most useful methods by which the nurse can identify health problems and the importance of 'scanning' children from head to toe cannot be underestimated. Much information can be gleaned about a child in an emergency situation, and so it is important that any observations are documented.

- What is the general demeanour of the child?
- How are they positioned when sitting or standing?
- Do they appear distressed or quiet, which may indicate severe respiratory problems?
- How is their behaviour? Abused children may exhibit a state of frozen awareness where they do not respond to the external environment.
- What is the behaviour of the parent to the child and vice versa?
- Any there any abnormal features that might suggest an inherited condition (these may not have been identified previously)?

This is not an exhaustive list, but identifies some issues the nurse needs to be aware of in combination with other assessments such as ABC.

Hearing/listening

Hearing can be differentiated into active and passive listening, both of which serve both therapeutic and assessment purposes. Active listening is concerned with the normal communication exchanges between the nurse and the child/family. Passive listening gives additional data about the child, their condition and interactions with parents and others.

- Children cry differently dependent on whether they are hungry, in pain, stressed or generally ill.
- Sighing or a very weak cry may indicate severe respiratory distress or the advanced stages of an infection.
- Variance in speech volume and tone may indicate differing degrees of pain, discomfort, or fear.
- Poor interactions with parents/caregivers might indicate neglect or abuse (along with other indicators).

Touch

Touch serves many purposes, including being therapeutic and comforting. However, it can also provide much useful data about a child's condition.

- Blood circulation to the skin is naturally altered with pyrexia or hypothermia.
- Peripheral shutdown occurs with shock, infections, and loss of blood volume, and leads to cold skin.
- Dry skin with limited elasticity may suggest dehydration.
- Dry, wrinkled skin can suggest malnutrition.
- Fractures may be obvious on touch.

Smell

Many smells which are emitted can provide clues to a possible disease or condition.

- Alcohol ingestion can usually be smelt on the breath.
- The smell of pears (acetone) in the breath potentially indicates diabetes/diabetic ketoacidosis.
- Faecal smelling breath may indicate intestinal obstruction.
- Foul smelling stools occur in conditions such as coeliac disease and cystic fibrosis.
- Diarrhoea can smell different with specific infections.
- Generalized smell might indicate an infected wound or abscess.

None of these assessments can be used on their own, but by developing your nursing skills in acknowledging and recording the data obtained through each one a more holistic view of the child and their status may be obtained.

Further reading

Glasper E. A., McEwing G., Richardson J. (eds) (2007) Oxford Handbook of Children's and Young People's Nursing. Oxford: Oxford University Press
Glasper A., Richardson J. (eds) (2006) A Textbook of Children's and Young People's Nursing. Edinburgh: Churchill Livingstone

⊙ **Safeguarding children**

One child dies each week in England and Wales from cruelty (Home Office 2008). It is every health professional's responsibility to take safeguarding of children into account.

What is child abuse?

A child
- Is anyone under 18 years of age.
- Can be abused by anyone who causes harm or fails to prevent harm.
- Can be abused by an adult or another child.

There are four categories of child abuse: neglect, physical, sexual, and emotional.
- Neglect is the ongoing failure to meet a child's basic needs which leads to an impairment to the child's health or development.
- Physical abuse is the actual or likely physical injury to a child or the failure to prevent physical injury.
- Sexual abuse is forcing or enticing a child to take part in sexual activities, or viewing material of a sexual nature.
- Emotional abuse is severe or persistent emotional ill treatment or rejection. All forms of abuse involve some emotional ill treatment.

What should you do if you are worried about a child?

If during the course of your work you have concerns about the well being of a child, you should discuss concerns with your line manager or an appropriately qualified colleague as soon as possible.

After a discussion you may still have concerns and a referral to the local children and young people's social care team should be made by the appropriate senior practitioner.

It is good practice to inform the parent that you are making a referral unless it could affect the child's safety or your own.

All conversations and actions must be written down; a telephone referral must be followed up with a written referral within 48 hours.

The following should be considered when you are concerned:
- Previous abuse within family
- Young carers
- Parental mental health issues
- Domestic violence
- Alcohol or drug use
- Attitude of parents or carers (inappropriate or mechanical behaviour)
- A withdrawn or unduly frightened child, or inappropriate interaction between the child and carer
- A changing story or history that does not fit with the examination findings or development of the child
- Odd time of presentation
- Delayed presentation
- Repeated attendances
- Any injuries (particularly fractures or head injuries) in non-ambulant children
- Child not in school
  Concerns should be raised if:

- An adult carer of children has attended following a domestic violence incident
- Main carer suffering from physical/mental health problems
- Children accompanying adult patient
- Children identified as at potential risk through discussion with carer/mother
- The family is involved in multi-agency working, e.g. social care, family support worker, HV, school nurse.

Practitioners who are working with families and children would be expected to share their concerns and intention to make a referral with the child's parents/carers.

Parents may request that a referral is not made; however, the needs of the child are paramount.

In cases where the practitioners are forewarned about receiving child protection information they should take care not to agree to accept a conditional confidence, e.g. promising not to disclose or act upon information, which could be detrimental to the child's welfare.

Further reading

HM Government (2006) Working Together to Safeguard Children. The Stationery Office: London
National Collaborating Centre for Women's and Children's Health (2009) When to suspect child maltreatment. NCCWCH: London.
www.everychildmatters.gov.uk/socialcare/safeguarding

⑦ Paediatric physiology

Introduction

Children are not small adults – their anatomy and physiology varies significantly in comparison to that of adults. Because of these variations in a child's anatomy and physiology which change during a child's growth, they can be classified in the following groups:

- Neonates: up to 28 days after birth
- Infants: up to one year
- Child: one year to onset of puberty
- Adolescents: up to 16 years of age

An overview of the changing physiology in each group will follow.

Respiratory system

Neonates are obligatory 'nose breathers'. They have narrow nasal passages that can become easily blocked with secretions and the presence of a nasogastric tube can provide problems.

The oxygen consumption is high at birth at 7mL/kg/min compared to an adult at 3–4mL/kg/min.

The airway and chest wall are compliant in infants as the diaphragmatic and intercostal muscles have no type 1 muscle fibres. These type 1 muscle fibres are 'fatigue resistant'. Any increase of work of breathing, due to infection or other, in infants is not well tolerated due to the deficit in these muscle fibres. The respiratory control centre in the brain is also poorly developed in neonates and infants and the presence of hypoxia and hypercapnia can lead to apnoea and eventually respiratory failure if the breathing is not supported by oxygen or ventilatory support.

See Table 1.3 for normal respiratory rates for different ages.

Table 1.3 Normal respiratory rates

<1 year	30–40 per minute
1–2 years	25–35 per minute
2–5 years	25–30 per minute
5–12 years	20–25 per minute
>12 years	15–20 per minute

Cardiovascular system

Fetal circulation begins its transition to normal circulation with the first breath. This breath decreases pulmonary vascular resistance, and the increase in oxygen and negative intrathoracic pressure diverts blood away from the patent ductus arteriosus, causing it to constrict and eventually close.

Normal heart blood flow consists of venous blood flowing into the right atrium from the inferior vena cava (body) and the superior vena cava (head and upper arms). The blood flows from the right atrium through the tricuspid valve into the right ventricle. The right ventricle pumps the blood through the pulmonary valve into the pulmonary artery, and on to the lungs to be oxygenated. From the lungs it flows into the left atrium via the pulmonary veins. It then flows through the mitral valve into the left ventricle. The left ventricle pumps the oxygenated blood up through the aortic valve into the ascending aorta and onwards to the systemic circulation.

Infants have a high cardiac output of 200mL/kg body weight/min progressively decreasing to 100mL/kg/min by adolescence.

Sixty per cent of the heart muscle in infants is non-contractile, compared to 30% in adults, and therefore the ventricle is less compliant. This means that in order to increase their cardiac output, infants have to increase their heart rate. Infants rely on increasing their heart rate to maintain their cardiac output, as they are unable to increase their stroke volume.

The systolic blood pressure at birth is low, about 80/50, increasing to 90/60 within the first month of life. Blood pressure reaches adult levels by the age of 16.

See Table 1.4 for normal systolic blood pressure values for different ages.

Table 1.4 Normal systolic blood pressure values

<1 year	70–90 mmHg
1–2 years	80–95 mmHg
2–5 years	80–100 mmHg
5–12 years	90–110 mmHg
>12 years	100–120 mmHg

Renal system

The kidneys are immature at birth and so glomerular filtration and tubular function are reduced. This can result in the inability to cope with large sodium loads, and therefore dehydration is poorly tolerated in the under twos.

Normal urine output is estimated at 1–2 mL/kg/h.

Complete maturation will occur at around 2 years of age.

Hepatic system

The liver is responsible for many functions, which can be categorized into three main groups:

- Metabolism: the liver metabolizes carbohydrates, fats, proteins, drugs and hormones. The liver is initially immature at birth, in that the liver enzymes, although developed, have not been 'stimulated' to function. Therefore the time taken to metabolize toxins or drugs (half life) is much longer and the effect of those toxins or drugs will be extended. As the infant grows, hepatic blood flow increases and liver enzymes are induced, so metabolism becomes quicker.
- Filtration: the liver contains Kupffer cells, which remove endotoxins, bacteria, and any other potentially harmful substances from the blood.

56996

- Storage: the liver can usually hold large amounts of blood (600mL in adults), and copes well during fluid shifts, vascular changes or other conditions causing similar. It also stores vitamins and minerals.

Central nervous system

The central nervous system is anatomically complete at birth, but myelination is still ongoing so function is reduced. Myelination is rapid though in the first 2 years of life and is completed by 7 years of age.

Cerebral autoregulation is present and functional from birth, and capable of rapid response in infants and young children.

The brain is totally dependent on glucose for its energy source, as it is the only molecule that can cross the blood–brain barrier. Other energy sources such as fatty acids cannot cross the barrier. The brain does not store glucose, and has only 3 minutes of energy supply to maintain normal cerebral function.

Further reading

Davies J, Hassell L (2001). Children in Intensive Care. London: Churchill Livingstone
Tortora GJ, Anagnostakos N (1990). Principles of Anatomy and Physiology (6th edn). London: Harper and Row

⑦ **Medicine administration**

Giving medication to children requires careful consideration in all circumstances; however, in the emergency care environment, where staff are under pressure or rushed, or in situations which require urgent action, the risk of error increases and therefore added vigilance and care are required.

As with all situations, using a system or tool to aid memory can support safe practice. Generally within the field of medicine administration the 5 'C's' (or 5 'Rights') are commonly used; these are:

- Correct Child
- Correct Drug
- Correct Dose
- Correct Time
- Correct Route

If we look at these areas more closely in regard to children within emergency situations we can consider where the additional dangers may occur.

Correct child

- Particularly problematic as formal identification measures are often missed in an emergency.
- Important to ensure that name bands are used to aid identification, even in an acute situation.
- Ensure that verbal verification of identity is also adhered to, either from the parent/carer or child him/herself.

Correct drug/correct route

- Identification of the correct drug and route is essential; however, when rushing it is easy to misread a prescription chart, ampoule, bottle, or label.
- *Beware*. It is also more common in an emergency for medication orders to be given as a verbal instruction; this practice should be avoided where possible, yet remains common practice in situations such as a resuscitation. In these circumstances, however, the medications to be given generally adhere to a clinical care algorithm; therefore if a request is unusual it must be questioned to ensure understanding and prescribed formally.
- **Ensure that any allergies have been identified.**

Correct dose

Medication calculations should not be rushed; therefore even in an emergency situation ensure that you are confident with your calculation. Some basic tips for good practice would include:

- **Find a quiet space** – move away from the patient and other practitioners in order to ensure that you can obtain a quieter environment to think about what you are doing.
- **Commit to the task** – do not juggle calculating a medication with other jobs, such as recording observations, instructions, etc. Commit to checking or calculating the medication and try not to allow interruptions.
- **Double check** – if in doubt ensure you use a second person, even if you work in a unit that advocates single person checking; never give a medication unless you are certain you are correct.

- **Use common sense** – the golden rule of any medicine calculation is to estimate first. Ensure that you have a clear idea of a sensible dose amount, i.e. not higher or lower than your available stock solution. By doing this you will identify potential errors of miscalculation quickly.
- **Use a calculator if needed** – even if only to check your calculation. The majority of medication calculation guides now advocate the use of a simple calculator to aid mental arithmetic skills in more complex sums (see below).
- **Understand the formula** – the understanding and conceptualization of the problem is of greater importance when performing calculations than the actual 'maths'. This is where a calculator can be used to aid mental arithmetic; however, a calculator is only as good as the information entered into it. Whichever formula you choose to use (Box 1.1 shows the most common), it is essential that you understand how it is constructed, and where you find the information to complete each section of the sum.

Box 1.1 Drug calculation formula

What you want (Prescribed dose) × **What it is in** (Stock solution) = **What you have got** (Stock dose)

Correct time

- Accurate documentation of drug administration should be rigorously followed.
- Potential problems arise if multiple pieces of documentation exist. Therefore, as an additional safety measure, ensure that you check all available notes to make certain that medications prescribed and administered from the emergency department paperwork are then transferred onto any subsequent prescription charts that are written for the baby or child.
- Documentation of the exact time of drug administration is essential to ensure accuracy of timing when additional doses of a drug are required.

Further reading

Hutton M, Gardner H (2005). Calculation Skills. *Paediatric Nursing* 17(2)
Nursing and Midwifery Council (2004). Standards for Medicine Management. NMC, London

ⓘ **Managing aggressive situations**

Although aggressive behaviours are seen as challenging and unwelcome, it is important to remember that such behaviours have a communicative function. It is our role as health professionals to be self aware, prioritizing safety first, and to react to the situation with a measured response which is encompassed within a legal and ethical framework.

The chapter provides guidance only and each individual area of employment will differ depending on their policies, but each will be in accordance with legal and ethical frameworks.

• Aggressive behaviour is behaviour that is deemed socially unacceptable, which may result in psychological or physical harm to self or others or damage to property.
• This could include destructive behaviours, disruptiveness, verbal abuse, physical attack, or self-injury.
• The contextual nature of the aggressive behaviour will be dependent on factors such as developmental stages of the child, social learning and personal experience, and whether other adults are involved. Such factors may also impact upon the mode of expression of aggression (e.g. biting, throwing objects, hitting) and also on the intensity, frequency and duration.

Organizations have a responsibility towards 'frontline' staff who may come into contact with an aggressive situation (see Fig. 1.2).

• It is the employer's responsibility to train practitioners to a standard that allows them to safely function within their role.
• Guidance and support should be available in all areas.

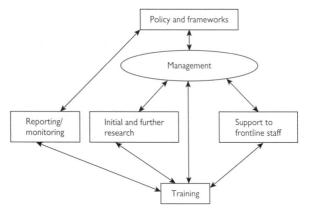

Fig. 1.2 Managing aggressive situations

Thinking about your own management and self awareness, consider these three key areas. Each will directly affect you and will subsequently have an impact on how you respond and engage with the situation (Fig. 1.3).

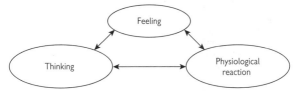

Fig.1.3 Key areas affecting individual response to an aggressive situation

Actions during an aggressive incident

For the purposes of this section we are focusing on the decision-making processes for a frontline member of staff who is involved in an escalating aggressive situation. The list below is not represented exactly as a sequential process nor does it present a panacea. Underneath each heading (consideration) will follow some suggested situational solutions.

Proximity

- If you are 'too close' then you are in danger of entering into another's personal space, which can be seen as an aggressive act in itself.
- If you are 'too close' you are in danger of escalating the behaviour further, reducing your reaction time, and reducing the effectiveness of your peripheral vision in assessing non-verbal behaviour.
- If you start from a position of being 'too close' be aware that this close proximity could be the trigger for the aggression, and therefore remove yourself quickly and politely to a safe distance.
- If you are 'too far' from the individual then your communication may be compromised and also misinterpreted. This can be due to the person not visually seeing you as being able to contribute to the solution of their situation. Also, your verbal communication may be lost within the environmental noise.
- A suggested safe distance would be out of a person's reach (out of their ability to make physical contact with you). Be aware of the person's ability to move and adjust your position accordingly.
- Avoid approaching anyone from behind.

Formulating a non-verbal response

- Facial and eye expressions – gentle relaxed gaze being at the same eye level whenever possible.
- Posture – relaxed, upright, well balanced and facing the other person directly at a distance acceptable to the other's cultural background and considering your own safety first.
- Gestures – open palm gestures.

Formulating a verbal response

- A practical tip is to take a deep breath before responding to the situation. This is beneficial for many reasons: it gives you time to think, physiologically provides your organs with oxygen (fight and flight response), and, by breathing out, can help you to present as less tense, e.g. lowering shoulders, thus looking more calm and assertive.
- Try where possible to maintain a conversational level of speech in relation to its tone, rate, rhythm, and volume. If your voice level rises, the other person may perceive this as aggressive on your part. If your voice level lowers then the other person may perceive this as submissive.
- Keep the dialogue open by using open ended questions – this has the potential benefit of gaining an understanding of the nature and causation of the person's aggression. Appraise a situation for its context:
  - Is the anger appropriate in proportion to the situation?
  - Is the anger directed at you personally, or are you the face of the institution?
  - Is this within limits of 'normal' or acceptable anger or is this aggression?
  - Is this behaviour likely to lead to harm towards you or others?

Other considerations

- Manage others around you (staff, parents, parental figures).
- Level of involvement of others in the immediate environment and reactions include:
  - silence, verbal interaction, some may attempt to bypass staff, some may offer to help, other people not (identifying potential allies and potential hindrances).
- Environmental factors (call button systems, objects, furniture, exits).
- Other factors (think about how you feel in terms of physical ability, e.g. exhausted from running to the situation, knowledge and skills to deal with the situation).

Actions after an aggressive incident

- Debrief – seek support, talk about it:
  - Document the incident and remain objective.
  - Have a professional supportive colleague with you while doing this.
- Do not go home carrying the emotional stress that the incident has caused.

Further reading

Lawrence C, Beale D, Leather P, Dickson R (1999) Violence in public houses: an integrated organisational approach. In Leather P, Brady C, Lawrence C, Beale D, Cox T (eds) Work Related Violence: Assessment and Intervention. Routledge, London

① Clinical holding

Definition

In children's nursing the terms holding, restraint, and immobilization are often used interchangeably, and further research is required to explore staff, parents', and children's perceptions.

The following definitions from the Royal College of Nursing (2003) are:

'Restraint' – use of force to overpower the child

'Holding still' or 'Immobilisation' – using limited force with the child's/parents' permission to manage a painful procedure quickly.

Care which may require clinical holding

Children are required to remain still to ensure accuracy of procedures and care, and to prevent injury to themselves and others. Holding usually occurs for the following reasons:

- Application of dressings/casts/splints
- Insertion of intravenous cannula/nasogastric tubes
- Administration of medication
- Suture insertion/removal
- Investigative procedures – lumbar puncture, X-rays

Potential complications

Complications may be immediate or long term. Although no longitudinal studies have explored the effects of restraint, the emerging knowledge of children's emotional development suggests it would be neglectful to dismiss the potential effect of the distress of clinical holding.

Short term effects may include:

- Anxiety
- Injury such as bruising or pressure sores
- Asphyxiation
- Regression in developmental milestones
- Alteration in behaviour during hospitalization

Long term effects of distress in childhood have been identified including anxiety disorders, post traumatic stress disorder, diabetes, heart disease, and immune disorders.

The role of the practitioner when holding the child

- The practitioner should be competent at holding techniques
- Care must be taken not to injure child
- Body, head and limbs must be held in a natural position
- Pressure must be avoided on face, neck, chest, abdomen and genitalia
- Ensure breathing and circulation are not compromised
- Reassure child throughout procedure and act as advocate if necessary

Factors to consider

A variety of factors may influence how or why an infant/child is held for a procedure; this list in not exhaustive:

- Age/cognitive ability
- Previous experience of hospital
- Presence/absence of parent
- Urgency of treatment and distress of injury

- Complexity of procedure necessary
- Experience of healthcare professionals involved
- Healthcare professionals' knowledge of emotional development/emotional needs of the infant/child
- Figure 1.4 offers key points to consider when caring for the infant/child in the ED.

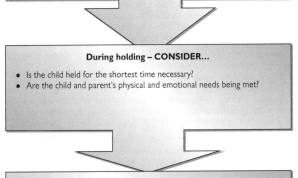

Pre holding – STOP...

- Why does this child need to be held still?
- Is this procedure urgent/necessary?
- Are there any alternatives to clinical holding that could be considered – distraction/imagery/sedation?
- Are you educated/experienced to competently hold this child?
- Are the parent(s) present? Have you considered what their input can be?
- Have you explained the rationale and proposed positioning to the child and parent(s)?
- Has consent been given by the parents and if possible by the child (RCN 2003)?

During holding – CONSIDER...

- Is the child held for the shortest time necessary?
- Are the child and parent's physical and emotional needs being met?

Post holding – REFLECT...

- Was there an appropriate rationale for clinical holding?
- Was the method/length of holding suitable in this situation?
- Are there any potential effects for the child/parents?
- Were they addressed and how can this be addressed in future?
- Debrief the child and parents
- Document events in detail

Fig. 1.4 Key points to consider when caring for the infant or child in ED

Further reading

Royal College of Nursing (2003). Restraining, holding still and containing children and young people: guidance for nursing staff. Royal College of Nursing, London.
Folkes K (2005) Is restraint a form of abuse? Paediatric Nursing 17:41–4.

ⓘ Performing an emergency X-ray on a child

Radiographers work under two laws designed to protect the patient, staff and others:
- Ionizing Radiation (Medical Exposure) Regulations 2000 (IRMER)
- Ionizing Radiation Regulations 1999 (IRR 99).

These aim to reduce the risks associated with medical radiation, while maximizing the benefits gained from diagnosis.

ALERT: incomplete request forms are one of the principal reasons that a request for imaging may be declined, causing delays to the procedure.

Radiographers are obliged to justify the exposures they make; hence the request form must contain enough information to enable them to do that.

Justification criteria for paediatric X-rays can be found in the Guidelines from the Royal College of Radiologists – 'Making the Best Use of Clinical Radiology Services' (RCR 2007).

Justification criteria for emergency mobile (portable) X-ray:
- Patient too ill or unstable to travel to department
- Patient immunosuppressed and/or barrier nursed
- Patient on invasive monitoring or therapy, e.g. nebuliser

X-rays are taken in various positions according to the information required and difficulty of the examination:
- X-ray supine if < 1 year or if injuries mean the child cannot be moved
- Erect antero-posterior (AP) projection until approx 5 years
- Postero-anterior (PA) projection for > 5 years or AP if sitting/trolley/etc.
- If querying perforation; child in erect or decubitus (right side uppermost) position for at least 5 minutes to allow free gas to rise.

Due to the projection, a mobile chest X-ray is rarely as diagnostic as a departmental image, and radiation protection for other patients, visitors, and staff in the vicinity of the patient is more difficult to achieve.

ALERT: requesting a mobile (portable) X-ray just to get it done quicker when the patient could otherwise travel to the department is not justified under IRMER, and the request may be declined, causing delays.

Management can and should be done co-operatively between nurse and radiographer. Consider all the following:
- Preparation of child and carer before X-ray (which can be done by nurse before radiographer arrives, thereby saving time) includes removal of clothing, necklaces, all leads, etc. that can be removed from area, also anything which might cause an artefact on the image, e.g. blankets, clothing, jewellery, long hair, bras.
- Clear and concise explanation of procedure, especially if the child must be moved as this may cause distress. It is important to use simple

language appropriate to the age of the child. Include an explanation of the 'big machine', and possible 'noise', but that it won't touch them.
- Consider 'play therapy' if time (unlikely in the emergency situation).
- It is important to follow radiographer's instructions regarding position, breathing, etc., so that the best image is achieved. If the child is ventilated, the child must lie straight for X-ray to show midline positioning of the endotracheal tube.
- Radiation protection of child, holder and other staff: a controlled area of 2 m exists around the X-ray machine – anyone who does not need to be present should leave the area. Anyone holding a patient must wear lead protection.
- The holder's hands MUST be out of the primary X-ray beam.
- Ensure privacy when undressing for all children.
- Special consideration should be given to mentally ill and physically disabled children: awareness of their limitations and physical needs such as that lying straight may be difficult and painful for some children.
- Liaison between radiographer and nurse for timing of X-ray, e.g. after feed so calmer, if practical.

Further reading

Ionising Radiation (Medical Exposure) Regulations (2000) accessible at: http://www.dh.gov.uk/en/ Publicationsandstatistics/Publications/PublicationsPolicyAndGuidance/DH_4007957
Ionising Radiation Regulations (1999) accessible at: http://www.hse.gov.uk

Critical events

:Ö: **Recognition of the sick child**

Recognition of the sick child can be difficult, and clues can be missed as infants/children are unable to describe their symptoms.

Therefore, it is important to use a structured approach. The European Resuscitation Council recommend using the airway, breathing, circulation (ABC) approach, to which may be added 'D' for disability.

Airway and breathing
- Respiratory rate—a raised rate may indicate lung or airway disease or metabolic acidosis.
- Recession—may be intercostal, subcostal or sternal.
- Inspiratory/expiratory noises—stridor or wheeze.
- Grunting—a sign of severe respiratory distress as it is an attempt to prevent airway collapse by generating a positive end expiratory pressure.
- Accessory muscle use—in infants this may cause head bobbing.
- Nasal flaring.

It should be remembered that if a child is in respiratory distress for a long period, then they will become exhausted and the signs of increased effort will decrease. Exhaustion is a pre-terminal sign and requires prompt attention.

Auscultation of the chest will indicate the amount of air being inspired and expired. Chest movement should be symmetrical and regular. A silent chest is extremely concerning.

Effects of respiratory distress on other organs
- Heart rate—initially produces tachycardia. Prolonged hypoxia leads to bradycardia—a pre-terminal sign.
- Skin colour—initially pale. Cyanosis is a pre-terminal sign.
- Mental status—hypoxia causes agitation and drowsiness.

Circulation
- Heart rate—increases in shock.
- Pulse volume—absent peripheral or weak central pulses are a sign of advanced shock.
- Capillary refill—should be less than 2 seconds.
- Blood pressure—children maintain their BP for long periods. Hypotension is a pre-terminal sign.

When assessing a sick child ABC takes priority and assessment of these should be repeated until normal parameters are reached.

Disability
A rapid assessment of level of consciousness is performed using:

A	Alert
V	Responsive to voice only
P	Responsive to pain only
U	Unconscious

If a child is at level P/U then it equates to a Glasgow Score of <8 and in-tubation should be considered to protect the airway (the paediatric Glasgow Coma Scale is applicable to infants too young to speak).

Further reading

Advanced Life Support Group (2005) Advanced Paediatric Life Support: The practical approach. 4th edn. London: BMJ Books (Wiley-Blackwell)
http://www.patient.co.uk/doctor/Glasgow-Coma-Scale-(GCS).htm

☼ Recognizing a seriously ill child

Early recognition of the seriously ill child is vital. Intervention given in the initial stages of illness improves outcome and stops the progression to cardiorespiratory arrest (Advanced Life Support Group 2005).

Rapid assessment using A = airway (cervical spine immobilization in trauma), B = breathing, C = circulation and D = disability can save lives.

See Table 2.1.

Table 2.1 Rapid assessment using ABC

ACTION	RATIONALE
A = AIRWAY	
Check patency/ maintain airway	• Partial/fully obstructed airway may be primary problem; opening airway may start breathing • Proceed to breathing when airway assessed as open and effective
B = BREATHING	
Assess rate	• Tachypnoea first sign of respiratory distress • Trends in rate over time more significant than single recordings • Bradypnoea highly significant: pre-terminal sign of exhaustion/central nervous system depression • Hypoxia: vasoconstriction/skin pallor
Assess air entry/ breath sounds	• Chest movement/air flow should be equal • Listen for breath sounds: Stridor = inspiratory noise, upper airway Wheeze = expiratory noise, lower airway Grunting = serious disease, exhalation against part closed glottis causing positive end expiratory pressure Silent/reduced noise = obstruction/exhaustion; a pre-terminal sign
Assess work of breathing	• Intercostals/subcostal/sternal recession/retraction: work of breathing • Accessory muscle use head bobbing/see-saw breathing implies inefficient respiration • Nasal flaring, seen in infants
Assess colour/ record saturations	• Central cyanosis: pre-terminal sign seen first on mucosa of mouth/nail beds

Table 2.1 Rapid assessment using ABC (*Continued*)

ACTION	RATIONALE
C = CIRCULATION	
Assess heart rate	• Tachycardia occurs to maintain tissue oxygenation; if this fails hypoxia/acidosis result, then bradycardia, a pre-terminal sign with cardiorespiratory arrest imminent
	• Trends in rate over time more significant than single recordings
Assess blood pressure	• Caution: hypotension is a late, pre-terminal sign of illness, cardiorespiratory arrest imminent
Assess peripheral/central pulses	• Peripheral pulse before central pulse; a diminished central pulse precedes cardiorespiratory arrest
Assess skin perfusion	• Capillary refill time >2 seconds is an early indictor of shock
	• Progressive line of coldness/mottling starts at digits and proceeds towards trunk; peripheral vasoconstriction
Monitor urine output	• 1mL/kg/hour = inadequate renal perfusion
D = DISABILITY	
Assess mental state	• Drowsy, agitated, lethargic indicates reduced cerebral perfusion, which will lead to reduced consciousness level
	• **Don't ever forget glucose**: BM-test using a blood glucose testing strip

An infant or child's vital signs should be appropriate to that child's age and condition. Normal vital signs are not always appropriate for a seriously ill child.

Further reading

Advanced Life Support Group (2005) Advanced Paediatric Life Support: The practical approach. 4th edn. London: BMJ Books (Wiley-Blackwell)

European Paediatric Life Support (2006) European Paediatric Life Support Course: Provider Manual for use in the UK. 2nd edn. London: Resuscitation Council (UK)

☼ Reasons why children arrest

The aetiology of cardiorespiratory arrest in children differs to that in adults. Physiological, anatomical and pathological differences more commonly lead to secondary cardiorespiratory arrest—resulting from respiratory and/or circulatory failure—rather than primary cardiorespiratory arrest, which results from cardiac dysfunction/arrhythmia (see Fig. 2.1 for common underlying causes for cardiorespiratory arrest).

Primary cardiorespiratory arrest

- Due to cardiac arrhythmia—commonly ventricular fibrillation or pulseless ventricular tachycardia.
- Onset abrupt and unpredictable, usually resulting from primary heart disease.
- Uncommon in children, but can be seen with existing cardiac disease, post cardiac surgery, with hypothermia, and following poisoning.
- Immediate defibrillation is required—delays reduce the chance of return to circulation by 10% every minute.

Secondary cardiorespiratory arrest

- Sequence more commonly seen in children—occurs due to the body's inability to cope with the underlying illness/injury.
- Pre-terminal rhythm is bradycardia—leading to asystole or pulseless electrical activity.
- Can arise from respiratory failure: inadequate oxygenation leads to hypoxia, hypercapnia, and acidosis, causing cell damage and death, and resulting in cardiac arrest.
- Can arise from circulatory failure: organs deprived of essential nutrients/oxygen are unable to remove waste products, causing hypoxia and acidosis. Inadequate circulation means the vital organs are underperfused.
- Body will activate physiological responses leading to compensated respiratory/circulatory failure. If no medical interventions, then progression to decompensated respiratory/circulatory failure occurs. If still no medical interventions, cardiac arrest follows.

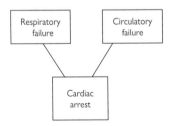

Fig. 2.1 Common underlying causes for cardiorespiratory arrest in children

- Respiratory and circulatory failure can occur separately or together—however, both will always unite as the body's condition worsens.
- Outcome of secondary cardiorespiratory arrest is very poor. Early recognition and intervention of the seriously ill child is vital, using the paediatric early warning system (PEWS).
- Knowledge of the underlying physiological and anatomical differences in children is important—these differences are often linked to the common illnesses/injuries that can lead to cardiorespiratory arrest.
- Always call for senior/specialist help as soon as possible.
- See reasons for cardiopulmonary arrest in Tables 2.2 a and b.

Table 2.2a Respiratory

Distress	Depression
Asthma	Convulsions
Croup	Head injury
Foreign body	Poisoning

Table 2.2b Circulatory

Fluid loss	Maldistribution
Blood loss	Septic shock
Gastroenteritis	Anaphylaxis
Burns	Cardiac disease

Further reading

Advanced Life Support Group (2005) Advanced Paediatric Life Support: The practical approach (4th edn). London: BMJ Books (Wiley-Blackwell)

European Paediatric Life Support (2006) European Paediatric Life Support Course: Provider Manual for use in the UK. 2nd edn. London: Resuscitation Council (UK)

Paediatric early warning tool: http://www.healthcareworkforce.nhs.uk/wtd_pilot_pages/liverpool_pilot/paediatric_early_warning_tool.html

:☠: **Paediatric basic life support (BLS)**

Definitions with reference to basic life support
Infant: birth to 1 year
Child: 1 year to puberty

Clinical signs
- Unresponsive
- Recent history of being generally unwell
- Evidence of trauma
- History of inhaling a foreign body
- Pale
- Cyanosed
- Pulseless
- Sudden onset of symptoms
- Congenital heart disease
- Recent history of breathing difficulties

The outcome from paediatric cardiac arrest is extremely poor. The anatomy and physiology of children affects both the cause and the management of paediatric disease and injury.

Application of the ABCD approach early in paediatric emergencies will improve outcome.

Immediate action
- Will be based on the Resuscitation Council Basic Life Support Guidelines
- Will depend on where the emergency has occurred
- Requires skilled help and equipment

Management
- Ensure safety of the victim and rescuer
- Stimulate
- Assess for signs of life
- Shout
- Alert others to the emergency

Airway
- Open the airway (Fig. 2.2):
  - neutral position: infant
  - head tilt/chin lift: child

Breathing
Check for breathing:
- Look at the chest
- Listen for expired air respiration
- Feel for exhaled breath
- If no signs of effective breathing attempt to deliver 5 effective breaths
- Call out for help

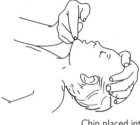

Chin placed into neutral position

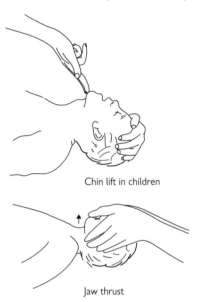

Chin lift in children

Jaw thrust

Fig. 2.2 Open the airway
Oxford Handbook of Children's and Young People's Nursing, Glasper et al., (2006), p.789, with permission from Oxford University Press

- If in hospital use a pocket mask or bag mask valve device. If out of hospital with no equipment deliver a slow steady breath lasting 1–1.5 seconds. To do this:
  - Seal your mouth over the infant's nose and mouth.
  - Pinch the child's nose and seal your mouth over the child's mouth.
  - As you deliver rescue breathing look for any gagging or coughing movements; such response, or indeed a lack of response, will form part of the assessment of C, circulation.

Circulation
- Are there signs of life?
- Is there a central pulse: in children, feel the carotid artery for 10 seconds, and in infants feel the brachial artery for 10 seconds.
- If no signs of life and no evidence of a central circulation, chest compressions will be required.
  However:
- If still alone with the victim and no breathing or signs of life, call for help—dial 2222 in hospital, if out of hospital dial 999 or 112.
- If alone go for help at this point.

Action
- In the chain of survival, basic life support is essential while help is coming.
- Chest compressions must be performed to circulate blood around the body, primarily to take oxygen to the brain.
- Expired air respiration is necessary to provide oxygen to the blood.

Basic life support
Child
- Place the child on a firm surface.
- Kneel by the side of the child's chest.
- Place the heel of one hand on the lower third of the chest and aim to depress the chest by 1/3 of the child's chest diameter. For a larger child this may require 2 hands to be used; if so place the heel of the other hand on top of the first hand.
- Interlock your fingers to avoid applying pressure over the child's ribs.
- Position yourself so that your shoulders are over the child's sternum.
- After each compression release the pressure and repeat at a rate of 100 compressions per minute.
- After 30 compressions return to the airway.
- The airway will need to be opened again.
- Close the child's nose by pinching the soft part of the nose using your thumb and index finger.
- Continue with chin lift and allow the child's mouth to open.
- Place your lips around the child's mouth and with a good seal blow steadily into the mouth, watching the child's chest rise.
- Take your lips away and allow the air to come out, and watch the chest wall fall.
- Take another breath and repeat to give a total of 2 effective breaths.
- Go back to the landmarks on the chest and repeat the 30 chest compressions.
  Basic life support must continue until:
- Help arrives to take over
- The child starts to breathe normally
- You are physically too exhausted to continue

Performing basic life support is very tiring; where possible share the work-load with another rescuer who can do the breathing and/or compressions with you, or get another rescuer to take over from you.

Infant
- Compress the mid lower-third of the sternum by approximately 1/3 of the depth of the chest using the tips of 2 fingers on the lower third of the sternum. This is good for the single rescuer.
- For a two-person rescue, chest compression may be better using the encircling technique whereby the person doing chest compressions places both thumbs flat side by side, on the lower third of the sternum with the thumb tips pointing towards the infant's head, spreads the rest of both hands, fingers together to encircle the lower part of the infant's rib cage, and presses down with the thumbs depressing the chest again 1/3 of the depth of the infant's chest.

Parents and carers
The resuscitation of any child is very distressing. For people with the child, care should be provided where possible. Ideally someone should support the parents or carers through the event, allowing them to stay if they wish.

Techniques practised throughout basic life support
- Airway opening
- Chest compressions
- Calling for expert help
- Paediatric resuscitation ratios

Further reading
Resuscitation Council (UK) (2010) Paediatric Basic Life Support. London: Resuscitation Council (UK).

☠ Paediatric advanced life support (ALS)

Resuscitation guidelines are produced to simplify treatment for managing medical emergencies.

Dealing with paediatric emergencies is always stressful. The incidence of paediatric cardiac arrest is small compared to the number of adult cardiac arrests.

The Resuscitation Council Guidelines are produced to provide a framework on which paediatric advanced life support (ALS) may be delivered.

Actions

Advanced life support
- Safety of rescuers
- Assess the patient
- Open the airway
- Assess respiratory effort: if not breathing deliver 5 rescue breaths
- Assess for signs of life and evidence of circulation: if not evident, perform chest compressions
- **Perform basic life support alternating 15 compressions with 2 breaths (15:2)**
- **Call resuscitation team**
- Bring cardiac arrest equipment to the victim
- This should include airway equipment including bag and mask, and intubation equipment
- Defibrillator/cardiac monitor
- Drug box
- Equipment to cannulate a vein or to insert an intraossious needle
- **Assess rhythm**
- The ALS treatment differentiates between a shockable rhythm (ventricular fibrillation, VF) or pulseless state (ventricular tachycardia, VT), and nonshockable (pulseless electrical activity/asystole) states.
- To monitor the rhythm place monitoring electrodes on the outer aspects of the chest. Place red tab to the right, lemon tab to the left and green tab over the spleen.
- If assessing the rhythm with defibrillator pads, place one pad below the right clavicle and one on the lower part of the rib cage on the left side of the chest.
- The pads should be 8–12cm in size for children and 4.5cm for infants.
- Check for a pulse for no more than 10 seconds.
- In children feel for a carotid pulse.
- In infants feel for a brachial pulse.

Nonshockable (asystole or pulseless electrical activity)
- More likely event in paediatrics.
- **Perform CPR.**
- Use high flow oxygen.
- When a bag mask unit is used deliver 15 compressions followed by 2 breaths.
- If the patient is intubated, chest compressions may be maintained at a rate of 100 per minute and 10–12 breaths delivered without interruptions.

- **Chest compressions and ventilation are vital to support cerebral perfusion and should only be interrupted for defibrillation**.
- Chest compressions are tiring and it is important that the team leader considers the team and changes the individuals performing CPR at regular intervals. It is therefore important that as many people as possible should be trained to perform good CPR.
- **Adrenaline** should be given every 3–5 minutes (N.B. this comes in two strengths and care must be taken to ensure correct strength used).
- Adrenaline 10 mcg/kg needs to be given (0.1 mL/kg of body weight of a 1:10,000 solution). The delivery of the drug may be by any of the following routes:
  - Venous access should be achieved with no more than 3 attempts to cannulate within 90 seconds.
  - Intraosseous access should be established if venous access is unsuccessful.
  - Endotracheal adrenaline may be given if neither intravenous nor intraosseous access has been achieved (although the evidence base for this is weak). When the tracheal route is used, adrenaline should be given at 100mcg /kg (0.1 mL/kg of a 1:1,000 solution).
- **Continue CPR 15:2.**
- During CPR consider the potential reversible causes of the collapse. The patient's medical history may provide big clues as to the cause and treatment of the cardiac arrest.
- Using the 4 H's and 4 T's can help in recalling the possible causes; these are:
  - Hypoxia
  - Hypovolaemia
  - Hyper/hypokalaemia (electrolyte disturbances)
  - Hypothermia
  - Tension pneumothorax
  - Tamponade
  - Toxic therapeutic disturbance
  - Thromboembolism
- Remember that in some cardiac arrest events the child may have a combination of a number of these problems. For example, a child with meningococcal septicaemia will be hypovolaemic, with hypoxia and probably electrolyte disturbances.
- If a cause of the problem is identified it should be treated accordingly, along with CPR and adrenaline following the ALS cycle plus fluids given at 20 mL/hr IV/IO.

Shockable (ventricular fibrillation and ventricular tachycardia)
- More likely in intensive care and cardiac units particularly in children with congenital heart defects
- **Perform CPR**
- **Perform defibrillation**
- Manual defibrillation: deliver 1 shock at 4 J/kg
- Automated external defibrillator
- For children aged 1–8 years use paediatric pads to deliver the shock
- For children over 8 years use the adult pads to deliver the shock

- After the shock do not reassess the rhythm or pulse, but go straight back to CPR 15:2
- CPR for 2 minutes
- Check the monitor: if still a shockable rhythm deliver a 2nd shock
- CPR for 2 minutes
- While doing so consider the 4 H's and 4 T's
- After 2 minutes check the monitor
- If still a shockable rhythm, give adrenaline 10 mcg/kg IV/IO followed by the 3rd shock
- CPR for 2 minutes
- If still showing a shockable rhythm give a bolus of amiodarone 5 mg/kg followed by the 4th shock
- If still a shockable rhythm continue with the CPR/shock sequence giving adrenaline every 3–5 minutes
- If at any point with the shockable or nonshockable pathways there is a return of spontaneous circulation stop CPR, check breathing, check pulse, and check for signs of life.

Further reading

Resuscitation Council (UK) (2010) Resuscitation Guidelines 2005. London: Resuscitation Council (UK).

:☠: **Newborn life support (NLS)**

Introduction

The Resuscitation Council provides a systematic approach to newborn resuscitation.

The majority of newborns will self resuscitate and establish normal breathing, have good tone, colour, and a good heart rate by 3 minutes of age.

NLS differs from other BLS

Newborn babies have the following potential complications:

- A large occiput that lends itself to flexion/extension of the neck so occluding the airway
- The length and shape of the pharynx and larynx make intubation more difficult
- Fluid filled lungs cannot exchange gas
- Cardiac compressions will be of no use without first achieving lung aeration
- Newborn babies are obligatory nasal breathers
- Newborn babies are small and wet, and so lose heat very quickly. Therefore, NLS's initial focus is airway management.

Newborn adaptation to these issues

- A newborn's first few breaths have to be sufficiently forceful to overcome massive intrapulmonary resistance, and to push the fluid out from the alveoli into the interstitia, to be absorbed by the lymph system. This allows air to enter the lungs, allowing for oxygenation and establishing a resting lung volume.
- The heart is packed with glycogen stores, allowing it to continue pumping effectively during this relative hypoxia imposed on it during the birthing process.

In cases where this does not apply—immediate action

- Dry the baby and wrap in a dry, warm towel.
- This stimulus helps initiate the first breath, as will the relatively cold environment and clamping of the cord.
- Assess colour, tone, heart rate, and breathing effort.

Do you need to intervene? Do you need to call for HELP?

- No: the baby is crying, has good tone and heart rate and is pinking up. Give to parents.
- Yes: the baby is not breathing, still blue, with slow heart rate and poor tone. Call for help, and perform the following NLS procedures.

Perform the following airway adjuncts, giving 5 inflation breaths and assessing for chest wall movement and an increase in heart rate after each intervention:

(Inflation breaths use pressures of 30 cmH$_2$O and each breath should last 2–3 seconds. These breaths are unique to newborn resuscitation as they are mimicking those first few breaths a baby would normally take.)

- Put the head in the 'neutral' position to open the airway.
- Reposition the airway with a 1 person jaw thrust.

- Try the 2 person jaw thrust.
- Look for an obstruction in the airway using a laryngoscope; you may find a clot of blood, meconium or vernix. Remove with a large bore suction catheter. (DO NOT SUCTION BLIND.)
- A Guedel airway can be inserted at this point as laryngeal tone is likely to be poor and it will help maintain the airway.
- If you successfully inflate the lungs and so move the chest wall, the heart rate generally increases, but some ventilatory breaths (lasting 1–2 seconds each at a rate of 30/minute) may be needed to assist full recovery.
- If the chest wall is not moving with inflation breaths and the heart rate is not increasing, DO NOT start chest compressions as the lungs have not been inflated.
- If this is the case then go back to the first airway adjunct and repeat the cycle, checking equipment is functioning correctly.
- If the chest wall is moving but the heart rate is not increasing, start cardiac compressions at a rate of 90 per/minute.
- Your thumbs, if hand encircling the chest, or 2 fingers if not, should be 1 finger breadth beneath the intra-nipple line; and should depress the chest 1/3rd its anterio-posterio diameter.
- The compression:breath ratio for newborn infants is 3:1.
- Reassess in 30 seconds and repeat if heart rate still below 60 or not rising.

Reassess
- If there is no increase in the heart rate but the chest is moving with the ventilatory breaths, consider drugs to aid resuscitation.
- IV access in the newborn is usually by means of an umbilical venous catheter, or if necessary an intraosseous needle.

Drugs and their doses (flushed in with 2 mL of 0.9% saline)
- Sodium bicarbonate: 2–4mL/kg of 4.2%
- Adrenaline: 0.1 mL/kg of 1:10,000 solution (up to 0.3mL/kg if needed on 3rd dose)
- Glucose: 2–5 mL/kg of 10% glucose (only if documented hypoglycaemia)
- Volume: 10 mL/kg of 0.9% saline or blood.

If no spontaneous breathing or heart rate occurs at 20 minutes, then the outcome is going to be poor, and a senior clinician will take the decision to stop resuscitative efforts.

Further treatment
- Documentation of the event (including times when each action was taken).
- Discussion with the parents, so that they have full understanding of the event and actions taken.

Further reading
Resuscitation Council (UK) (2010). Newborn Life Support. http://www.resus.org.uk/pages/nls.pdf

☠ **Witnessed resuscitation**

Introduction

Within child health the concepts of family-centred care and partnership with parents are widely supported; therefore the notion that a parent should be forced to be separated from their child at a time of crisis, such as resuscitation, directly conflicts with the key principles of children's nursing. Back in 1996, the Resuscitation Council (UK) first published guidance on the presence of relatives in the resuscitation room and since then, although reservations remain, the practice of supporting parents within the resuscitation room has become more widely recognized, with the introduction of guidance both at a national and, in a few cases, local level. It is fair to say that parental presence at the resuscitation of children is not yet standard, as generally the decision remains at the discretion of the individual resuscitation team/team leader; however, the practice is becoming increasingly more common.

Arguments for

The arguments supporting witnessed resuscitation result from empirical evidence following studies, primarily within North America, but also worldwide, examining the responses from parents who had been present with their child during cardiopulmonary resuscitation (CPR). These included:

• Parents being able to see that everything possible was being done.
• Parents felt that they were included in the decision making process, even if that may be the decision to stop a futile attempt.
• Parents felt they were able to maintain some level of a parental role.
• Parents had the opportunity to prepare for possible death.
• Parents felt that they were able to continue to support their child, at a time when their child really needed them.
• Parents felt they were given the opportunity to say goodbye to their child prior to resuscitation ceasing.
• The suggestion that the grieving process is aided by having witnessed CPR.
• Most crucially the main argument for parents witnessing their child's resuscitation is that of parental right, and supporting the parent's wishes, as, for many, they do not want to be anywhere else!

Arguments against

Rather than supported by evidence, the majority of arguments against witnessed resuscitation are anecdotal fears from medical practitioners, many of which are discounted by the evidence available; however, they include:

• The sensory disturbance for the parent; resuscitation is potentially both visually and audibly disturbing.
• Lack of consent, as there is no way for medical staff to know whether the patient wishes for the relative to be present. Although key for the adult patient, this argument is counterbalanced by the rights of the parents when the patient is a child.
• Parent's emotional responses and the fear that the parent will interfere with the resuscitation process.
• Staff responses—concern regarding the ability to perform when being 'watched', and fear of complaint or reprisal.

Standards for supporting parents

As support for parents witnessing resuscitation continues to become more widely recognized, key factors must be observed:

- Choice—do not make assumptions. Not all parents wish to remain present, and of those who do, many may not know to ask. Therefore it is the nurses' responsibility to determine the parent's wishes, and then endeavour to support them where possible.
- Support person—in order for witness resuscitation to be successfully managed and appropriate, a support person must be available solely caring for the needs of the parent/s. A variety of models exist suggesting whose role this should be; however, in the majority of cases a senior experienced nurse is recommended. Should a parent choose not to witness their child's resuscitation their distress will not be eased, and therefore their need for support remains a priority.
- Consider the terminology used when talking to relatives: simple, repeated explanations are required.
- Understand that everyone is different, and therefore various emotional responses and coping mechanisms will be observed. Controlled crying, even sobbing, does not necessarily indicate that a parent is unable to cope or that their presence is inappropriate.

Further reading

Resuscitation Council (UK) (1994) Should relatives witness resuscitation? Available at: www.resus. org.uk/pages/witness.pdf

Royal College of Anaesthetists, The Royal College of Physicians of London, The Intensive Care Society & The Resuscitation Council (UK) (2004) Cardiopulmonary Resuscitation: Standards for Clinical Practice and Training, a joint statement. Resuscitation Council, London

Royal College of Pathologists and The Royal College of Paediatrics & Child Health (2004) Sudden unexpected death in infancy. Available from: www.rcpath.org or www.rcpch.ac.uk

Royal College of Nursing (2002) Witnessing resuscitation: guidance for nursing staff. Royal College of Nursing. Available from: http://www.rcn.org.uk/__data/assets/pdf_file/0006/78531/001736.pdf

ⓘ **Withholding and withdrawing curative treatment**

Introduction

- The child health team and parents have a duty to act in the best interests of the child, including life sustaining treatment. There are, however, times when treatment that merely saves life does not restore health or offer other benefits, and can be considered no longer in the best interests of the child.
- There is no legal obligation on health professionals to provide treatment that is not in the child's best interests.
- Withholding—decision from the onset is that any curative treatment would not be in the child's best interests, and no resuscitative action is taken.
- Withdrawing—decision is taken after treatment intended to prolong life has started, and involves the active withdrawal of life saving treatments.
- BUT withholding or withdrawing treatment does not mean that a child will receive no care. It is never acceptable to withdraw procedures that alleviate pain or promote comfort.
- The Royal College of Paediatrics and Child Health (2004) identifies five circumstances for withholding/withdrawing life saving treatments:
  - Brain dead child
  - Permanent vegetative state
  - 'No-chance' situation
  - 'No-purpose' situation
  - 'Unbearable' situation

Immediate action

- Acute life threatening events include:
  - Major trauma
  - Violence including homicide
  - Suicide
  - Sudden unexplained death in infancy
  - Drowning
  - Poisoning
  - Burns
  - Medical emergency in children with pre-existing conditions
  - Infection/respiratory disease resulting in respiratory and cardio-vascular collapse and multi-organ failure
- Life sustaining treatment should always be initiated, and is often commenced prior to arrival in the emergency department, by parents, the public or emergency services.
- Current protocol directs emergency practitioners to begin resuscitation unless contraindications are very clear, e.g. rigor mortis, injuries incompatible with life.
- Children should be taken to the emergency department, even if already dead, unless the circumstances of death require the body to remain at the scene for forensic examination.
- The dignity of the child should be protected at all times.

Emergency department

- Emergency department staff expecting the child should continue these efforts and call the paediatric cardiac arrest team.
- Resuscitation should continue until more information is available—for a minimum of 20–30 minutes with no evidence of a pulse, respiratory effort, cardiac output or cerebral activity.
- If cardiac arrest has occurred, usually secondary to respiratory acidosis and hypoxia, survival rates are only 3–17%.

Withholding/withdrawing life sustaining treatment

- The role of the paediatric resuscitation team leader is to decide if the attempt should be abandoned—taking into account the cause, pre-existing conditions, effectiveness and duration of basic life support and associated special circumstances including drugs and hypothermia—child's core temperature must rise to 32°C before discontinuation.
- Initial response to resuscitation may occur, and the child is transferred to a paediatric intensive care unit (PICU), where, following developments, the decision to withdraw treatment may still occur—withdrawal of life sustaining treatment accounts for between 43 and 72% of child deaths in PICUs.
- Where treatment is likely to be withdrawn or withheld, it is important to prepare parents and members of the health care team, informing them of the poor outcome, and to allow parents to be present during resuscitative efforts and be supported by a senior team member.
- The decision to withdraw/withhold life sustaining treatment needs to be made with the consent of the parents, where possible, but the child health team must take the main responsibility for the decision, which will help alleviate the burden of guilt some parents feel.
- Withdrawal/withholding of curative treatments do not always lead to death and the lives of those who survive, even with severe disability, should be respected and cared for appropriately.
- Resuscitation is not always appropriate: for some children with life-limiting or incurable conditions it may be argued that any attempt to resuscitate is not in the best interests of the child.
- Record all communication with parents; 'do not resuscitate' orders and discussions to withdraw/withhold life sustaining treatments should also be clearly recorded.

Legal and ethical framework

- Where health care professionals and parents do not agree with withholding/withdrawing life sustaining treatment, legal and ethical frameworks are in place to assist with this process, including:
  - United Nations Convention on the Rights of the Child
  - Legal duty
  - Children Act
  - Human Rights Act
  - Duty of Care

Further reading

Royal College of Pathologists and Royal College of Paediatric and Child Health (RCPath & RCPCH) (2004) Sudden unexpected death in infancy: A multi-agency protocol for care and investigation (Kennedy protocol), London, Royal College of Pathologists, Royal College of Paediatrics and Child Health. http://www.rcpch.ac.uk/Publications

RCPCH (2007) Services for Children in Emergency Departments. RCPCH, London. http://www.rcpch.ac.uk/Publications

Royal College of Paediatrics and Child Health (2004) Withholding or withdrawing life sustaining treatment in children: A framework for practice, 2nd edn. http://www.rcpch.ac.uk/Publications

⚠ **Post mortem examination and organ donation**

Background information

- Post mortem examination and organ donation may be post-death considerations following sudden death after a critical injury or medical emergency.
- These procedures are embedded in law. In the United Kingdom, for instance, the request for post mortem examination and organ donation is underpinned by the principles of informed consent in the Human Tissue Act of 2004. The Act also sets out a hierarchy of individuals who may be approached for consent in the case of a deceased child or adult.
- Each country has a national system for coordinating the organ donation process; for instance, in the United Kingdom, UK Transplant is the organization tasked with the responsibility of training transplant coordinators, allocating donor organs, and keeping statistics for the transplant community.

Post-mortem examination

- Mandatory post-mortem examination may be carried out as part of a coronial or criminal investigation. In this circumstance consent of the person/s that have guardianship of the child is not required.
- In some cases parent/s or guardian/s may be asked to consent to a 'hospital' post-mortem examination as a means of answering questions that might be important to the family, such as information about inherited conditions, the cause of death, or to inform clinical knowledge.
- In the case of a 'hospital' post-mortem the doctor with responsibility for the treatment of the child at the time of death, or a person trained to request post mortems, and designated with this task, should approach the decision makers to discuss the request and arrange appropriate support for the family.

Organ donation

- Organ donation should be considered as part of high quality end of life or bereavement care, as families are known to attribute importance to it. Therefore in all cases of donor suitability parent/s or guardian/s of the deceased child should be approached and the request discussed with them.
- Approaches to the bereaved parent/s or guardian/s should only be carried out by knowledgeable professionals who are trained to carry out this request and who are confident and comfortable with their role, and who can remain available to the family during their decision-making process, to support them and answer their questions.
- The discussion should ensure that families make a decision that is right for them; one they will remain happy with and will not regret later.
- Agreement to organ donation has been found to be most successful in cases where a transplant coordinator has had early involvement

with the family and where the discussion about donation has been carried out collaboratively with a member of the medical team and the transplant coordinator. Early referral to a transplant coordinator is therefore crucial to a positive donation outcome.

Effective systems for organ donation include

- Being familiar with the hospital's organ donation policy.
- Early identification of a potential donor, which depends on a severe injury or illness that is incompatible with life.
- Agreed clinical triggers, such as a score of 5 or less on the Glasgow Coma Scale, to initiate early identification of potential donors.
- Rapid, early referral and linkage of a transplant coordinator or hospital in-house coordinator with the family of a potential donor.
- Early collaboration between hospital staff caring for the child and their family and transplant coordinator/s, which should result in a jointly developed plan for approaching the family to request consent to donation. All concerned should feel comfortable and that they can effectively participate, as their roles in the process have been clearly defined.
- Ongoing assessment of the family, the family dynamics and recognition of the main decision-maker/s. Individualized, ongoing assessment is crucial to personalize the approach, fulfil the family's needs, evaluate their ability to process and use information, and ensure the decision is timely.
- Every effort to determine the family's willingness to donate should be made. If consent is initially withheld, reapproaching the family after they have had time to reflect upon the request can provide them with the opportunity to ensure that they have made the right decision.
- Timely follow-up of families is important to answer any questions they have about the donation process.
- Evaluation and feedback after each donation, by hospital staff and transplant coordinators, about the donation and its outcomes may be helpful in confirming that their efforts have been worthwhile, serves to keep them enthusiastic about donation, defines needs in the system, provides an opportunity to make modifications, builds team relationships, and identifies learning opportunities.
- Support mechanisms are advisable so staff can process any issues they may have about a particular death and donation.

Further reading

Department of Health (2008) Organs for transplants: a report from the organ donation taskforce. Department of Health Publications, London.

Shafer TJ, Wagner D, Chessare J, Zampiello FA, McBride V, Perdue J, (2006). Organ donation breakthrough collaborative: increasing organ donation through system redesign. *Critical Care Nurse*, 26(2), 33–49.

Sque M, Long T, Payne S, Allardyce D. (2008) Why do relatives not donate organs for transplants: 'sacrifice' or 'gift of life'? *Journal of Advanced Nursing* 61:134–44.

ⓘ Last offices

Introduction
- Last offices is the care delivered to the deceased patient and should include the patient's and family's wishes.

Background information
- The family's wishes may include how the deceased's body is to be laid out, spending time with the deceased, and the appropriate religious rituals, if applicable.
- Important ethical and legal guidelines need to be adhered to depending on the environment in which the child dies.
- Holistic care to the deceased child should be given.
- There may be special considerations with regard to the religious and cultural rituals of the deceased.

Management

Last offices in a hospital setting
- The hospital environment is an acute setting; for most, the death of a child here is unexpected, and at times initially unexplained.
- Recent changes have occurred through the H.M. Government document 'Working together to safeguard children' (2006).
- This document sets out guidelines for the death review process for hospital trusts to follow in the event of an unexpected death.
- The Local Safeguarding Children for Board (LSCB) ensures different phases occur immediately after death.
- These phases and evidence are gathered to be presented to the Death Overview Panel, which reviews all unexpected children's deaths in the country to attempt to prevent further deaths and ensure safety to the family.
- Within the emergency department (ED) and ward environment, the most important aspect of last offices is the care of the family/carers.
- Clear evidence shows parents are able to start the grieving process better if they witness the resuscitation and they can see first-hand the efforts made to try to resuscitate their child.
- The coroner is informed immediately after an unexpected death; the body then falls under his/her jurisdiction.
- All actions regarding samples required and management of the body will be agreed with the coroner.
- The consultant or most senior doctor involved in the resuscitation must speak with the family and explain what interventions were undertaken to save their child and the subsequent processes post-death.
- The police, in most cases of children brought into the ED, will be in attendance.
- Decisions will be made as to removal of clothes, nappies, and other invasive equipment such as cannulas or intubation tubes.
- The consultant paediatrician may be required to accompany the police to the child's home; this will enable the evidence to be gathered from a paediatrician's/medical perspective as well as a forensic one.
- The parents will be informed of the situation.

- The process may change if the family request donation of organs. In the case of unexplained death, or if there are safeguarding issues, the coroner would need to agree to the organ donation. If there are no objections then the organ donation would take place prior to the post mortem.
- The caring and washing of the child's body takes place under the instruction of the family and coroner.
- At the time of death the family should be asked if they would like the hospital chaplain or a member of their faith contacted to support them.
- Another aspect that may affect last offices is infection control. Hospital policies must be followed where cross contamination may occur.
- Families should be allowed the opportunity to spend time with their child in a quiet, protected area.
- For preservation purposes, the temperature in the hospital is not ideal. After 3–4 hours it will be necessary to remove the child's body, wrap the body in sheets, and take it to the mortuary with the appropriate documentation and samples. The family can make arrangements to see the child again.

NB: last offices arrangements for children in the community and hospice settings may differ significantly.

Advice

- Last Offices is an extremely complex topic, which is further complicated by legal guidelines and ethical considerations dependent on the environment of the child's death.
- Fulfilling the family's wishes, whether they are non-religious, religious or spiritual, is essential.
- As a healthcare professional in an emotionally charged situation, it is possible that caring for a deceased child may affect you, and therefore adequate support is needed for both the family and healthcare professionals involved.

Further reading

Kent, H. and McDowell, J. (2004) Sudden Bereavement in Acute Care Settings. *Nursing Standard.* 19:38–42

Komaromy, C. (2004) Cultural Diversity in Death and Dying. *Nursing Management* 11:32–6

H.M. Government (2006) Working together to safeguard children. Available at http://www. everychildmatters.gov.uk.

Neuberger, J. (2004) Caring for Dying People of Different Faiths. Radcliffe Medical Press, Abingdon

① **Post-bereavement care**

Introduction

- The Royal College of Paediatrics and Child Health defines sudden unexpected death as 'the death of a child that was not anticipated as a significant possibility 24 hours before death, or where there was a similarly unexpected collapse leading to or precipitating the events that led to the death'.
- The sudden, unexpected death of a child has a devastating effect on the family: with no warning, no time to understand the inevitability of their child's death, the news will change the lives of the whole family forever.
- Following childhood death in the emergency department, health care professionals will need support from colleagues; many feel failure or guilt.
- Post-bereavement care is complicated by the need for a multiagency response to the child's death, in line with the death review process, and the need to balance forensic enquires and medical requirements with support for the family.
- Parents may have witnessed resuscitation or they may have been in a suitable, private waiting area, but they must be supported by an experienced member of staff.

Management

Immediate aftercare

- Information should be given to both parents together by a senior member of the paediatric team in a warm, sympathetic and supportive manner. Avoid euphemisms, clearly include the word 'dead'. Say sorry, use touch.
- Parents will be in the first stages of grief and be shocked; they may appear numb, withdrawn, angry or emotional.
- The child must be referred to by their name throughout.
- Ensure religious needs are met, including prayers or a blessing for the child.
- Organ donation must be asked about sensitively.
- Explain that cases of sudden, unexpected death require investigation by specialist pathologists, the coroner's office, and the police.
- Where possible, drips, drains, etc. should be removed from the child's body, but record their positions on a chart for the pathologist.
- Allow parents to spend unhurried time with their child's body.
- Help parents touch, hold and talk to their dead child—guide them in this process.
- Mementos—e.g. a lock of hair, foot or palm print, or photograph—should be offered, but never do anything without the parents' permission, just as if the child were alive.
- Allow the parents to be involved in providing the child's 'final care' including washing, using the child's own toiletries and clothes (unless the case is referred to the coroner, when the body must not be washed).
- Return the child's original clothes (unless requested by the coroner).

Before parents leave the emergency department

- Provide access to a telephone, privacy, and tea/coffee.
- Help parents contact other family members, and discuss breaking the news to siblings and other children in the family.
- Explain process for obtaining death certificate, registering death (within 5 days, unless coroner involved), releasing the child to the funeral directors, and funeral arrangements.
- Paediatricians need to gain consent for a hospital post mortem, but this is not needed for a coroner's post mortem, which is a legal requirement—explain the process and who it involves.
- The coroner will need consent for retaining any organs/tissues at post mortem, and instructions for their disposal at a later date.
- Explain the process for seeing their child in the mortuary chapel, where they can bring family and religious support, and see the child before and after the post mortem.
- Explain that for 48–60 hours after death the child will not look very different, but after that their appearance will change.
- Provide written information about what to do when a child dies including details of support groups such as the Compassionate Friends (www.tcf.org.uk), and contact details in case they have questions later.

Follow-up care

- The emergency department needs to notify the child's GP, medical records, the health visitor and any other professionals involved with the child.
- When death is unexplained there will be a joint home visit by the police and paediatrician.
- Parents will usually be provided with the results of the post mortem if available.
- The paediatrician should arrange a further follow-up visit 4–12 weeks later, either at home or at the hospital to explain medical facts, new information, answer questions/concerns, support parents and siblings in coping with the psychological effect of the death, organize referral to counselling/bereavement services if needed, and provide opportunity to revisit the place where the child died.

Further reading

Child Bereavement Trust: http://www.childbereavement.org.uk/for_professionals/supporting_ families

Cook P, White DK, Ross-Russell RF (2002) Bereavement support following sudden unexpected death: Guidelines for care. *Archives of Disease in Childhood* 87:36–38

RCPath and RCPCH (2004) http://www.rcpch.ac.uk/Publications/Publications-list-by-date#2004)

☼ Apnoea/apparent life threatening event (ALTE)

Introduction

Definition of apnoea: 'an unexplained episode of cessation of breathing for 20 seconds or longer, or a shorter respiratory pause associated with bradycardia, cyanosis, pallor, and/or marked hypotonia' (AAP 1978).

Immediate identification

- An episode that is frightening to the observer
- Apnoea
- Colour change—pallor to mucous membrane cyanosis
- Change in muscle tone, usually limpness
- Notable episode of coughing, choking or gagging
- Bradycardia may begin 1.5–2 seconds after the onset of apnoea
- Pulse oximetry may reveal significant desaturation, typically with a delay in recording the event

If an infant's caregiver reports that an infant has stopped breathing, this is an apparent life threatening event (ALTE) and the child should be admitted for investigation and review.

Immediate action

- Prehospital, carers should attempt simple manual stimulation of the infant.
- Brisk rubbing along the back, patting the feet and thumping the feet may all be tried.
- Commence resuscitation if necessary and emergency transport to nearest emergency department.

Management

The infant who appears ill

- All infants with ALTE should receive cardiac and respiratory monitoring.
- If the infant appears ill, treat as needed on basis of clinical condition. This may include resuscitation or treatment of sepsis.
- Observe the child carefully for any deterioration.

The infant who appears well

- The well-appearing infant will need a physical examination, careful history taking and close observation.

History should include

- Did the infant vomit?
- Was any coughing/choking associated with the event?
- Was there any associated colour change? Cyanosis suggests more significant episode than infants seen to turn red.
- Was the infant making respiratory efforts?
- Did the infant make any movements during the event, such as unusual limb or eye movements?

- How long did the event last?
- Was stimulation required to end the event?
- If episode occurred during home apnoea monitor use, was there a malfunction or improper use?

Risk factors
- Prematurity (apnoea of prematurity).
- Infants 8–14 weeks old.

Causes
Well-appearing infant
- Idiopathic central apnoea (most common)—often presumed to be immaturity of the respiratory centre.
- Toxin-related central apnoea (carbon monoxide poisoning, drug exposure/maternal illicit drug use).
- Obstructive apnoea (laryngomalacia, tracheomalacia, gastroesophageal reflux).
- Cardiac arrythmias (less likely to present with primary apnoea).
- Neonatal seizures (apnoea usually not the only symptom).

Ill-appearing infant
- Infection (sepsis, meningitis, infant botulism).
- Inborn error of metabolism.
- Dehydration.
- Bronchiolitis.

Consider safeguarding issues, including aborted infanticide, fabricated and induced illness, and physical abuse (raised intracranial pressure).

Investigations
- Blood glucose monitoring
- Urinalysis
- SaO_2
- ECG
- Full blood count and differential
- Urea and electrolytes
- Lumbar puncture

Further investigations depending on history and condition
- CT scan of head
- Chest X-ray
- Full skeletal survey
- Carboxyhaemoglobin level
- Toxin screen
- Methaemoglobin level
- Theophylline/caffeine therapeutic levels in infants with diagnosed central apnoea on drug treatment

Infants who may be safe to discharge
- Carers have misinterpreted the infant's normal breathing pattern (normal infants have respiratory pauses up to 20 seconds).
- Isolated choking episode during feeding.

Discharge instructions

- Return if further episodes occur
- Return if new symptoms occur (fever, vomiting, lethargy)
- Give feeding instructions to carers of infants following choking episode (slower flow teat, interrupt feed, and burp more frequently)
- Offer families CPR training

Further reading

American Academy of Pediatrics (1978) Prolonged Apnoea Task Force on Prolonged Apnoea. *Pediatrics* 61:651–2. http://www.pediatrics.org

American Academy of Pediatrics (2003) Apnea, sudden infant death syndrome, and home monitoring. *Pediatrics* 111:914–17.

Jones, E (2007) Pediatrics, Apnea. Available at: http://www.emedicine.com/emerg/topic362.htm. Accessed 30/07/08

☠: Sudden unexplained death in infancy (SUDI)

Any death of an infant which remains unexplained after post mortem may be registered as sudden unexplained infant death (SUDI) (formerly known as sudden infant death syndrome, SIDS, or cot death).

Occurrence of SUDI is rare under one month of age, with a peak incidence in the second month. As the baby grows older the likelihood of SUDI diminishes, with over 90% of deaths occurring prior to six months and very few over one year. Since the 1991 'Reduce the Risk' campaign, the death rate from SUDI has dramatically decreased by 75%, from 1367 recorded deaths in 1991 to 328 in 2004; however, at over 300 deaths per year, SUDI continues to be the leading cause of death of babies over one month of age in the UK.

The 'Reduce the Risk' campaign and subsequent research findings dictate the advice given to parents to help reduce the death rate further, which are:

- Stop smoking in pregnancy (fathers too). Don't let anyone smoke in the same room as your baby.
- Place your baby on their back to sleep.
- Do not let your baby overheat and keep their head uncovered when indoors.
- Place the baby's feet at the foot of the cot, as this can prevent them wriggling down under the covers.
- Never sleep with your baby on a sofa or armchair.
- For the first six months the safest place for your baby to sleep is in a crib or cot in a room with you.
- It is more dangerous for your baby to sleep in bed with you, if you (or your partner):
  - Are a smoker, even if you do not smoke in bed or at home.
  - Have been drinking alcohol
  - Take medication or drugs that make you drowsy
  - Feel very tired
- Or if your baby:
  - Was born before 37 weeks
  - Weighed less than 2.5kg (5.5 lb) at birth
  - Is less than 3 months old.

More recently, additional research has suggested breast fed babies also have a reduced risk of cot death, with some research claiming the risk to a formula fed baby doubles. Although the evidence is conflicting with regard to statistics, the recommendations support breast-feeding as a preventative measure.

The Foundation for the Study of Infant Deaths (FSID) advocates the use of a dummy from the age of one month to approximately six months, as it is believed that using a dummy to settle your baby can reduce the risk further, even if it falls out while the baby is sleeping.

Further reading

Care of family in the Emergency Department

The management of Sudden Unexplained Infant Death within the Emergency Department is discussed in Unexpected Death (see pp 100).

Foundation for the Study of Infant Deaths (2006) Cot death facts & figures. Available at: www.fsid.org.uk/facts-figures.html

Foundation for the Study of Infant Deaths (2003) Sudden unexpected death in infancy: suggested guidelines for Accident and Emergency Departments. Available from: www.fsid.org.uk

Royal College of Pathologists & The Royal College of Paediatrics & Child Health (2004) Sudden unexpected death in infancy. Available from: www.rcpath.org or www.rcpch.ac.uk

Taylor RC, McClure RJ, Acerini CL (2008) Oxford Handbook of Paediatrics. Oxford University Press, Oxford

☠ Unexpected death

Introduction

The sudden, unexpected death of an infant or child is an inevitably difficult situation for all concerned. Once the death of a baby or child has been confirmed, the primary role of the nurse within the emergency department is to provide support for the child's family. Alongside this objective, emergency department staff must also balance the need to ask questions about the child's death, to ensure that evidence is collected that might aid the determination of a cause of death, but also to ensure compliance with the law and any forensic requirements that exist.

Although the majority of child deaths will be due to tragic, unpreventable occurrences, it must not be forgotten that a small percentage of children will be brought into the emergency department following a sudden, unexpected death resulting from suspicious circumstances requiring investigation. It is therefore essential that all unexpected deaths of infants and children are managed professionally, but with an open mind.

The coroner

Once any unexpected death has been pronounced, the responsibility for the body, and any subsequent measures or actions affecting it, comes under the jurisdiction of the coroner. Before proceeding with any actions, consent from the coroner must be sought, either through direct consultation or via longstanding agreement in the form of local policy or guidance. The procedures permitted will vary according to the individual coroner, and therefore advance planning is advisable.

Planning

In addition to negotiation with the local coroners, preplanning of facilities, equipment, and information needed following a sudden death aids staff at a stressful time. These considerations should include:

- A suitable room where the family can go, either during the resuscitation, should they choose not to remain present (see witnessed resuscitation, pp 82–3) or immediately following death.
- A suitable room in which the infant or child can be visited once death has been confirmed.
- A range of appropriate clothing, nappies, bedding and shawls in which the baby or child can be dressed or wrapped prior to viewing.
- A box containing: a camera (and preferably facilities to provide instant pictures), along with other items to collect mementoes, such as memory books, cards and ink pads for footprints, and sealable pockets for locks of hair.
- An information folder containing contact details of all relevant personnel, local guidelines, documentation checklists, and information on support agencies for parents.

Immediate actions

- On confirmation of death the lead doctor should report the case to the coroner or the coroner's officer, confirming agreement to proceed with other measures.

- Depending on local policy the police may also be informed at this stage, either routinely or only if circumstances warrant suspicion.
- Ensure the paediatric consultant on call is in attendance, or en route.
- A history of preceding events, past medical history, recent illness, etc. must be obtained from the parent/s; this information is usually gathered by a member of the paediatric medical team.
- An experienced paediatrician must then perform a physical examination of the infant/child. This will include:
  - General appearance, markings to the skin, including those obtained through invasive procedure or resuscitation, rashes, bruises, abrasions, etc.
  - Examination of the eyes, mouth and genitalia.
  - Some post mortem samples may also be obtained at this time, such as blood, urine and nasopharyngeal swabs (depending on local policy, these may be obtained later).
  - Arranging for skeletal X-ray survey.

Additional actions

With the consent of the coroner, once the procedures above have been followed the following actions can then be considered, in order to prepare the baby or child for viewing by their parent/s. It is essential, however, that clear documentation is made of all actions taken including:

- Cleaning the baby/child's face, and if necessary changing their nappy.
- Removing, bagging, and labelling their clothes if needed for forensic examination, or soiled. This must be explained to the parent, and consent obtained to either re-dress the infant/child in alternative clothing, or wrap them gently in a clean shawl, sheet or blanket.
- If authorized, record then remove all equipment such as invasive lines, ET tubes, monitoring electrodes, etc.
- Arrange the collection of personal mementos for the parents. Although often thought of for the parents of infants, remember that these precious items may be as essential for the parent of an older child. These may include:
  - Photographs—these should be taken as early as possible, and offered to the parent. Regardless of the child's age, photographs are important; the parents of an older child may not have a recent picture, and therefore the photo may be as precious as for a newborn. Unless a parent expresses a strong wish that photographs are not taken, it is worth ensuring one is obtained that can be made available to a parent at a later date, as many who initially decline later change their minds.
  - Locks of hair—try to obtain a lock from the back of the child's head, where it will not be obvious when viewing.
  - Foot and hand prints—for infants, memory books are available which can have a hand or foot print applied to; alternatively a supply of plain coloured card should be available for use with the older child, with ink pad or roller.
  - Prior to obtaining mementos, it is advisable to discuss your plans with the parent/s, and in some instances this may be something that they wish to be part of and do with you, rather than be excluded from.

- Support the parent/s and other family members while you allow them to spend some time with their baby or child. A nurse should be present to support them at all times; some coroners may require a police officer to also be present, and it would be unusual for the parents to be left alone with the baby/child. Generally a parent should be allowed to hold their child at this time; however, in suspicious circumstances, they may be prevented from holding their child, and in these circumstances you will be guided by the police in attendance. A parent should never be excluded from viewing their child.
- Finally, ensure that all appropriate people have been informed of the child's death following the local policy for death notification. This will include the baby/child's:
  - GP
  - Health visitor, school nurse or midwife (depending on age)
  - School.

Further reading

Child Bereavement Charity (2007) Best Practice Guidance for the care of a family when their baby or child dies in the Neonatal, Paediatric or the Accident and Emergency Units. Available from: www.childbereavement.org.uk

Foundation for the Study of Infant Deaths (2003) Sudden unexpected death in infancy: suggested guidelines for Accident and Emergency Departments. Available from: www.fsid.org.uk

Royal College of Pathologists & The Royal College of Paediatrics & Child Health (2004) Sudden unexpected death in infancy. Available from: www.rcpath.org or www.rcpch.ac.uk

Your Local Safeguarding Children Board website is usually found within Local Council web pages.

:☠: **Multiple trauma**

Trauma is the leading cause of death and disability worldwide in children over 1 year. Blunt trauma is seen in 80% of paediatric cases; of these two thirds are associated with brain injury.

Injury patterns in children vary from those seen in adults, owing to the different physiological and anatomical responses to trauma. Children have relatively smaller muscle mass, less subcutaneous tissue, and increased elasticity of the ribs and other bones. This means that in most children the impacting energy is transmitted to the underlying organs such as the lungs (often without rib fracture) or abdomen (with damage to the visceral organs); internal injury therefore must always be considered, as there may have been significant force involved without external signs being present.

Primary survey

- Airway compromise and respiratory and circulatory failure can coexist following trauma. A systematic rapid evaluation (the primary survey) identifies life threatening problems. It can be completed in the first few minutes of the initial assessment of the child.
- When dealing with an injured child the following algorithm should be applied:
  Ac—Airway and cervical spine
  B—Breathing
  C—Circulation
  D—Disability
  E—Exposure

Airway and cervical spine

- Head tilt/chin lift is not recommended following trauma, because cervical spine injuries may be made worse. Under these circumstances use the jaw thrust technique.

Assessment of airway

- The airway is opened using jaw thrust. Use the look, listen, and feel technique to asses airway patency; cervical spine immobilization must be simultaneously maintained.
  - Place your head close to the child's face and look down the body. **Look** for movement of the chest (include the abdomen in infants)
  - **Listen** for respiratory noises
  - **Feel** for breath against your cheek

An obstructed airway may be the primary problem, and correction of the obstruction can result in the recovery without further intervention.

- If the child is breathing spontaneously and effectively they should be allowed to remain in a comfortable position.
- In an unconscious child with spontaneous breathing the main problem is an insecure airway as the tongue may fall back and occlude the airway. The child may also be unable to clear secretions such as vomit or blood. Under these circumstances consider using suction and airway opening adjuncts.
- An airway opening adjunct is used to maintain airway patency. There are two main devices: the oropharyngeal (Guedal) and

nasopharyngeal airways. (N.B. Do not use a nasopharyngeal airway if a fractured base of skull is suspected.)

Cervical spine in-line immobilization

- Cervical spine injury in childhood is uncommon; however, if it is missed or incorrectly managed, there can be tragic consequences such as paralysis, quadriplegia, or death.

Sizing the cervical collar

- The cervical collar must fit exactly; too small and the head may become flexed on the spine, too large and the neck may be free to move in any direction and therefore not immobilized.
- Measure the distance from the top of the patient's shoulder to the angle of the jaw with your hand while the child's head is in the neutral position. Then compare the number of fingers that can be comfortably inserted within this space to the markers on the cervical collar.
- **Once a decision is made to immobilize the patient, the hard collar should remain in place until the cervical spine is cleared**.

Breathing

- Assess breathing once the airway is open!
- Oxygen must be administered at the highest available concentration through a flow meter capable of delivering at least 15 L/min.
- If the airway opening techniques described do not result in the resumption of adequate breathing within 10 seconds, resuscitation should commence as per basic life support (BLS) guidelines.
- If the chest does not rise then the airway is not clear!

Assessment of breathing

- Effort
- Rate
- Recession
- Inspiratory/expiratory noises
- Grunting
- Use of accessory muscles
- Flare of the nostrils

Indications for bag valve mask (BVM) and recourse to tracheal intubation

- Inadequate oxygenation
- Respiratory arrest
- Respiratory failure
- GCS of <8/15 or P or U on the AVPU scale
- Prolonged ventilation required
- Controlled hyperventilation required
- Flail chest
- Inhalation burn injury
- Bronchioalveolar lavage required

Intubation is a specialist skill, and anaesthetists often require an assistant to control the cervical spine during intubation.

Circulation

Once any breathing problems have been corrected attention should be turned to the circulation.

Assessment of circulation
- Palpate the pulse for 10 seconds
- Brachial pulse—infants
- Carotid pulse— children/adolescents

If on assessing circulation there is no pulse, or a pulse of less than 60 beats per minute (1 beat per second) in the infant, resuscitation should commence as per basic life support (BLS) guidelines.
- Heart rate: tachycardia that suddenly turns bradycardic is a pre-terminal sign
- Pulse volume
- Capillary refill: a capillary refill time of greater than 2 seconds may indicate circulatory insufficiency
- Blood pressure: a child's body can tolerate a loss of 20–25% in circulating volume prior to a drop in blood pressure and cardiac output.

On assessing cardiovascular status
- Control blood loss (blood loss is the most common cause of shock in injured children).
- Pain can exacerbate shock and should be managed accordingly.
- Secure vascular access. Consider the intraosseous route as a first choice if the patient is in cardiorespiratory arrest or a decompensated failure state.
- Blood samples for cross match and laboratory studies must be taken at this point.
- Treat hypovolaemic shock:
  • In mild to moderate hypovolaemic shock (Grades I–II) a bolus of **20mL/kg of crystalloid or colloid** is given. Once reassessed, if signs of shock remain a **second bolus of 20mL/kg** is administered. If the child remains shocked, **10mL/kg of whole warmed blood** should be given.
  • A urethral catheter should be inserted and strict fluid balance maintained.
- Surgical involvement is essential in all trauma cases.

Disability
- Neurological assessment should only be performed after A, B and C have been assessed.
- Remember that both respiratory and circulatory failure will have central neurological effects.

Assessment of disability
A rapid assessment of conscious level can be made by assigning the patient to one of the categories below.
- A–Alert
- V–responds to Voice
- P–responds to Pain
- U–Unresponsive

N.B. Glasgow Coma Score <8/15 or P or U on AVPU score are indications for intubation and assisted ventilation. For a complete neurological assessment see page 135 on head injury in children.

Posture

Stiff posture such as decorticate (flexed arms, extended legs) or decerebrate (extended arms, extended legs) posturing is a sign of serious brain dysfunction.

Pupils

- Many drugs and cerebral lesions have effects on pupil size and reaction.
- The most important signs to seek are:
  - Dilation
  - Unreactivity
  - Inequality

  These may indicate serious brain disorders.

Exposure (secondary survey)

The secondary survey should only be attempted once all immediately life threatening injuries have been treated.

- In the secondary survey a full examination of the child takes place to detect hidden injuries.
- In order to assess a seriously injured child fully, it is necessary to take their clothes off.
- Although exposure is necessary the time taken for it should be minimal, and a blanket provided at all times.
- Use the log roll technique to keep the child's spine in line with the rest of the body whilst the back is examined.
- If there is any deterioration go back to the beginning of the primary survey.

Nursing care

- Pain should be assessed using an appropriate tool and managed according to local protocol.
- The child and family's psychological needs must be addressed by providing adequate explanations and reassurance.
- Continue to communicate with the child verbally as the child's sense of hearing is the last sense to be compromised during deepening loss of consciousness.
- Consent—in the absence of the parents the emergency team may need to act in loco parentis following local protocol.
- The child's dignity must be maintained throughout all procedures and care.
- Good note-taking and appropriate referral are essential in providing optimal treatment.
- Consideration should be given to further care being taken in a specialist centre.

Further reading

European Resuscitation Council (2006) European Paediatric Life Support (2nd edn). Resuscitation Council (UK), London

Wilkie, M (2007). Airway adjuncts, uses, sizing, and potential hazards. In: Oxford Handbook of Children's and Young People's Nursing. Oxford: Oxford University Press, pp. 960–961

Kelly, M (2007). Multiple Traumas. In: Oxford Handbook of Children's and Young People's Nursing. Oxford: Oxford University Press, p. 949

☼ Infectious disease outbreaks

Introduction
Infectious disease outbreaks may be described as:
- Two or more **associated** cases of a communicable disease or infection. Single cases of severe or potentially highly infectious diseases such as diphtheria, rabies or polio should be treated as an outbreak.
- A rate of infection greater than that usually expected for a particular place and time.

Infectious disease incidents may include:
- Contamination of food or water by microbes or chemicals.
- Exposure or suspected exposure to an infectious agent (e.g. HIV infected healthcare worker, release of biological agent).

Causes
- Pandemic influenza occurs when a new influenza A virus subtype emerges which is able to infect humans and spread efficiently from person to person. There is a possibility of epidemic waves in the UK within a few months of the emergence of a pandemic virus.
- Clinicians should remain aware of the possibility of covert release of biological agents through food, water or air. Intentional and natural outbreaks of disease may be impossible to differentiate at first.

Signs and symptoms
- Some forms of accidental or intentional chemical poisoning may mimic some infections.
  Have a high index of suspicion for the unusual, unexpected and cases that 'do not fit'.
- Unusual illness
- Unusual number of patients with same symptoms
- Unusual time of year for particular illness
- Unusual clinical signs
- Unusual illness progression
- Unusual place to acquire an illness

Immediate management
- Effective isolation of symptomatic individuals in a single room; restrict access to essential personnel only.
- Adherence to standard infection control principles, especially hand hygiene and containment of respiratory secretions.
- Use of personal protective equipment (PPE) appropriate to the task if aetiology uncertain.
- Discuss with senior medical staff and on call medical microbiologist for immediate assessment.
- Ask other patients/relatives/staff/visitors to remain in department until diagnosis confirmed or excluded if high risk illness/outbreak suspected.
- Separate or cohort patients and their contacts to reduce risk of disease transmission.
- Inform infection control team, senior nursing staff, and management.

During the peak of an epidemic/pandemic

- Display signs on entrance to A&E instructing patients with specific epidemic symptoms to inform reception immediately on arrival.
- If feasible have a separate entrance and exit from the rest of the hospital.
- Triage practitioner on reception to manage patient flow.
- Deferral of patients not requiring emergency care.
- Segregated waiting area for patients with epidemic symptoms with signage and physical barriers to reduce wandering around department.
- Cohort children according to age groups or separately if coinfected with another pathogen (e.g. RSV).
- Communal areas such as playrooms should be closed.
- Ensure immunocompromised patients are segregated with different teams of staff to provide care.

Outbreaks are usually investigated by infection control teams or the health protection unit (HPU). Ensure:

- Early detection and reporting to HPU or the Consultant in Communicable Disease Control (CCDC) following local policies.
- Educate children and their families in good hygiene measures such as covering nose and mouth when coughing and sneezing, use of disposable tissues, and hand washing afterwards.

Follow up

- Identify case contacts for follow up and post-exposure prophylaxis or vaccination of patients and staff.

Specific management of suspected chemical, biological, radiological or nuclear (CBRN) incidents is described at http://www.hpa.org.uk/webw/HPAweb&Page&HPAwebAutoListName/Page/1158934607980?p=1158934607980.

History

Decisions will need to be based on a focused history and physical assessment in order to identify patients with significant signs and symptoms.

- Contacts, family, nursery, school peers with similar symptoms
- Travel abroad, dates, countries, antimalarial measures, immunizations
- Unusual events (animal, insect bite)
- Recreational activity, contact with pets, animals, food
- Recent medication (e.g. antibiotic use)

Investigations

- Use standard precautions when taking specimens
- Label specimens as high risk and inform laboratory staff in advance
- Pre-label specimen containers and avoid contaminating the outside of specimen containers

Complications

- Potential for large numbers of patients
- Large numbers of healthcare workers at risk of exposure to the infection
- Potential limited availability of control measures

Background information

Under the Public Health (Control of Diseases) Act 1984 and the Public Health (Infectious Diseases) Regulations 1988, it is a legal requirement to report specific infectious diseases. The senior clinician suspecting these diagnoses is required to notify the proper officer of the local authority, usually the lead in CCDC. Statutorily notifiable diseases in England and Wales are indicated in Table 2.3.

Table 2.3 Statutorily notifiable diseases in England and Wales

Anthrax	Meningococcal septicaemia	Smallpox
Cholera	Mumps	Tetanus
Diphtheria	Opthalmia neonatorum	Tuberculosis
Dysentery	Paratyphoid fever	Typhoid fever
Encephalitis	Plague	Typhus
Food poisoning	Poliomyelitis	Viral haemorrhagic fever
Leprosy	Rabies	Viral hepatitis
Malaria	Relapsing fever	Whooping cough
Measles	Rubella	Yellow fever
Meningitis	Scarlet fever	

For the above conditions, always consult with the local HPU for advice on management.

Other diseases readily transmittable or with public health implications if diagnosed or suspected in particular within schools or child care settings include:

• Chickenpox (risk to pregnant contacts and those children vulnerable to infection)
• Conjunctivitis (if an outbreak consult HPU)
• Diarrhoea/vomiting with suspected infective cause
• *E. coli* 0157 (always consult with HPU)
• Hand, foot and mouth (contact HPU if a large number of children affected)
• Influenza including swine flu (vulnerable children may require immunization)
• Legionnaires' disease
• Pyrexia of unknown origin
• Scabies (contact HPU if further information required)
• Severe soft tissue infection
• MRSA (contact HPU if further information required)

Further reading

Department of Health (1984) Public Health (Control of Diseases) Act. HMSO. At: http://www.statutelaw.gov.uk/legResults.aspx?LegType=All+Primary&PageNumber=43&NavFrom=2&activeTextDocId=1468798. Accessed 1/08/08
Department of Health (1988) Public Health (Infectious Diseases) Regulations. HMSO. At: http://www.opsi.gov.uk/si/si1988/Uksi_19881546_en_2.htm. Accessed 1/08/08

Department of Health (2005) Guidance for Pandemic Influenza: Infection Control in Hospitals and Primary Care Settings. At: http://www.dh.gov.uk/en/Publicationsandstatistics/Publications/PublicationsPolicyAndGuidance/DH_4121752. Accessed 10/02/09

Department of Health (2006) Immunisation against infectious. 'The Green Book'. At: http://www.dh.gov.uk/en/Publichealth/Healthprotection/Immunisation/GreeN.B.ook/DH_4097254. Accessed 10/02/09

Health Protection Agency (2006) *Guidance on Infection Control in Schools and other Child Care Settings.* At: http://www.hpa.org.uk/web/HPAwebFile/HPAweb_C/1194947358374. Accessed 01/08/08

Health Protection Agency. At: http://www.hpa.org.uk/webw/HPAweb&Page&HPAwebAutoListName/Page/1191942172947 www.dh.gov.uk/en/Publichealth/Flu/Swineflu/index.htm

Further information on notifiable diseases is available at: http://www.hpa.org.uk/webw/HPAweb&Page&HPAwebAutoListName/Page/1191942172947

Neurological problems

☠ Unconsciousness

Unconsciousness is a natural response to trauma or to disease that involves the cerebral neurons or any change in the constituents of the skull (Advanced Paediatric Life Support Guidelines, 2010).

Immediate identification
- Person is unaware of his/herself and his/her surroundings
- Person lacks the ability to understand what is happening at that moment in time
- Person is unable to respond to external stimuli

Immediate action: emergency situation
- Initial assessment–ABC
- Commence basic life support algorithm
- Consider c-spine immobilization and management if situation indicates potential c-spine injury
- Place person in recovery position if their breathing can be considered to be adequate to maintain life

Ongoing assessment
Breathing
- Frequency, depth and pattern of respirations.
- Noisy breathing.
- Oxygen saturation levels: hypoxia and hypercarbia can cause acid-base changes and worsen the unconsciousness.

Circulation
- Assess heart rate and systolic arterial pressure. Blood pressure changing is a very late sign.
- Check limb perfusion and capillary refill, and central and peripheral pulses.
- Electrocardiogram (ECG) assessment.

Disability
- Glasgow Coma Scale/AVPU.
- Skeletal muscle response, spontaneous or in response to stimulation (where muscle relaxants have not been administered). Look for purposeful movement of all four limbs.
- Duration and depth of unconsciousness.
- Changing nature of unconscious state; periods of being lucid.
- Pupil size and reactivity to light.
- Sweat and tear production (often used more to assess depth of anaesthesia).

Exposure: assess core and peripheral temperature.
Glucose: assess blood glucose status.

Further assessment
- Ascertain history of situation, e.g. environmental factors such as smoke, tablets, syringes, alcohol, recent illnesses. Ascertain preceding symptoms, e.g. confusion, headache, and any recent trauma.

- Blood tests: urea/electrolytes, full blood count, glucose, blood gas analysis, liver function tests, ammonia levels, blood cultures.
- Urinalysis: collect for laboratory analysis.

Measuring

- Use relevant, age/cognition specific, coma scale (see Coma section).
- Using an electroencephalogram (EEG), unconsciousness can be defined objectively; however:
  - This is often of no practical value in the acute, emergency situation
  - It can be time-consuming to set up
  - Traces produced can be very difficult to interpret accurately, to ensure meaningful information can be used for the individual patient.

Causes of unconsciousness: unexpected (includes)

- Trauma: head injury, concussion, contusion
- Infection: meningitis, encephalitis, toxic shock syndrome, sepsis, cerebral abscesses
- Vascular causes: aneurysms, cerebrovascular accident (CVA), syncope, cerebral bleeds
- Metabolic causes: hypoglycaemia, diabetic ketoacidosis, inborn errors of metabolism, electrolyte abnormalities, renal failure, encephalopathy, hormonal abnormalities
- Poisoning: from medicines or ingested poisons
- Neoplasm: brain tumours
- Hypoxic: ischaemic brain injury following respiratory or circulatory failure
- Hypothermia and hyperthermia
- Seizures and epilepsy
- Hydrocephalus

Causes of unconsciousness: elective

- Anaesthesia aims to provide sedation, analgesia and paralysis, ensuring the person is sufficiently unconscious so as not to be aware of their surroundings or feel pain during procedures and surgery. Awareness of events occurring whilst unconscious can be extremely psychologically traumatizing and can cause long-term effects.
- Using sedation aims to relax the child's responses to external stimuli sufficiently to allow them to cope with a situation (weaning ventilation/ procedural sedation), and is particularly useful in the emergency situation.
- General anaesthesia aims to ensure the child reaches a state of unconsciousness whereby the child will not be able to respond to external stimuli.

Management

- Protect airway: adjuncts, suction.
- C-spine immobilization (if mechanism of injury suggests sufficient force to potentially affect c-spine in addition to the unconsciousness).
- Support breathing: provide oxygen to keep oxygen saturation levels high, over 95% in children. Consider intubation.

- Maintain circulation: IV access, fluid management (NB: neurological considerations if giving fluid for hypovolaemic shock).
- Definite management depends on the cause of unconsciousness.

Specific nursing considerations

Immobility issues:
- Position to minimize risk of c-spine and respiratory issues, if indicated by the situation/cause, i.e. maintain alignment of body, with child's head in a neutral position, in line with the spine.
  If no c-spine injury suspected:
- Position comfortably noting neurological issues and developmental considerations (infants).
- Regular pressure area assessment.
- Prevent muscle contractions, e.g. ankle extension.
- If immobility needs to continue, collaborate with specialist children's physiotherapists.

Background information

- Unconsciousness can be sudden and is often unexpected.
- Lasts a few seconds to months.
- There is a continuum of consciousness, with altered levels of consciousness from drowsiness, confusion, disorientation, and unawareness of surroundings to fully unconscious.
- If intracranial pressure increases as a result of the cause of unconsciousness, e.g. in acute injuries, then the cerebral perfusion pressure can fall.
- If diminished cerebral perfusion pressure is left untreated, changes would potentially culminate in Cushing's triad or Cushing's reflex (Munroe–Kellie doctrine).

Physiological mechanism of consciousness

- Consciousness depends on the ability of the brain to function fully, comprising alertness and cognition.
- The reticular activating system (RAS) relays sensory impulses up to the cerebral cortex.
- Some of these impulses travel via the thalamus prior to reaching the cerebral cortex.
- The thalamus produces an arousal state, related to the amount of acetylcholine present (this is increased in the conscious person).
- In an unconscious/asleep person, levels of acetylcholine fall, and feedback mechanisms to the RAS slow or are inhibited. As a result, sensory stimuli do not get through to the cerebral cortex.

Further reading

Fisher JD, Brown SN, Cooke MW (eds) (2006). UK Ambulance Service Clinical Practice Guidelines (2006). London: Edexcel.

The Paediatric Accident and Emergency Research Group (2008). The management of a child (aged 0–18 years) with a decreased conscious level – an evidence-based guideline for health professionals based in the hospital setting. Available at: www.nottingham.ac.uk/paediatric-guideline

☠ Meningitis

Meningitis is an acute inflammation of the meninges, the lining around the brain and spinal cord.

Incidence

Meningitis occurs far more commonly in children than in adults, with incidence peaking in children under 5 years of age. Meningitis is bacterial or viral in origin. The onset is usually insidious, and the younger the child, the more difficult the diagnosis.

Causes

Causes of meningitis vary with age.

Neonatal period

- Group B (or beta) streptococcus (GBS) infection is the main cause of meningitis, with *Escherichia coli* and *Listeria monocytes* more uncommon causes.

Over 1 month in age

- Meningococcal (*Neisseria meningitidis*) infection accounts for most bacterial meningitis cases in the UK.
- Pneumococcal (*Streptococcus pneumoniae*) infection was the second most common cause of bacterial meningitis; however, the pneumococcal conjugate vaccine (PCV) was introduced into the UK Childhood Immunization Programme in 2006. Pneumoccoccal meningitis does carry high mortality and morbidity rates, especially for neurological sequelae.
- *Haemophilus influenzae* has become rare in the UK following the introduction of the HiB vaccine.
- Viral meningitis is almost never life threatening, but does have important morbidity, with antibiotic administration not indicated. Most commonly associated with mumps, enteroviruses, Epstein–Barr virus.
- Very rarely, fungal meningitis, such as *Cryptococcus neoformans*, *Candida albicans*, or Histoplasma, can occur in children who are immunocompromised. Other classes of organism can also cause inflammation of the meninges, and furthermore there can be chemical causes of meningitis.

Signs and symptoms

- Early symptoms of meningitis are nonspecific and may include fever, poor feeding, vomiting, muscle aches, irritability and drowsiness.
- More specific signs in infants include a tense or bulging fontanelle, and a high pitched or moaning cry.
- In older children, headache, neck stiffness, and photophobia may be present.
- Kernig's sign (inability to extend the knee when the leg is flexed at the hip) and Brudzinski's sign (bending the head forwards results in flexion movements of the legs) may be present.
- Seizures may also occur at any age.
- Meningococcal infection can also present with a characteristic non-blanching rash if septicaemia is present.

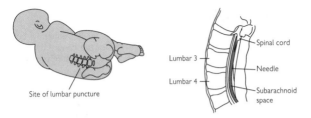

Fig. 3.1 Lumbar puncture
Oxford Handbook of Children's and Young People's Nursing, Glasper et al., (2006), p.267, with permission from Oxford University Press

Immediate management and diagnosis

- Acute bacterial meningitis is a life-threatening condition, which requires early recognition and prompt treatment with IV antibiotics.
- A lumbar puncture (Fig. 3.1) is the definitive diagnostic test, but is contraindicated if there are signs of cardiovascular instability and/or raised ICP. Cerebrospinal fluid (CSF) will need to be sent for protein, glucose and bacteriology and virology.
- In bacterial meningitis there is a raised WBC (mainly lymphocytes), increased protein and reduced glucose (<2.2mmol/L) in the CSF. In viral meningitis there is a raised WBC (mainly lymphocytes), normal or slightly raised protein and CSF glucose is normal. Organisms may be seen on Gram stain. Blood cultures may also indicate the causative agent.

Nursing management

- Management includes both treatment of the cause and prevention of secondary complications, and depends upon the condition of the child.
- Initial assessment includes patency of the airway and adequacy of breathing and circulation, in line with APLS guidelines.
- Closely monitor and assess the child's cardiorespiratory and neurological function to detect early signs of deterioration in conscious level, rising ICP and shock.
- Administer IV antibiotics.
- Many children with bacterial meningitis may be fluid restricted until the risks of developing the syndrome of inappropriate anti-diuretic hormone hypersecretion (SIADH) and associated cerebral oedema are excluded.
- Maintain optimal hydration through IV therapy or oral fluids. Measure accurately and record fluid balance, including urinary output.
- If at all possible, keep the child in a quiet room with reduced light and environmental stimuli.
- Support and reassure parents; give clear explanations of their child's progress and all treatments and procedures.
- All children will require a hearing assessment 6–8 weeks after discharge, or sooner if hearing loss is suspected.

Further reading

Meningitis Research Foundation. http://www.meningitis.org/
Meningitis Trust. http://www.meningitisuk.org/
Isabel–a clinical decision support system. http://www.isabelhealthcare.com/home/default

☠ Encephalitis

Encephalitis is a severe inflammation of the brain, more frequently, but not exclusively, caused by a virus. Any infection of the central nervous system is potentially life threatening and requires early identification and treatment.

Incidence/causes
- Uncommon: a typical district general hospital may see 5 cases a year
- Caused by common viruses, often the herpes simplex virus (HSV) in children in the UK

Signs and symptoms
- High temperature, >38.5°C
- Severe headache
- Vomiting
- Drowsiness/disorientation/confusion/loss of consciousness
- Abnormal behaviour
- Stiff neck and back
- Sensitivity to light
- Seizures
- Muscle weakness or paralysis

ALERT: Many children with viral encephalitis may initially present with minor symptoms such as headache, fever and irritability.

Immediate management
- Stabilization of child to include control of seizures
- Intravenous access
- Commencement of antiviral medication, aciclovir, intravenously (NHS Library)
- Commencement of antibiotics, if in any doubt of diagnosis
- Mental assessment to ascertain encephalitis not meningitis:
  - severe mental state changes
  - motor or sensory deficits
  - behaviour or personality changes
  - difficulties with speech
  - partial paralysis on one side of the body
  - paresthesias of the extremities.

ALERT: For young children parents/carers are the most accurate source of reference when assessing mental status.

History
- Any insect bites or foreign travel, which may indicate tick borne encephalitis.
- Ingestion of contaminated food or inhalation of respiratory droplets from infected person.
- History of rashes to include measles, mumps, varicella or rubella.
- Any other relevant history, e.g. immunocompromised children.
- Social history to include HIV contacts.

Examination

- Full neurological assessment to include behavioural changes
- Rashes
- Meningism and signs of raised intracranial pressure

Investigations

- Blood tests including full blood count and cultures
- Lumbar puncture when safe to do so: analyze cerebrospinal fluid for viral particles, particularly herpes simplex virus, and also to exclude bacterial meningitis
- Brain scan to ascertain extent of inflammation, while also excluding other neurological causes such as tumours or haemorrhage
- An electroencephalogram may show subtle motor seizures

Nursing management

- Anti-convulsants to control seizures
- Steroids may be effective against cerebral oedema
- Frequently assess child's neurological status, checking for changes in level of consciousness and for signs of nerve damage such as ptosis or double vision
- Maintain adequate fluid balance; support with intravenous fluids if required
- Avoid fluid overload to prevent cerebral oedema
- Administer analgesia for head and neck pain as required
- Consider transfer to a Paediatric Intensive Care Unit

ALERT: Encephalitis is a statutory notifiable disease and must be reported to the Department of Health.

Complications

- Full recovery may be slow and fatigue is common
- Developmental delay/problems with gross motor skills and balance
- Speech delays and a lack of concentration
- Ongoing seizures and headaches

Further reading

NHS Library. http://cks.library.nhs.uk/patient_information_leaflet/Encephalitis
Kneen R, Solomon T (2007). Management and outcome of viral encephalitis in children. *Paediatrics and Child Health* 18:7–16

:☠: Poisoning

Poisoning is the introduction of a noxious substance to an infant, child or young person by means of ingestion, absorption or inhalation.

Poisoning may be:
- Accidental
- Intentional (self)
- Drug abuse (including solvent inhalation)
- Iatrogenic
- Deliberate (others)

Immediate management

Key information required
- Event and supporting information, e.g. if ingestion of medicine, the drug involved and preparation.
- Time of event.
- Time elapsed since event.
- Amount of ingestion (include all medication that was potentially in the bottle or packet when calculating).
- Weight of child (actual weight preferable).

Ask yourself
- Is event potentially harmful?
- Is there a possibility of a mixed overdose?
- Is there a possibility of inaccurate dose reporting on history taking?

If mixed or undetermined ingestion of either paracetamol or aspirin, levels should be tested.

Assessment and management
- Airway
- Breathing
- Circulation

Removal of poison (if necessary)

Activated charcoal
- This is the treatment of choice for most ingestions.
- Most effective when given within first hour.
- May need instillation through naso-gastric tube.

Contraindications
- Patients with altered conscious state
- Or if the following have been ingested:
  - Ethanol/glycols
  - Alkalis
  - Boric acid
  - Lithium
  - Iron compounds
  - Potassium and other metallic ions
  - Fluoride

- Cyanide
- Petroleum distillates
- Mineral acids
- Clofenotane (dicophane, DDT)

Gastric lavage has a very limited role in treatment and should not be used without consultation.

Specific antidotes may be available, and serum drug levels may help in treatment decisions.

If no explanation for presenting symptoms, a urinary drug screen may be indicated.

Advice

For specific advice in the UK

- Utilize TOXBASE (http://www.toxbase.org/) via NHS web or internet as first point of access.
- Contact the National Poisons Information Service telephone service for clinically complex cases. Use regional centre contact.

BELFAST
Royal Victoria Hospital
Grosvenor Road
Belfast, BT9 7BL
02890 632032

EDINBURGH
Royal Infirmary of Edinburgh
Little France Crescent
Edinburgh, EH16 4SA
0131 242 1381
www.spib.scot.nhs.uk

BIRMINGHAM
City Hospital
Dudley Road
Birmingham, B18 7QH
0121 507 4123
www.npis.org

NEWCASTLE
Wolfson Unit
Claremont Place
Newcastle-upon-Tyne, NE2 4HH
0191 260 6180

CARDIFF
Llandough Hospital
Penarth
Cardiff, CF64 2XX
029 2071 5554

Other countries

Reciprocal National Poisons Information Services.
Australia: Contact details at http://ausdi.hcn.net.au/poisons.html
United States of America: Contact details at http://www.dorway.com/poisons.html

Ongoing management of intentional harm

- Local policy and guidelines with regard to safeguarding children must be initiated when appropriate.
- Ensure that contemporaneous documentation that is timed, dated and signed occurs for all aspects of management and care.

Ongoing assessment and management of self harm
- Children and young people under 16 who have self harmed should be:
  - Assessed and managed by appropriately trained children's nurses and doctors.
  - Be admitted overnight and assessed fully by practitioners experienced in the assessment of children and young people who self harm.

(NICE 2004)

Further reading
Advanced Life Support Group (2005) Advanced Paediatric Life Support – The Practical Approach, 4th edn. BMJ Books, Blackwell Publishing Ltd, Oxford
BNF for Children 2008 (2008) BMJ Group, RPS Publishing, RCPCH Publications Ltd, London
NICE (2004) Self-harm. Clinical Guideline CG16. www.nice.org.uk

⑦ **Role of the national poisons centres**

Poisons information centres are established to provide expert advice in the diagnosis, treatment, and management of patients who have been poisoned. Services exist internationally within all countries, usually in major cities, and are also able to access specific advice for the locality.

Healthcare facilities are able to access the services directly through internet access or telephone link, often with a two-tier system that provides expert general advice on specific poisons through an internet database, with advice for complex cases being provided via a consultant-led information service by telephone.

Within the UK this facility is provided by the National Poisons Information Service (NPIS), whereby information on actual or suspected cases of poisoning is accessed initially through the TOXBASE database.

See Table 3.1 for UK regions and contacts, and Fig. 3.2 for flowchart.

Table 3.1 UK regions and contacts

Area/region	Centre	Contact
Northern Ireland	BELFAST	02890 632032
West Midlands, Trent and Oxfordshire medical deaneries	BIRMINGHAM	0121 507 4123
South Western and Wessex medical deaneries and Wales	CARDIFF	029 2071 5554
Scotland	EDINBURGH	0131 242 1381
Northern Yorkshire, North Western and Mersey medical deaneries	NEWCASTLE	0191 260 6180

Ensure information available

- Time of event/ingestion
- Substance name and quantity/dose (actual or suspected)
- Sex of patient
- Age of patient
- Weight of patient
- Presenting symptoms

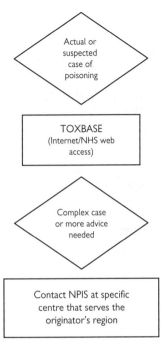

Fig. 3.2 Actual or suspected case of poisoning

Further reading

National Poisons Information Service – http:/www.npis.org
TOXBASE–http://www.toxbase.org/
Advanced Paediatric Life Support Guidelines (2010). http://www.resus.org.uk/pages/pals.pdf

ⓘ **Epilepsy**

Introduction

Epilepsy is defined as a neurological condition characterized by more than one seizure unprovoked by any immediately identifiable cause.

Seizure

- Refers to the neurological event where there is a change of awareness or behaviour, e.g. blankness or absences, strange sensations or involuntary movement.
- Occurs due to an interruption in cerebral function brought about by excessive neuronal activity.

Incidence

- One of the most common neurological conditions in adults and children, epilepsy affects at least 456,000 people in the UK, and 1 in 280 children.

Causes

- Genetic defects directly contribute to epilepsy, and seizures are the core symptom of the disorder.
- Structural or metabolic insult or disorder of the brain.
- In other cases the cause is unknown and might be genetic, structural, or metabolic.

Signs and symptoms

Seizures can be:

- Partial, sometimes referred to as focal or local, where one hemisphere or lobe is affected. Can be simple or complex. Consciousness not impaired.
- Generalized, where the whole of the brain is affected. Loss of consciousness and no memory of occurrence are common. These seizures include:
  - Absences
  - Tonic: stiffness
  - Atonic: loss of muscle control
  - Myoclonic: muscle contractions (jerking)
  - Tonic-clonic: rhythmical contraction and relaxation of muscles
  - Status epilepticus: prolonged seizure

Immediate management

Nurse's role

- Ensure child is safe
- Time seizure
- Stay until fully recovered
- Do not restrain
- Do not put anything in child's mouth
- Care of family

A child who presents with a seizure lasting more than 5 minutes should be treated the same as a child in 'established status' to stop the seizure and prevent the development of status epilepticus.

Nurse's role
- Call for help
- Secure airway
- Give oxygen
- Assess cardiac and respiratory function
- Secure intravenous (IV) access as a first line treatment
- Care of the family

Also see Resuscitation, p. 72 and Unconscious child, p. 114.

History and examination
- Based on detailed description of events by the person/witness. Recording the episode on a phone or video camera is useful.
- Clinical examination and referral to a specialist.

Investigations
- Electroencephalogram (EEG), which records electrical function in the brain, where appropriate.
- Neuroimaging using computed tomography (CT) or magnetic resonance imaging (MRI) scans that visualize the brain and identify structural abnormalities.
- Blood and urine biochemistry, to exclude other diagnoses.
- 12 lead ECG in cases of diagnostic uncertainty.

Nursing management and treatment
- Child-centred self-management education advocated.
- Anti-epileptic drugs (AEDs). There are a number of medications used to control seizures, successful in around 70% of cases.
- Diazepam/lorazepam is prescribed to stop prolonged seizures.
- Psychological interventions.
- Ketogenic diet: a high fat, low carbohydrate diet is useful in many children. NB: it is important for the nurse to ascertain this, as the giving of sugar, e.g. in certain medications, may undermine the ketogenic control.
- Vagal nerve stimulation.
- Brain surgery (NICE 2004).

Complications/prognosis
- Overall prognosis good
- Risk of injury during seizure
- Sudden death in epilepsy (SUDEP) occurs in approximately 1 in 100,000 cases; this is minimized by optimizing seizure control

Further reading
National Society for Epilepsy. http://www.epilepsysociety.org.uk/Forprofessionals

⊙ Febrile convulsion

Introduction
Febrile seizures, despite being a common childhood event, are very traumatic experiences for parents, and can be a symptom of various acute illnesses.

Incidence
Febrile seizures affect around 3% of children between six months and five years of age (Pang et al, 2005).

Signs and symptoms
- Pyrexia (temperature >38°C)
- The child may appear hot and flushed
- Altered level of consciousness, which may include body stiffness, limb jerking, eye rolling and unresponsiveness, usually lasting less than 5 minutes.

Immediate management
- Assessment of airway, breathing and circulation
- Monitoring of clinical observations: temperature, heart rate and respiratory rate (NICE 2007).
- Administration of anti-pyretic medication. Please note that anti-pyretic agents do not prevent febrile convulsions, and they should not be used specifically for this purpose. However, preparatory preparations such as paracetamol may relieve pain and discomfort (NICE 2007).
- Reassurance of child and family.

History
- History from the parent as to preceding circumstances should be accurately documented.

Examination
- Physical examination of the child.
- Consider colour, activity, respiratory, and hydration aspects of child's condition.
- Determine presence of any serious underlying illness.

Investigations
- Urinalysis
- Blood investigations/chest X-ray if clinically indicated
- Observation of the child's response to treatment

Treatment and nursing management
- If an underlying condition is diagnosed that may have contributed to the febrile seizure, it must be managed appropriately to prevent further episodes of febrile seizure, which can reoccur in 30% of cases.
- Oral antibiotics to manage infections may be commenced as soon after confirmation of diagnosis as possible.

- Close monitoring of the child's temperature during the acute phase of the illness.
- Nurse in minimal clothing in a room of appropriate temperature.
- Education of parents regarding future management of similar episodes, for example, safe use of anti-pyretics, environmental issues and when to access medical assistance.

Complications/prognosis

- Despite being a traumatic event, febrile convulsions are not usually dangerous, with most children having a fully recovery without after-effects.
- It is important to reassure parents that having a febrile seizure does not cause their child to develop epilepsy.

Further reading

NICE (2007) Feverish illness in children: assessment and initial management in children younger than 5 years. London: NICE
Pang D, Newson T, Budd C, Gardiner M (2005) Paediatrics (2nd edn). Edinburgh: Mosby

⊙ Head injury in children

Introduction

Head injury is the leading cause of trauma-related death in children aged 1–15 years.

The commonest cause is road traffic accidents (pedestrian, cyclist, passenger), followed by falls. In infants, head injury associated deaths are primarily due to nonaccidental injury.

Primary brain injury

Primary brain injury occurs at the time of impact, potentially causing irreversible brain damage.

Secondary brain injury

Secondary brain injury can occur within minutes, hours, or days after the head injury due to adverse physiological effects including:

- Hypoxia
- Hypotension
- Intracranial hypertension
- Seizures
- Fever
- Hypo/hyperglycaemia
- Raised intracranial pressure due to intracranial haematoma or cerebral oedema
- Infection (later)

Assessment

Head injuries vary from minor to severe to fatal. Children with serious injuries must be identified promptly and managed appropriately. The National Institute for Health and Clinical Excellence (NICE) (2007) has produced evidence based guidelines for the triage, assessment, investigation, and early management of head injury in infants, children, and adults. Any patient presenting with impaired consciousness should be assessed immediately, and all head injured patients seen within 15 minutes of arrival to determine their individual risk of clinically important brain injury.

Immediate management

The key priority in head injury management is to prevent secondary brain injury by maintaining adequate oxygenation, ventilation, and circulation, and avoiding raised intracranial pressure.

Primary survey

The primary ABC survey is an immediate, rapid, systematic assessment to promptly identify and treat any life threatening problems following paediatric life support principles.

ALERT: Cervical spine injury may be associated with head injury. C-spine immobilization must be achieved as a priority.

• Assess conscious level using the AVPU scale:

A–Alert

V–responds to Voice

P–responds to Pain

U–Unresponsive

ALERT: If you are concerned or if patient scores V or below contact resuscitation team for support.

In addition assess conscious level using the Glasgow Coma Scale (GCS), or paediatric modified GCS in children under 4 years old. If GCS < 8, immediately involve anaesthetist to support airway management.

• Assess pupil size, equality and reaction.

Secondary survey

The secondary survey involves a detailed history of the injury, the child's condition following the injury and a full examination.

• Examine the head for bruising, scalp lacerations, depressed skull fracture, or tense/bulging fontanelle in infants.
• Look for evidence of basal skull fractures including:
  • CSF leakage from nose or ear
  • Haemotympanum
  • Panda eyes
  • Bruising to the mastoid process behind the ear (Battle's sign).
• Re-examine pupils for size, equality and reaction.
• Examine ophthalmic fundi. In infants retinal haemorrhages may indicate a nonaccidental injury.
• Assess motor function by examining facial/limb movements, and limb tone and reflexes.

Nursing management

Neurological assessment

Conduct frequent neurological assessments to promptly detect early signs or symptoms of raised intracranial pressure.

Assess conscious level using the Glasgow Coma Scale (GCS) or paediatric modified GCS (<4 years).

• Continue frequent reassessment of GCS, every few minutes if GCS level is changing.
• Monitor respiratory rate, heart rate, blood pressure, temperature, and blood oxygen saturation.

Frequency of assessment

• At least half-hourly observations until GCS of 15 is obtained.
• When GCS is 15 then:
  • Half-hourly for 2 hours
  • Hourly for 4 hours
  • 2-hourly thereafter
• If patient deteriorates to GCS <15, revert to half-hourly observations and follow original frequency schedule.

Investigations
- Arterial blood gas analysis should be performed in severely head injured patients. Check pH and base deficit and carefully control PaO_2 and $PaCO_2$.
- CT scan is the investigation of choice for the detection of brain injuries. NICE guidelines provide criteria indicating the need for urgent CT imaging in children.
- Skull X-ray may be useful as part of the skeletal survey if nonaccidental injury is suspected.

Neurosurgical opinion/referral
- The care of patients with persistently abnormal neurological signs or abnormal CT scans should be discussed immediately with a regional neurosurgeon.

Pain management
Pain must be managed effectively because it can lead to agitation and raised intracranial pressure.
- Splint any limb fractures and administer appropriate analgesia.
- Treat severe pain with intravenous opioids titrated against clinical response.

Admission to hospital
NICE recommendations:
- Abnormal CT scan
- GCS remaining less than 15
- Continuing worrying signs such as: persistent vomiting, severe headaches, drug or alcohol intoxication, other injuries, shock, suspected nonaccidental injury, meningism, cerebrospinal fluid leak.

Transfer to definitive care
- Children with serious head injuries (GCS <8) should be transferred to a specialist paediatric neurosciences unit by staff experienced in the transfer of critically ill children. Local guidelines should be available to guide care in this situation.

Discharge
- No head injured patients should be discharged until GCS of 15 (or normal consciousness assessed on paediatric GCS) is achieved.
- Verbal and written head injury advice should be given to the person responsible for the continued observation of the child at home. Suitable discharge advice is available on the NICE website (www.nice.org.uk/CG056).
- Warn parent/carer that some head injured patients make a rapid recovery, but may later develop delayed complications.
- When nonaccidental injury is suspected a full child protection assessment will be undertaken prior to discharge.

Further reading

Trengove, R (2008). Neurological Assessment (Chapter 10). In: Clinical Skills in Child Health
    Practice. Kelsey J, McEwing G (eds). London: Churchill Livingstone Elsevier.
Advanced Life Support Group (2005). Advanced Paediatric Life Support: The Practical Approach
    (4th edn). London: Blackwell Publishing Ltd.
National Institute for Health and Clinical Excellence (NICE) (2007) Head Injury: Triage,
    Assessment, Investigation and Early Management of Head Injury in Infants, Children and Adults.
    Clinical Guideline 56. London, NICE. http://guidance.nice.org.uk/Cg56

☠ Trauma induced raised intracranial pressure

Introduction
Cranial sutures close at 12–18 months of age. After this age the skull is a rigid, unyielding structure with no space to accommodate expanding lesions such as cerebral oedema or haematoma. Such lesions may cause a rise in intracranial pressure, which compresses cerebral blood vessels and compromises cerebral perfusion. This increased pressure can lead to brain death or herniation of the brain through the foramen magnum causing death (coning).

Causes
In head injured children, raised intracranial pressure is most commonly caused by cerebral oedema. If caused by an expanding cerebral haematoma, rapid neurosurgical intervention is required.

Signs and symptoms
- Deteriorating level of consciousness (exclude hypoglycaemia as the cause)
- Headache, nausea, vomiting
- Confusion, agitation, drowsiness
- Pupils – sluggish/unequal/unreactive/dilated
- Abnormal motor activity/reflexes/posturing
- Cushing's triad (hypertension, bradycardia, decreasing respiratory rate with altered breathing pattern)

ALERT: Cushing's triad is a late and preterminal sign.
ALERT: In infants, unfused cranial sutures initially allow for increased cranial volumes and large cerebral bleeds may occur before neurological signs or symptoms develop. A significant fall in haemoglobin concentration should alert the practitioner to such bleeds in infants.

Immediate management
- Raised intracranial pressure should be prevented, or rapidly identified and the cause treated promptly.
- Urgent CT scan and an immediate neurosurgical referral are indicated.
- Initiate measures to increase cerebral perfusion pressure:
  - Nurse patient in 20° head-up position to aid venous drainage
  - Ventilate patient and maintain $PaCO_2$ between 4.0 and 4.5 kPa
  - Treat hypotension with colloid infusion
  - Maintain mean arterial pressure above normal value for child's age
  - Administer IV mannitol infusion 0.25–0.5g/kg
  - Control seizure activity
  - Maintain normal glycaemic state

Further reading

Advanced Life Support Group (2005). Advanced Paediatric Life Support: The Practical Approach (4th Edition). London: Blackwell Publishing Ltd.
European Resuscitation Council and Resuscitation Council (UK) 2006 (2nd Edition) European Paediatric Life Support. London: Resuscitation Council (UK)

☠ Raised intracranial pressure (nontraumatic)

Introduction

The intracranial volume comprises the brain (80%), intravascular blood (10%), and cerebrospinal fluid (CSF) (10%). If any of these three components increases in volume, another component must decrease to maintain equilibrium. This is known as the Munro–Kellie hypothesis.

Raised ICP is a symptom rather than a disease, but if left untreated it will result in local ischaemia, coma, brain herniation and eventually death.

Causes

Disturbance to CSF

- Obstruction to CSF flow (due to obstructive hydrocephalus)
- Decreased absorption of CSF (due to communicating hydrocephalus, subarachnoid haemorrhage, meningitis)
- Increased production of CSF (due to tumours of the choroid plexus)
- Increase in venous pressure (due to heart failure)

Increase in brain volume

- Cerebral oedema (due to head injury, ischaemic-toxic states, Reye's syndrome)
- Space occupying lesion (tumour, haematoma, abscess)

Increase in blood volume

- Obstruction of venous outflow
- Hyperaemia
- Hypercapnia

Idiopathic

Acute liver failure

Signs and symptoms

- Headache
- Vomiting
- Decreased level of consciousness
- Pupillary abnormalities (enlarging and/or unequal pupils)
- Cushing's triad: hypertension, bradycardia and abnormal respiratory pattern, comparatively late sign in young children and infants
- Visual disturbances
- Papilloedema (if chronic raised ICP)
- Motor dysfunction
- Aphasia
- Increased head circumference will occur in babies and infants if the fontanelles are still open

Investigations
- CT (computed tomography)
- Cranial ultrasound (babies)
- X-ray ('copper beaten skull')
- MRI (magnetic resonance imaging)
- Lumbar puncture (following safety clearance by CT/MRI that reducing the ICP will not result in coning)

Immediate management
- This depends on the aetiology, but management of acute raised ICP must be rapid to avoid resulting morbidity and mortality.
  - A. Management of airway
  - B. Management of breathing
  - C. Management of circulation
  A+B+C = Adequate oxygenation is essential in avoiding hypoxia and consequent cerebral oedema.
  - D. Management of seizures: seizure activity increases cerebral metabolism and hence cerebral requirements, so must be avoided if possible. Paediatric GCS chart must be used to assess and score any deterioration in level of consciousness.

In addition to the immediate management above, the following measures may be utilized as appropriate:
- Pharmacological agents
- Fluid restriction and osmotic agents
- Normalization of serum electrolytes
- Temperature control
- Surgery: CSF drainage (external ventricular drain); craniotomy/ craniectomy for removal of space occupying lesion.

Further management and prognosis
This will depend on the cause of the raised ICP.

Further reading
Hickey J (1997) The Clinical Practice of Neurological and Neurosurgical Nursing. Philadelphia: Lippincott-Raven
May L (2001) Paediatric Neurosurgery – a handbook for the multidisciplinary team. London and Philadelphia: Whurr

☼ Encephalopathy

Introduction
Encephalopathy is a generalized diffuse disorder of the brain that alters function and structure. It is a general categorization that includes a number of syndromes and diseases. Encephalopathy presents with a manifestation of a primary illness, can occur at any age, and has no preference for gender or race.

Causes
There are three main causes of encephalopathy, where the primary disorder stems from hypoxia, liver, or kidney disease. Other factors also include:
• Infective agents such as viruses, bacteria or prions
• Metabolic or mitochondrial dysfunction
• Brain tumour or raised intracranial pressure
• Prolonged exposure to toxic elements
• Chronic progressive trauma
• Poor nutrition

Hypoxic encephalopathy
Hypoxic encephalopathy may occur when the cerebral circulation is starved of oxygen; this can occur as a result of:
• Drowning
• Hypotension
• Birth injuries
• Cardiac arrest/respiratory failure
• Strangulation
• Asphyxiation
• Smoke inhalation
• Severe haemorrhage
• Carbon dioxide poisoning
• High altitudes
• Choking
• Complications of anaesthesia

In the newborn, a combination of hypoxia and ischaemia as a result of birth trauma is termed hypoxic-ischaemic encephalopathy. Although the immature brain is able to tolerate a level of asphyxia, it does start a process of abnormal biochemical events that may lead to neuronal injury or death. A complex pathway of damage to the cerebral circulation, free radical generation, excess calcium entry, and apoptosis will result in cerebral damage (Levene et al. 2008).

Hepatic encephalopathy
Encephalopathy may occur due to liver failure and an inability to detoxify waste products. Hepatic encephalopathy occurs as a result of the liver's inability to convert ammonia to urea. Ammonia acts as a neurotoxin that damages and destroys brain tissue when it enters the cerebral circulation. This may occur in diseases such as:
• Hepatitis
• Cirrhosis

Renal or uraemic encephalopathy
Any reduction of renal function will result in the accumulation of waste products and an increase in circulatory volume. This mechanism is poorly understood, but may result in the build-up of toxic organic acids and electrolyte imbalances such as sodium imbalance (Porth 2007). Regardless of the cause, this has a detrimental effect on cerebral function. Diseases that may ultimately cause renal encephalopathy include:

- Diabetes mellitus
- Chronic renal failure
- Analgesic nephropathy
- Polycystic kidney disease
- Pyelonephritis
- Glomerulonephritis
- Renal artery stenosis
- Lead poisoning

Signs and symptoms

The nature and the extent of clinical features are dependent on the primary cause of the encephalopathy. Cerebral oedema as a result of cerebral ischaemia and intracranial hypertension (raised intracranial pressure) progress quickly if the primary cause of the illness is not treated effectively. This will result in cerebral circulatory collapse, the breakdown of the blood–brain barrier, brain stem herniation, and possibly the leaking of neurotoxins that will ultimately result in death.

Common neurological features include:

- Progressive loss of memory and cognitive ability
- Subtle personality changes and the inability to concentrate
- Lethargy and the progressive loss of consciousness.

Other clinical features include:

- Myoclonus (involuntary twitching of muscles)
- Nystagmus
- Tremor
- Muscle atrophy and weakness
- Dementia
- Seizures
- Dysphasia and dysphagia.

Diagnosis

Diagnosis of encephalopathy is dependent on the primary cause, but the common diagnostic tests include:

- Complete blood count
- Liver and renal function tests
- Lactate levels
- Blood gases
- Blood cultures
- Virology testing
- Neuroimaging studies and ultrasound
- Lumbar puncture

Immediate management

In addition to treating symptoms as they progress, the main focus of treatment will be to cure or at least control the primary disease. Prognosis is dependent on this being successful. More acute disease presentations that can be promptly treated have relatively good outcomes. If the primary illness results from advanced chronic disease that responds poorly to treatment then outcome will be poor. Often, supportive and palliative nursing care are fundamental requirements.

Further reading

Levene MI, Tudehope DI, et al. (2008). Essential Neonatal Medicine. Oxford: Blackwell Publishing.
Porth CM (2007). Essentials of Pathophysiology: Concepts of altered health states. Philadelphia: Lippincott, Williams & Wilkins.
http://bestpractice.bmj.com/best-practice/monograph/294/treatment/guidelines.html

Respiratory problems

:☼: **Recognizing respiratory distress**

Introduction
Respiratory distress is a common end set of symptoms caused by a variety of underlying conditions.

Incidence
Respiratory distress accounts for nearly 10% of paediatric emergency department visits for all children.

Possible causes of respiratory distress
- Respiratory conditions, e.g. bronchiolitis, asthma, allergic reaction, cystic fibrosis, bronchietasis, bacterial tracheitis, croup, inhaled foreign body, respiratory distress syndrome, pneumonia, pneumothorax.
- Congenital respiratory defects, e.g. bronchopulmonary dysplasia, diaphragmatic hernia, pulmonary hypoplasia, cystic malformation of the lung, congenital surfactant deficiency.
- Congenital cardiac defects, e.g. transposition of the great vessels, hypoplastic left heart syndrome, pulmonary atresia, tetralogy of Fallot, tracheoesophageal anomalies.
- Neurological conditions, e.g. meningitis, intracranial haemorrhage or hypertension
- Haematological conditions, e.g. sepsis, polycythemia, severe anaemia, blood loss.
- Metabolic disorders, e.g. hypoglycaemia.
- Trauma.
- Foreign body.

Anatomy and physiology of a child's chest
- Compliant chest wall (develops recession easily)
- Airway collapse at low lung volumes (e.g. laryngomalacia, stridor)
- Low functional residual capacity (FRC)
- High oxygen consumption (less reserve, desaturates quickly)

History
A full history from parents or caregivers will help determine cause and diagnosis.

Examination/signs and symptoms
Conduct the physical exam when the child is least distressed, e.g. in a caregiver's arms and/or after nasal suctioning.
- Respiratory rate:
  - Too fast for age? (increasing work of breathing initially)
  - Too slow for age? (decreasing work of breathing, with exhaustion)
  - Take more than one measurement; trends in measurement are the most useful indicator of improvement or deterioration
  - See Table 4.1 for normal paediatric respiratory rates

Table 4.1 Normal paediatric respiratory rates

<1 year: 30–40 breaths/minute
1–2 years: 25–35 breaths/minute
2–5 years: 25–30 breaths/minute
5–12 years: 20–25 breaths/minute
>12 years: 15–20 breaths/minute

- Tachypnoeic or apnoeic episodes?
- Observe for noisy breathing. What kind of noise?
- Wheeze (asthma, foreign body)
  - Inspiratory stridor (croup) may be expiratory when severe
  - Expiratory grunting (→ severe respiratory distress, characteristically seen in infants with pneumonia or pulmonary oedema; also a sign of raised intracranial pressure)
  - Gasping (→ sign of severe hypoxia and may be preterminal)
  - Inability to speak or cry/silent (ominous if distressed)
- Nasal flaring? (→ especially seen in infants with respiratory distress)
- Use of accessory muscles? (leads to 'head bobbing')
- Observe for subcostal, intercostal or sternal recession and/or retractions (→ shows increased work of breathing). More common in infants due to compliant chest wall; if seen in children >6 years, this suggests severe respiratory distress.
- Observe position:
  - Lying?
  - Sitting forward (if old enough), tripod
- Note colour of child (late and unreliable)
  - Pale, blue or grey
- Observe feeding
  - Infant tires with feeding/not tolerating feeds
  - Post-tussis emesis
  - Signs of dehydration
- Use pulse oximetry
  - Low/decreased oxygen saturation (<95%)

Immediate management

- Removal of foreign body following correct procedure
- Immediate hospitalization of infant/child
- Maintain a patent airway as a key component of supportive care
- Place the infant in a supine or lateral position (avoid prone positioning)
- Suction mucus from nasal and oral passages
- Isolate infants admitted to the hospital with respiratory tract infection, or if isolation facilities are not available, test for respiratory syncytial virus (RSV) as appropriate
- Provide supportive care, such as oxygen therapy
- Continue to monitor oxygen saturation levels
- Hydrate the patient with oral and/or intravenous fluids as appropriate

Rationale
- Nasal suctioning increases the capacity for upper airway patency, especially in young infants, who are obligatory nose breathers.
- Infants who are in severe respiratory distress, causing a decrease in oxygen saturation of less than 94% in air, will benefit from oxygen therapy.
- Hydration avoids metabolic decompensation in the face of respiratory distress. (BMJ Advanced Life Support Group (2005) Advanced Paediatric Life Support: The Practical Approach. 4th Edition. Blackwell Publishing Ltd.)

Investigations
- Chest X-ray and other imaging as appropriate (e.g. following trauma)
- Viral and bacterial screen
- Arterial blood gases if appropriate

Treatment
Depends on cause of respiratory distress! Any or all of the treatments below may be necessary:
- High-flow oxygen therapy; may require continuous positive airway pressure (CPAP) or intubation and ventilation
- Bronchodilators (although not for infants with bronchiolitis) (SIGN, 2006.)
- Steroids (although not for infants with bronchiolitis) (SIGN, 2006)
- Antibiotics (although not for infants with bronchiolitis) (SIGN, 2006)
- Nasogastric feeding

Complications/prognosis
If unrecognized, respiratory distress may lead to respiratory arrest and death.

Further reading
Baumer JH (2007). SIGN guideline on bronchiolitis in infants. *Arch Dis Child Educ Pract Ed* 92:149–51.
Scottish Intercollegiate Guidelines Network (2006). 91: Bronchiolitis in children. Available at: www.sign.ac.uk
Scottish Intercollegiate Guidelines Network (2008). 101: British Guideline on management of asthma. Available at: www.sign.ac.uk

☠ Acute epiglottitis

Acute epiglottitis is an inflammation of the epiglottis, commonly caused by the bacteria *Haemophilus influenzae* B.

The epiglottis is a lid-like flap of elastic cartilage tissue covered with a mucous membrane, attached to the root of the tongue. It covers the entrance of the larynx during swallowing. (See Fig. 4.1)

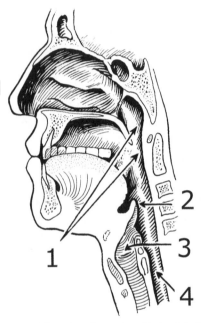

Fig. 4.1 The epiglottis (donated to public domain by Pearson Scott Foresman). 1–Pharynx; 2–Epiglottis; 3–Larynx; 4–Oesophagus

Incidence/causes

- Acute infection with *Haemophilus influenzae* B results in severe swelling of the epiglottis and surrounding tissues and ultimately obstruction of the larynx.
- Most common in children aged between 1 and 6 years, but can occur in adults and infants.
- Routine immunization of infants in the UK with HiB vaccine (*Haemophilus influenzae* type B) has reduced the incidence of acute epiglottitis dramatically, and it is now a rare condition.

- However, it can still occur in cases of vaccine failure and unimmunized children.
- It can be a severe, life threatening disease of the upper airway. Mortality is approximately 2% secondary to airway obstruction.

Signs and symptoms

These children appear toxic and very unwell.

- Acute and rapid onset, over 3–6 hours
- Inspiratory stridor
- High fever (> 39° C)
- Pallor
- Tachypnoea
- Tachycardia
- Poor peripheral circulation (cool extremities)
- Delayed capillary refill time (>2 seconds)
- Lethargy
- Drooling saliva (unable to swallow)
- Reluctant to talk or muffled speech, due to an intense sore throat
- Classically the child sits immobile, with the chin raised slightly and the mouth open
- Cough is rare

Diagnosis

- Diagnosis of acute epiglottitis is made from the distinctive history and clinical findings.
- Lateral radiographs (X-rays) of the neck are occasionally used to confirm diagnosis, but should be avoided as they upset the child and may precipitate total airway obstruction.
- Tracheal intubation will reveal the classic sign of a 'cherry red' epiglottis.

Management

- The overriding management aims are to keep the child calm and to avoid examination of the throat. Disturbance must be kept to a minimum, as if the child becomes distressed and cries this can cause further swelling of the airway and possible total obstruction.
- Most children with acute epiglottitis are septic with acute airway compromise.
- Rapid diagnosis is vital and appropriate treatment must be commenced at the earliest opportunity, otherwise total airway obstruction may occur, resulting in death.

(American Academy of Paediatrics, American College of Emergency Medicine 2005)

- Take child to the resuscitation room.
- Do not separate the child from their parent/carer.
- Keep child on parent/carer's lap.
- Do not lie the child flat.

- Do not insert a venous cannula.
- Do not attempt to examine the child's throat.
- Give high flow oxygen, but remove if it distresses the child.
- Try to distract the child and keep them calm.
- Reassure parents/carers, keeping them well informed of procedures.
- A senior experienced paediatric anaesthetist should be contacted urgently.
- Ideally, the child should go immediately to theatre for tracheal intubation; however, this may be done in the emergency department in cases of severe respiratory distress and near or complete airway obstruction.
- Preparations should be made in advance for a surgical airway, should orotracheal intubation fail.
- Once intravenous access has been secured, blood cultures can be taken and intravenous antibiotics commenced.

Further reading

(ALSG 2005) Advanced Life Support Group (2005) Advanced Paediatric Life Support. The Practical Approach. 4th edition. London. Blackwell Publishing

American Academy of Pediatrics, American College of Emergency Medicine (2005) The Pediatric Emergency Medicine Resource. 3rd edition. Available from: www.APLSonline.com. (Accessed 3 October 2008)

Kelsey J, McEwing G (2006). Respiratory Illness in Children. In: A Textbook of Children's and Young People's Nursing. Glasper A, Richardson J (eds). Edinburgh: Churchill Livingstone. pp. 434–35

London M, Ladewig P, Ball J, Bindler R (2006). The Child with Alterations in Respiratory Function. In: Maternal & Child Nursing Care (2nd Edition). New Jersey: Pearson. pp.1403–4

⚙ Management of pneumonia

Introduction

Pneumonia is an inflammatory illness of the lungs, in particular the alveoli. See Fig. 4.2. Pneumonia can be caused by viruses, bacteria, fungi and parasites.

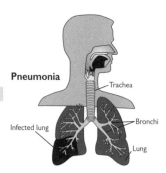

Pneumonia

Trachea

Infected lung

Bronchi

Lung

Fig. 4.2 Respiratory system

The common causes of pneumonia
- Chlamydia, especially in babies
- Viruses such as adenovirus and RSV (in infants)
- Bacteria such as *Streptococcus pneumoniae, Mycoplasma* and *Haemophilus influenzae* (in children)

Immediate identification in infants
- Presents as bronchopneumonia
- May have had upper respiratory tract infection recently
- Pyrexia usually over 38°C; may have had febrile convulsions
- Lethargy
- Tachypnoea, and signs of respiratory distress, may also have apnoeas
- Grunting
- Do not always have a cough
- Abdominal distension due to swallowed air
- Signs of dehydration
- Colour change; pale or cyanotic mucous membranes

Immediate identification in children
- Presents as lobar pneumonia
- Usually have had a recent upper respiratory tract infection
- Rigors, high temperature
- Restlessness
- Unproductive cough
- Tachypnoea

ALERT: Check child has no underlying chronic disease or congenital abnormality.

Immediate action

www.brit-thoracic.org.uk

- Ensure adequate oxygenation of the infant/child.
- This will be dependent upon severity of condition of infant/child.

Nursing management

The child who is cyanosed

- Administer oxygen. Monitor oxygen saturations continuously.
- Monitor pulse and respiratory rate hourly.
- Observe for uneven/abnormal chest movement.
- Rule out underlying condition such as cystic fibrosis or cardiac condition.

All other children

- Blood test for full infection screen, including blood cultures.
- Chest X-ray.
- Correct dehydration. Some infants may require IV fluids.
- Antibiotics if indicated.
- Analgesia if indicated.

Complications/prognosis

Children and infants should make a complete recovery. Complications are rare but may include:

- Empyema
- Septicaemia
- Pneumothorax
- Lung abscess

Further reading

Candy D, Davies G, Ross E (2001). Clinical Paediatrics and Child Health, Chapter 23 Respirology. Oxford: Elsevier.

Rudolph M, Levene M (2006). Chapter 9 Respiratory symptoms. In: Paediatrics and Child Health. (2nd edn). Oxford: Blackwell Publishing

:Ø: **Bronchiolitis**

Bronchiolitis is the most common severe lower respiratory infection in infants and children under the age of 18 months. Most common in the winter, it occurs in association with viral infections: 75% of cases are caused by respiratory syncytial virus (RSV) (SIGN 2006). Other pathogens implicated include adenovirus, parainfluenza, and rhinovirus.

Pathophysiology

- Inflammation of small airways (bronchioles).
- Infection of the bronchiolar and ciliated epithelial cells → increased mucous secretion, cell death, and sloughing.
- Peribronchiolar lymphocytic infiltrate and submucosal oedema.
- Distal airway obstruction → decreased airflow, air trapping, and impaired gas exchange.
- Impaired ventilation, together with ventilation perfusion imbalance, increases the effort of breathing. This often leads to exhaustion, hypoventilation, and apnoea with resultant hypoxaemia and hypercapnia.
- Recovery of pulmonary epithelial cells occurs after 3–4 days, but cilia do not regenerate for approximately 2 weeks.
- See Table 4.2 for the risk and environmental factors related to the incidence of bronchiolitis.

Table 4.2 Risk and environmental factors related to bronchiolitis

Risk factors	Environmental factors
Prematurity	Crowding
Infection at <6 months of age	Poverty
Chronic respiratory disease	Exposure to tobacco smoke
Congenital heart disease	Malnutrition, body mass <5 kg (Nichols et al, 2008)
Neurological disorders	Ethnicity and male sex also important factors
Immunodeficiency	

Signs and symptoms

Diagnosis of bronchiolitis is based on presenting clinical features and typically begins with upper respiratory tract infection with symptoms as follows:

- Initial coryza (cold symptoms)
- Fever
- Harsh dry cough becoming more productive
- Coughing spasms lasting several minutes
- Increasingly rapid, irregular, distressed breathing
- Wheeze
- Subcostal and intercostal recession

- Apnoea may be a presenting feature
- Cyanosis/pallor
- Fatigue leading to feeding difficulties
- Vomiting.

Differential diagnosis
- Cystic fibrosis, aspiration pneumonia
- Congenital cardiac defects, immunodeficiency
- Asthma, inhaled foreign body
- Septicaemia, pneumonia

In the first 72 hours of the illness, infants with bronchiolitis may deteriorate clinically before symptoms improve (SIGN 2006).

Clinical features of severe disease in bronchiolitis (SIGN 2006)
- Respiratory rate >70/minute
- Oxygen saturations < 94% or = 94%
- Presence of nasal flaring and/or grunting
- Severe chest wall recession
- Cyanosis
- History of apnoea
- Poor feeding: intake is less than 50% of usual intake in preceding 24 hours
- Lethargy

Indications for high dependency/intensive care
- Failure to maintain oxygen saturations >92% with increasing oxygen therapy
- Deteriorating respiratory status with signs of increasing respiratory distress and/or exhaustion
- Recurrent apnoea (SIGN 2006)

Investigations
- Analysis of nasopharyngeal secretions for RSV and other likely causative organisms.
- Chest X-ray is only required if infant is to have assisted ventilation or where there is diagnostic uncertainty.

Management of acute illness
Treatment and care are largely supportive, paying attention to maintaining satisfactory oxygenation, hydration, and infection control. Initial and ongoing assessment and evaluation of all interventions must be strictly recorded.
- Isolation, strict hand washing, and restricted visiting in order to prevent cross-infection, as RSV spreads easily through direct and indirect contact.
- Nurse in upright position and administer humified oxygen as prescribed. Infants with O_2 saturation levels ≤ 92%, or who have severe respiratory distress, should receive supplemental oxygen to prevent hypoxia. Method of administration will depend on concentration required.
- Nasal suctioning, to clear secretions in infants who exhibit respiratory distress due to nasal blockage.

- Nasogastric feeding, to be considered in infants who have difficulty feeding due to increased work of breathing, nasal secretions and exhaustion to ensure fluid balance and adequate hydration.
- Nebulized β-2-receptor agonists, nebulized adrenaline, and steroids should not be used as there is no evidence of their efficacy.
- Ventilatory support: bronchiolitis can cause severe respiratory compromise so ventilatory support with continuous positive airway pressure (CPAP) or full ventilation in an intensive care setting may be required.

Preventative treatments/vaccinations

A number of treatment regimens have been employed to reduce infection with RSV bronchiolitis, namely RSV immunoglobulin and palivizumab. Vaccination is currently a high research priority.

Further reading

Meatos-Dennis M (2005) Best practice bronchiolitis. *Archives of Disease in Childhood, Education and Practice* 90: 81–86

Scottish Intercollegiate Guidelines Network (2006) Bronchiolitis in children. A clinical guideline. NHS Scotland. Available at: www.sign.ac.uk

Floues G, Horwitz RI (1997) Efficacy of beta 2 agonist in bronchiolitis; a reappraisal and meta-analysis. *Pediatrics* 100:233–239

☼ Croup

What is croup?

Croup is a viral respiratory illness caused by the influenza virus; it may also be referred to as 'viral croup' or 'laryngotracheobronchitis (LTB)' and is commonly seen in children aged 6 months to 2 years.

The virus causes the inflammation and swelling of the larynx of the upper airway. Quick recognition and treatment is important in the younger child, due to their smaller airway and susceptibility to swelling and inflammation.

Signs and symptoms

- Hoarseness
- 'Barking' cough
- Inspiratory and expiratory stridor
- Recession (sternal and intercostal)
- Use of accessory muscles
- Tracheal tug
- Agitation due to hypoxia
- Increased heart rate
- Increased respiratory rate
- Pyrexia (<39°C)
- Coryzal symptoms

ALERT: Stridor may be heard only when the child is upset or hyper-ventilating; however, inspiratory and expiratory stridor, when the child is at rest, may indicate an increased narrowing of the airways (Advanced Life Support Group 2005) and increasing degree of obstruction due to inflammation.

Management

Airway/breathing

Maintaining the airway is vital and medical help should be sought immediately on admission.

Less than 5% of children require intubation (Advanced Life Support Group 2005). Despite this figure being relatively low, airway management equipment needs to be readily available in case the child needs assistance to maintain their airway and breathing on arrival at hospital.

Steroids (inhaled, oral or IV) are commonly used as treatment for croup, and relief of symptoms should be seen within 30 minutes (Advanced Life Support Group 2005).

- Dexamethasone (oral) 150mcg/kg (twice a day) or 600mcg/kg (once a day)
- Budesonide (nebulizer) 2mg (single dose)
- Adrenaline (nebulizer) 1–5mL of 1:1000 (single dose) – child will need ECG and oxygen saturation monitoring
  (Advanced Life Support Group 2005)

Circulation
Administration of antipyretics may be required; they can also be used for pain relief for any discomfort the child may have.

The **Westley clinical scoring system** classifies cases into mild, moderate or severe (see Table 4.3).

Table 4.3 Westley croup score

Total score ranging from 0 to 17 points. Five component items make up the score:

• Stridor (0 = none, 1 = with agitation only, 2 = at rest)

• Retractions (0 = none, 1 = mild, 2 = moderate, 3 = severe)

• Cyanosis (0 = none, 4 = cyanosis with agitation, 5 = cyanosis at rest)

• Level of consciousness (0 = normal [including asleep], 5 = disorientated)

Mild croup: Occasional barking cough, no stridor at rest, and no to mild suprasternal, intercostal indrawing (retractions of the skin of the chest wall), or both, corresponding to a Westley croup score of 0–2.
Moderate croup: Frequent barking cough, easily audible stridor at rest, and suprasternal and sternal wall retraction at rest, but no or little distress or agitation, corresponding to a Westley croup score of 3–5.
Severe croup: Frequent barking cough, prominent inspiratory and – occasionally – expiratory stridor, marked sternal wall retractions, decreased air entry on auscultation, and significant distress and agitation, corresponding to a Westley croup score of 6–11.
ALERT: Respiratory failure may develop regardless of the severity of the symptoms and evidence of the following signs should be seen as an emergency:
• Change in mental state, such as lethargy and listlessness or decreased level of consciousness.
• Pallor.
• Dusky appearance.
• Tachycardia.
• Breathing may be laboured, a barking cough may not be prominent, stridor at rest may be hard to hear, and sternal wall retractions may not be marked.
• A child who appears to be deteriorating but whose stridor appears to be improving has worsening airway obstruction and is at high risk of complete airway occlusion.

Nursing interventions on admission
• Keep the child calm, and nurse in the presence of parents/main care provider. An upset child increases the risk of them developing further respiratory distress and subsequently increases the risk of hypoxia. Try to keep child upright, e.g. sitting on parent's lap. Reassure family, and explain to both child and family what is happening.
• Provide oxygen, and maintain oxygen saturations >92% with oxygen therapy. The child may appear distressed with having the mask on their face, but remember that they may not be distressed due to the mask,

but agitated due to hypoxia. Involve the parents, explain to them the importance of the oxygen and gain their cooperation with holding the mask in place.

- Observations – respiratory rate, heart rate, temperature, oxygen saturations (in air and in oxygen) – using correct saturation monitor probe for age of child and ensure a good 'trace' is noted on the monitor before documenting the reading.
- Assess and record stridor – awake and at rest.
- Assess and record recession, use of accessory muscles, tracheal tug.
- Assess level of consciousness of child – AVPU.
- Weight (for steroid treatment doses).

Further reading

Advanced Life Support Group (2005) Advanced Paediatric Life Support–The Practical Approach, 4th edition. Oxford: Blachwell Publishing

BMJ Clinical evidence – http://clinicalevidence.bmj.com/ceweb/conditions/chd

Firth M (2007). Croup Syndromes. In: Glasper E A, McEwing G, Richardson J (eds). Oxford Handbook of Children's and Young People's Nursing. Oxford: Oxford University Press

Nichols WG, Peck Campbell AJ, Boeckh M (2008) Respiratory viruses other than Influenza Virus: Impact and Therapeutic Advances. *Clin Microbiol Rev* **21**, 274–90.

Rudolf, Levene (2008) Paediatrics and child health (2nd edn). Oxford: Blackwell Publishing

⚙ Pertussis (whooping cough)

Introduction
- Pertussis is a very infectious disease that can cause death in infants; those under 6 months old are most vulnerable.
- Widespread vaccination against *Bordella pertussis* has led to a notable reduction in the number of notified cases of whooping cough.
- Sporadic cases still occur in unimmunized infants and children, with a significant morbidity in very young infants.
- After a 2 week incubation period, a coryzal phase of 7–10 days is followed by the spasmodic phase: bursts of coughing without inspiratory pauses followed by a 'whoop' as air is drawn into the lungs.
- This disease is notifiable in the UK under the Public Health Infectious Diseases Regulations 1988.

ALERT: Apnoea, cyanosis and seizures as a result of cerebral anoxia may occur.

Signs and symptoms
- Runny nose, sneezing, mild cough, and a low grade fever (at this stage, culture of a pernasal swab may detect pertussis bacteria and a characteristic absolute lymphocytosis on full blood count).
- During a coughing spell which can last for more than 1 minute, the child may turn red or purple. At the end of a spell some, but not all, children make a characteristic whooping sound when breathing in, or vomit.
- High fever, rapid pulse and respirations, pale and lethargic.
- Extreme anxiety and agitation.
- **ALERT: It is important to nurse these children near oxygen and suction.**

Immediate management
- If whooping cough is suspected, take a pernasal swab.
- Isolate the child as soon as possible.
- Antimicrobial therapy may be required. (Erythromycin if commenced early may reduce the period of infectivity, otherwise treatment is supportive).
- Some children may require increased oxygen and humidity.
- In the most severe cases, intubation may be necessary.

Nursing management
Reduce anxiety
- Act quickly and calmly to provide support and guidance
- Provide a suitable environment to allow the child to rest
- Give clear explanations to the child and parents before ANY procedure is carried out

Maintain airway
- Increased oxygen and suction may be required
- Keep emergency equipment available

Maintain and monitor respiratory function
- Allow the child to adopt a position that is comfortable for him/her
- Continue monitoring of respiratory status
- Pulse oximetry to monitor overall oxygen status

Nutrition
- Encourage fluids; offer small amounts of fluid regularly

Prevent spread of infection
- Use universal precautions/procedures

Complications
- Pneumonia
- Bronchiolitis
- Convulsions
- Weight loss and dehydration

Prevention
- Routine pertussis vaccine at 2, 3 and 4 months of age and later at 3 years and 4 months to 5 years old
- Pertussis is a notifiable disease and should be reported to the local health protection team.

Further reading
www.immunisation.org.uk

Trigg E, Mohammed T (2006). Practices in Children's Nursing: Guidelines for Hospital and Community (2nd edn). Oxford: Churchill Livingstone Elsevier

☠ Anaphylaxis and angio-oedema

Anaphylaxis

Anaphylaxis is an allergic response to a substance to which the body has become sensitized. It is usually marked by the sudden onset of rapidly progressive urticaria (angio-oedema) and normally accompanied by respiratory distress.

Angio-oedema

There are varying degrees of urticaria. It is a common skin condition characterized by the acute development of an itchy rash resulting from the release of histamine by mast cells. This produces individual swellings commonly recognized as hives, weals and nettle rash. These swellings tend to develop acutely over a few minutes and occur anywhere on the skin.

Patients who are having an anaphylactic shock also have severe urticaria with cutaneous/subcutaneous involvement, which can present as a soft tissue swelling (angio-oedema) in areas of the skin. Most commonly this affects the areas around the eyes, the lips and the hands. Rarely, the mucosal area such as the mouth and larynx are involved. Angio-oedema can lead to respiratory distress, and the combination of skin and respiratory problems is known as anaphylactic shock.

Causes of anaphylaxis

Anaphylaxis can be caused by a number of triggers (allergens), e.g. foods, drugs or venoms. Below is a list of the most common allergens.
- Foods, e.g. nuts, fish, milk
- Antibiotics, e.g. penicillin
- Anaesthetic drugs, e.g. suxamethonium, vecuronium and atracurium
- Stings, e.g. wasps and bees
- Venoms, e.g. snakes
- Substances, e.g. latex, hair dye and aerosol deodorants

Symptoms and recognition of anaphylaxis

A diagnosis of an anaphylactic reaction is likely if the patient is exposed to an allergen and develops sudden illness within minutes to the exposure. This sudden illness includes progressive skin changes and severe life-threatening changes to their airway, breathing and circulation (Resuscitation Council 2008).

The most common problems for anaphylactic patients are their airway, breathing, and circulation. Patients suffer with either all or a combination of the above.

Table 4.4 describes the different problems in a patient with anaphylaxis.

NB: anaphylaxis is likely when the following three items are met (Resuscitation Council 2008):
- Sudden onset and rapid progression of symptoms
- Life threatening airway and/or breathing and/or circulation
- Skin and mucosal changes (flushing, urticaria and angio-oedema)

Table 4.4 Symptoms of anaphylaxis

Airway	Throat swelling
	Tongue swelling
	Patient can't swallow
	Patient feels throat is closing up
	Hoarse voice
	Stridor (inspiratory noise)
Breathing	Shortness of breath
	Increasased respiratory rate
	Wheeze (expiratory noise)
	Cyanosis
	Respiratory arrest
Circulation	Signs of shock: pale and sweaty
	Tachycardia
	Hypotensive
	Low conscious level
	Cardiac arrest
Disability	Confusion by patient usually caused by hypoxia
Exposure	Signs of urticaria
	Signs of angio-oedema
	Flushing, hives and weals

Treatment of anaphylaxis

Figure 4.3 is adapted from the 'Anaphylaxis Reactions Treatment' guide by the Resuscitation Council (2008). This is a guide to treating an anaphylactic patient appropriately.

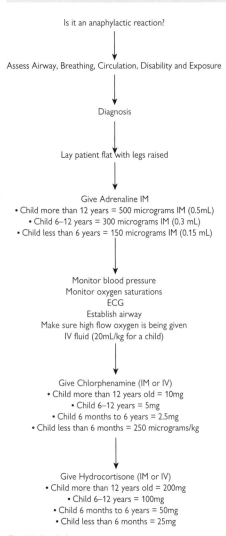

Is it an anaphylactic reaction?

↓

Assess Airway, Breathing, Circulation, Disability and Exposure

↓

Diagnosis

↓

Lay patient flat with legs raised

↓

Give Adrenaline IM
• Child more than 12 years = 500 micrograms IM (0.5mL)
• Child 6–12 years = 300 micrograms IM (0.3 mL)
• Child less than 6 years = 150 micrograms IM (0.15 mL)

↓

Monitor blood pressure
Monitor oxygen saturations
ECG
Establish airway
Make sure high flow oxygen is being given
IV fluid (20mL/kg for a child)

↓

Give Chlorphenamine (IM or IV)
• Child more than 12 years old = 10mg
• Child 6–12 years = 5mg
• Child 6 months to 6 years = 2.5mg
• Child less than 6 months = 250 micrograms/kg

↓

Give Hydrocortisone (IM or IV)
• Child more than 12 years old = 200mg
• Child 6–12 years = 100mg
• Child 6 months to 6 years = 50mg
• Child less than 6 months = 25mg

Fig. 4.3 Anaphylaxis treatment
(Adapted from the Resuscitation Council (UK) (2008) Anaphylaxis algorithm; www.resus.org.uk/pages/pchkalgo.pdf)

Further reading

Kumar P, Clark M. (2002) Clinical Medicine (5th edn). London: W.B. Saunders

Resuscitation Council, Emergency Treatment of Anaphylatic Reactions (2008). http://www.resus.org.uk/pages/reaction.pdf

Schilling, J. (2007) Emergency Nursing. London: LW&W.

:⚙: Acute asthma

Introduction
Asthma is a chronic inflammatory condition of the airways.
- Hyperresponsiveness of the airways is induced by a trigger.
- Presents as a lower airway obstruction; the wheezing is generated by turbulent airflow causing oscillation of the bronchial wall.
  Three factors are involved in the asthmatic response:
- Bronchospasm: narrowing of the bronchial walls due to contraction of the smooth muscle this is more severe in the smaller bronchi and bronchioles.
- Inflammation: causes the airways to become hyperresponsive and narrow easily in reaction to a wide range of stimuli. Further narrowing of the airways results from the invasion of the mucosa, submucosa and muscle tissue by inflammatory cells.
- Inflammatory cells cause vasodilation and increased capillary permeability resulting in mucus production and oedema.

The lumen of the airways is therefore narrowed by contraction of the smooth muscle, mucosal oedema, and the hypersecretion of mucus (see Fig. 4.4).

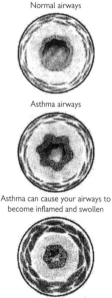

Normal airways

Asthma airways

Asthma can cause your airways to become inflamed and swollen

In addition, the airway walls can become 'twitchy' and thicker, making the airways narrower

Fig. 4.4 Cross section of bronchiole demonstrating narrowing lumen due to constriction and inflammation
Oxford Handbook of Children's and Young People's Nursing, Glasper et al., (2006), p.279, with permission from Oxford University Press

Incidence/causes
- Personal or family history of asthma
- Triggers, e.g. allergens, dust, exercise, viruses, chemicals, changes in weather, irritants, and smoke.
- Obesity
- Prematurity and low birth weight
- Maternal smoking
- Exercise
- Smoking around children increases the risk of developing asthma. It also increases the severity and the frequency of attacks.

Signs and symptoms
- Wheeze: present in expiration, in severe cases also during inspiration
- Cough: may be the only presentation in children, especially during exercise
- Chest tightness, particularly at night and during exertion
- Breathlessness, varies according to severity

Principles of immediate management
- 2–4 puffs of a β_2-agonist, via a spacer and face-mask or mouth piece; repeated every 2 minutes as necessary.
- This may be sufficient for a mild asthma attack.
- If the child has not improved after 10 puffs they should be taken to hospital immediately (British Thoracic Society/Scottish Intercollegiate Guidelines Network 2009; BTS/SIGN).
- When waiting for transfer to hospital the child can continue to have puffs of β_2-agonist as necessary. During the transfer by ambulance the child should be given oxygen and nebulized β_2-agonists.
- A bolus of intravenous salbutamol can be effective in cases of severe asthma.
- The early use of steroids is recommended; therefore oral soluble prednisolone should be given early in the attack as it can prevent the relapse of symptoms and reduce the need for hospital admission (BTS/SIGN 2009).

Assessment
Correct treatment depends on accurate assessment.
Accurate observations are required to assess severity.
(SIGN/BTS 2009):
- Pulse rate: increasing tachycardia generally denotes worsening asthma; a fall in heart rate in life threatening asthma is a preterminal event
- Respiratory rate and degree of breathlessness: too breathless to complete sentences in one breath or to feed
- Use of accessory muscles of respiration, best noted by palpation of neck muscles
- Amount of wheezing, which might become biphasic or less apparent with increasing airway obstruction
- Degree of agitation and conscious level: always give calm reassurance.

Moderate exacerbation of asthma
Signs and symptoms
- Still able to talk in sentences
- SpO_2 ≥92%
- Peak flow >33% best or predicted

- Tachycardia
  - >140 in children aged 2–5 years
  - > 125 in children aged > 5 years
- Tachypnoeic
  - >40 breaths/min aged 2–5 years
  - >30 breaths/min aged 7–5 years

ALERT: Clinical signs correlate poorly with the severity of airways obstruction.

Some children with acute severe asthma do not appear distressed.

Decisions about admission and treatment should be made by trained clinicians after repeated assessment of the response to bronchodilator treatment.

Immediate management

Administration of β_2-agonist bronchodilators (salbutamol) in aerosol form, via a spacer (with or without a mask). Spray in individual puffs, inhalation being by tidal breathing. Allow 2 puffs every 2 minutes according to response, up to 10 puffs.

Observation and management

Moderate asthma: on a ward.

- Position in way most comfortable for child: may be supported by parent, or lean forward with arms supported on a pillow on bed table.
- Observation frequency determined by child's/young person's response, initially hourly.
- Oxygen by nasal prongs/humidified oxygen via facemask to maintain normal SpO_2.
- β_2-agonist bronchodilator regularly; if in response to assessment these are required hourly for more than 4 hours then give nebulized bronchodilators.
- Corticosteroid orally once daily.

Severe life threatening asthma

Worsening of asthma symptoms over a short period of time can lead to a life - threatening situation, where rapid assessment and management are crucial.

Signs and symptoms

- Unable to talk in sentences, too breathless to talk/feed
- Silent chest
- Cyanosis
- Poor respiratory effort/use of accessory muscles
- Hypotension
- Exhaustion
- Confusion/reduced level of consciousness/agitation
- SpO_2 <92%
- PEF <33% best or predicted
- Tachycardia
  - >140 in children aged 2–5 years
  - > 125 in children aged > 5 years
- Tachypnoeic
  - >40 breaths/min aged 2–5 years
  - >30 breaths/min aged 7–5 years

Immediate management

- Present with a calm reassuring approach to both child/young person and family.
- Assess airway, breathing, and circulation.
- Assess and record the above parameters hourly, and before and after bronchodilator administration.
- Oxygen should be given when SpO_2 <94% via a tight fitting mask or nasal cannula at a sufficient flow rate to achieve normal saturations.
- β_2-agonist bronchodilators (salbutamol) in nebulized form, administered with oxygen, may be given every 20–30 minutes.
- If poor response, combine with nebulized ipratropium bromide.
- Discontinue long-acting β_2-agonists when giving short-acting ones more than 4-hourly.
- Cardiac monitoring is essential, because salbutamol will produce a sinus tachycardia and hypokalaemia (monitor serum potassium and supplement as necessary).
- Management should continue either within a High Dependency Unit or an Intensive Care Unit.

Nursing care on a High Dependency Unit or an Intensive Care Unit

- Position most comfortable for child.
- Humidified oxygen via facemask to maintain SpO_2 above 95%.
- Continuous monitoring.
- Bronchodilators nebulized.
- β2-agonist bronchodilators intravenously if necessary in addition to nebulizer.
- Corticosteroids intravenously.
- Management of intravenous therapy.
- Preparation of equipment to enable intubation and subsequent ventilation.
- Children may require intravenous fluids to avoid dehydration if severe asthma is prolonged and they are not tolerating oral fluids.
- In some hospitals, during severe and life threatening asthma not responding to maximum dose of bronchiodilators and steroids, *aminophylline* may be used. An intravenous loading dose is given over 20 minutes (with cardiac monitoring for tachycardia and arrhythmias) followed by continuous infusion. Check theophylline levels when already receiving oral therapy or when treatment prolonged.

Magnesium sulphate by slow infusion has shown some benefit in patients unresponsive to other therapies; however, there is inconclusive evidence as to its place in routine management of asthma.

Complications

- Infection of the lungs (pneumonia)
- Collapse of part, or all, of the lung
- Respiratory failure
- Severe asthma attacks that do not respond to treatment (status asthmaticus) can lead to death

Further reading

British Thoracic Society/Scottish Intercollegiate Guidelines Network (2008) (revised 2009) British guideline on the management of asthma – A national clinical guidance. www.sign.ac.uk

☼ Management of fractured ribs

Background information

- Rib fractures are rare in young children.
- The relative elasticity of the rib cage means that the ribs can be compressed without causing rib fractures, but still causing damage to the underlying lung.
- As the child gets older, the bony rib cage ossifies, and fractures become more common.
- Rib fractures in children indicate a significant mechanism of injury.
- Pulmonary contusion may be present in the absence of rib fractures.
- Pulmonary contusion (with or without rib fractures) is the most common significant chest injury in children.
- An isolated chest injury is rare in children. Check carefully for other injuries.
- A flail segment occurs if two or more adjacent ribs are broken in two or more places.
- This results in a segment of the chest wall being free-floating, moving inwards with inspiration and outwards with expiration. This is called paradoxical movement.
- Flail rib segments are rare in children, but may lead to severe respiratory compromise.

ALERT: Children can have severe internal chest injuries with minimal or no evidence of external injury.

Causes

- Infants and children are most commonly victims of passive blunt trauma, e.g. road traffic collision (RTC) and nonaccidental injury (NAI).
- In the age group 0–3, NAI should be a paramount concern.
- School age children often have transport-related mechanisms of injury, e.g. skateboards, scooters, bicycles, etc.
- Teenagers are more likely to be involved in RTCs, sports injuries, and personal violence.

Signs and symptoms

- History of injury
- Pain
- Crepitus may be felt over fracture site
- Hypoxia, respiratory distress and haemoptysis may be present

Immediate management

- Supportive measures; ensure adequate analgesia and breathing exercises
- Patients with pulmonary contusion require supplemental oxygen and close monitoring

Immediate management of patients with flail segments

- High flow oxygen should be given via face mask with reservoir bag
- Minor cases may simply need good pain relief and supplemental oxygen

- Intermediate cases may benefit from additional CPAP (continuous positive airway pressure)
- Close observation for signs of increasing respiratory compromise
- If child is compromised, intubation and ventilation should be considered immediately
- Pain relief via titrated IV opiates initially; local or regional blocks may be considered

Investigations

- Multiple rib fractures and pulmonary contusion can be diagnosed by chest X-ray (CXR).
- May be little evidence of lung contusion on initial CXR, although findings may progress over a few hours.
- A CT scan can distinguish pulmonary contusion from other diagnoses, but is not warranted for this purpose alone (Advanced Life Support Group 2005).
- Single rib fractures are very difficult to see on CXR; children who are well, with simple isolated injuries, are therefore often not X-rayed but are instead treated supportively.

Further reading

Advanced Life Support Group (2005). Advanced Paediatric Life Support. The Practical Approach, 4th Ed. Blackwell Publishing Ltd: Oxford

Inan M, Ayvaz S, Sut N et al (2007) Blunt Chest Trauma in Childhood. *ANZ J Surg.* 77:682–685

Kemp AM, Dunstan F, Harrison S, Morris S, Mann M, Rolfe K, Datta S, Thomas DP, Sibert JR, Maguire S. (2008) Patterns of skeletal fractures in child abuse: systematic review. BMJ. 337:a1518

Resuscitation Council (UK) (2005) Resuscitation Guidelines 2010. London: Resuscitation Council (UK).

:☀: Management of pneumothorax

Simple pneumothorax

Introduction
- An accumulation of air in the pleural space, which results in some degree of lung collapse.
- Signs will vary depending on the size of the pneumothorax, and coexisting injuries.
- Pneumothorax may be associated with a small amount of blood in the pleural space (a haemopneumothorax).

Signs and symptoms
- Increased respiratory rate
- Decreased oxygen saturation
- Increased work of breathing
- Decreased chest movement on affected side
- Decreased breath sounds on affected side
- Surgical emphysema may be palpable
- Increased pulse rate
- Diagnosis usually made on CXR, although small anterior pneumothoraces are commonly missed

Immediate management
- High flow oxygen via nonrebreathe mask
- Regular monitoring of respiratory rate, oxygen saturation, pulse rate and blood pressure

Treatment
- Traumatic pneumothoraces do not usually resolve spontaneously, so a chest drain will be inserted as a planned procedure
- Spontaneous pneumothoraces, although rare in childhood, may be managed conservatively

ALERT: If the child needs positive pressure ventilation the chest drain should be inserted as a matter of urgency to prevent a simple pneumothorax developing into a tension pneumothorax (ALSG 2005).

Tension pneumothorax

Introduction
- Air collects progressively under pressure in the pleural space as a consequence of a 'flap-valve' mechanism in the underlying injured lung.
- As the intrapleural pressure increases, the lung on the affected side collapses and the mediastinum is deviated to the opposite side. This can cause the inferior vena cava to kink at the diaphragm, leading to profound impairment of venous return to the heart, which if not treated will lead to a cardiac arrest.
- Higher incidence of tension pneumothorax in children because of the more mobile mediastinum.
- Tension pneumothorax is a particular complication in patients with chest injuries who are ventilated, as air is forced into the pneumothorax by positive pressure ventilation.

Signs and symptoms
- Child will be hypoxic and shocked
- Respiratory distress
- Decreased chest movement on affected side
- Decreased breath sounds on affected side
- Surgical emphysema may be palpable
- Distended neck veins may be visible in thin child

Immediate management
ALERT: This is a life threatening emergency and immediate treatment takes priority over performing a chest X-ray
- High flow oxygen via nonrebreathe mask
- Summon senior skilled help
- Immediate insertion of large bore cannula into second intercostal space to release the tension
- Insertion of a chest drain into 5th intercostal space to treat the pneumothorax

Open pneumothorax

Introduction
- An open or sucking wound in the chest wall with associated pneumothorax.
- If the diameter of the wound is greater than about 1/3 of the diameter of the trachea, air will preferentially enter the pleural space via the defect rather than be drawn into the lungs via the trachea. This will lead to severe hypoxia unless the defect is sealed with a one way valve.
- The one way valve dressing or chest seal allows air to flow out on expiration, but prevents air entering the wound on inhalation. This ensures air is drawn into the lungs via the trachea.

Signs and symptoms
- Wound to the chest (remember to check under the arms and over the back of the chest)
- Air may be felt moving in and out of the wound
- Child will be hypoxic
- Signs of pneumothorax

Immediate management
ALERT: This is a life threatening emergency
- High flow oxygen via nonrebreathe mask
- Cover the wound with an occlusive dressing secured on three sides only or apply an Ascherman chest seal
- Insertion of a chest drain in a site away from the wound

Further reading

Advanced Life Support Group (2005). Advanced Paediatric Life Support. The Practical Approach, 4th Ed. Blackwell Publishing Ltd: Oxford
National Patient Safety Agency (2008) Rapid Response Report: Risk of Chest Drain Insertion. http://www.npsa.nhs.uk/nrls/alerts-and-directives/rapidrr/risks-of-chest-drain-insertion/
British Thoracic Society (2008) Guidance for the implementation of local Trust policies for the safe insertion of chest drains in children. www.brit-thoracic.org.uk

☠: Management of haemothorax

Introduction
- A haemothorax is a collection of blood in the pleural space that most commonly occurs after trauma. Signs will vary dependent on the size of the haemothorax and coexisting injuries
- A haemothorax may be associated with air in the pleural space (a haemopneumothorax).

Signs and symptoms
- Increased respiratory rate
- Decreased oxygen saturation
- Increased work of breathing
- Decreased chest movement on the affected side
- Decreased breath sounds on the affected side
- Increased pulse rate
- Diagnosis usually made on chest X-ray, although a small haemothorax may be missed

Immediate management
- High flow oxygen via nonrebreathe mask
- Ensure venous access has been obtained
- Ensure fluid replacement is ongoing
- Prepare for insertion of a chest drain through the 5th intercostal space. The drain will be the biggest one that can fit between the child's ribs

Investigations
- Chest X-ray

Massive haemothorax

Introduction
- Haemorrhage into pleural cavity and compression of lung may cause hypoxia.
- The chest can hold a significant proportion of child's blood volume causing haemorrhagic shock.

ALERT: This is a life-threatening emergency.

Signs and symptoms
- Child will be hypoxic and shocked
- Decreased chest movement on the affected side
- Dullness to percussion on affected side
- Decreased breath sounds on the affected side

Immediate management
- High flow oxygen via nonrebreathe mask
- Ensure venous access has been obtained (two IV or IO lines)
- Ensure fluid replacement is ongoing
- A blood transfusion may be needed, so ensure blood samples have been taken for crossmatching

- Prepare for emergency insertion of a chest drain through the 5th intercostal space; the drain will be the biggest one that can fit between the child's ribs
- Accurate monitoring of the blood loss will be required

Investigations
- Diagnosis may be clinical or may be following a chest X-ray.
- Because injured children are initially managed with spinal protection in place and are therefore lying flat, the chest X-ray may show the haemothorax as a 'white out' in the affected lung.

Further reading

Advanced Life Support Group (2005). Advanced Paediatric Life Support. The Practical Approach 4th Ed. Oxford: Blackwell Publishing

Inan M, Ayvaz S, Sut N et al (2007) Blunt Chest Trauma in Childhood. *ANZ J Surg*. 77:682–685

☠ Thoracic trauma

Sternal fracture

Background information
- Uncommon injury
- May be caused by relatively minor blunt trauma
- Often an isolated injury

Causes
- Direct injury, e.g. striking anterior chest falling off a bicycle.
- Indirect injury caused by hyperflexion of the thoracic spine, e.g. falling off trampoline onto upper back.

Signs and symptoms
- Sternal tenderness

Immediate management
- Analgesia
- Observations
- ECG if history suggestive of significant trauma, e.g. RTC

Investigations
- Lateral X-ray of sternum
- Examination of the spine in indirect injury
- ECG monitoring if significant trauma caused sternal fracture, because of potential for cardiac contusion

Ruptured diaphragm

Background information
- This is a rare injury following blunt trauma, but can also occur following penetrating trauma.
- Often associated with other intra-abdominal injury and possible vertebral injury (e.g. Chance fracture).

Causes
- Most common cause is RTC with children who are wearing lap belts
- Has been reported following injury with bicycle handlebars

Signs and symptoms
- May be stable, but with degree of respiratory distress proportional to amount of abdominal contents in pulmonary space.
- May be shocked due to distortion of mediastinal structures affecting venous return or injury to surrounding structures.
- Bruising across abdomen and flanks.

Immediate management
- Resuscitation as needed
- High flow oxygen via nonrebreathe mask
- Regular monitoring of respiratory rate, oxygen saturation, pulse rate and blood pressure

- Placement of nasogastric tube to decompress stomach
- May need ventilation depending on degree of respiratory distress

Investigations
- CXR
- CT scan

Laryngeal and tracheobronchial injury

Background information
- Possible mechanisms include rapid rise in airway pressure on impact caused by reflex closure of the glottis.

Causes
- May occur after blunt or penetrating injury
- Falls where the neck or chest strikes a hard object
- 'Clothes line' injuries when on motorbikes
- Strangulation

Signs and symptoms
- Subcutaneous emphysema is main clinical sign
- Hoarseness if laryngeal injury
- Possible inability to speak
- May have a stridor
- Dyspnoea
- Dysphagia/drooling
- Haemoptysis
- May have associated pneumothorax

Immediate management
- Airway management is a priority.
- Resuscitation as needed.
- Do not distress a currently 'stable' child as crying can make injury worse, and reduce airflow.
- Keep child in position in which they are most comfortable, often sitting up unless other injuries prevent this.
- High flow oxygen via nonrebreathe mask.
- Regular monitoring of respiratory rate, oxygen saturation, pulse rate and blood pressure.

Investigations
- CXR
- Laryngoscopy/bronchoscopy (probably under general anaesthetic)

Further reading

Advanced Life Support Group (2005). Advanced Paediatric Life Support. The Practical Approach (4th edn). Oxford: Blackwell Publishing

Ferguson LP, Wilkinson AG, Beattie TF (2003) Fracture of the sternum in children. Emerg Med J 20:518–520

Losek JD, Tecklenburg FW, White DR (2008) Blunt laryngeal trauma in children: Case Report and Review of Initial Airway Management. Pediatric Emergency Care. 24:370–373

Soundappan SV, Holland AJ, Cass DT, Farrow GB. (2005) Blunt traumatic diaphragmatic injuries in children. Injury. 36:51–4.

☠ Thoracic cardiovascular injury

Cardiac tamponade

Background Information
- This is a life threatening emergency where blood fills the pericardial sac and impairs cardiac filling during diastole.

Causes
- Most commonly caused by penetrating injury

Signs and symptoms
- High index of suspicion
- The child will be in shock
- Tachycardia

Immediate management
ALERT: This is a life threatening emergency and immediate treatment takes priority over investigation
- High flow oxygen via nonrebreathe mask
- IV fluid replacement
- Emergency needle pericardiocentesis

Cardiac contusion

Background information
- The most common cardiac injury after blunt trauma
- Rare, but may be overlooked
- Usually has minimal clinical significance
- Often associated with injury to at least one other body area

Causes
- RTC either as passenger or pedestrian
- Other blunt trauma

Signs and symptoms
- Chest wall tenderness
- Generalized chest pain
- Tachycardia
- Other ECG changes or dysrhythmias may occur
- Patient may be shocked

Immediate management
- High flow oxygen via nonrebreathe mask
  - Regular monitoring of respiratory rate, oxygen saturation, pulse rate and blood pressure
  - Cardiac monitor

Investigations
- ECG

Commotio cordis

Background information
- A rare cause of sudden death
- A nonpenetrating blow to the chest may cause sudden death to children engaged in sports, such as cricket, hockey, etc.

Causes
- The impact to the precordium gives rise to disturbances of cardiac rhythm of varying type, duration and severity.
- The circulatory arrest is due to atrioventricular block or ventricular fibrillation (VF) because the projectile struck the chest during the ventricular vulnerable period.
- There is no evidence of any structural damage to the heart.

Signs and symptoms
- Disturbances of cardiac rhythm
- May be in cardiac arrest (commonest rhythm is ventricular fibrillation)

Immediate management
- CPR as appropriate
- Cardiac monitor

Disruption of great vessels

Background information
- Rare injury usually caused by deceleration
- In almost all cases is a part of multi-system injuries

Causes
- High speed RTC
- Pedestrian hit by car

Signs and symptoms
- Often fatal at scene
- If tear has tamponaded itself patient may be shocked with poor peripheral pulses
- Symptoms generally nonspecific

Immediate management
- Resuscitation as necessary

Investigations
- CXR
- CT scan

Further reading

Advanced Life Support Group (2005). Advanced Paediatric Life Support. The Practical Approach (4th edn). Oxford: Blackwell Publishing

Baum VC (2002) Cardiac trauma in children. Review article. *Paediatric Anaesthesia*. 12:110–117

Nesbitt AD, Cooper PJ, Kohl P (2001) Rediscovering commotio cordis. *The Lancet*. 357:1195–1197

☠ Choking

Introduction

A child presenting with a choking episode or foreign body airway obstruction (FBAO) is an airway emergency; if not dealt with effectively this could have a potentially fatal outcome.

Immediate identification
- Previously well child
- Sudden onset of symptoms
- May have been witnessed, e.g. during meal
- Suggestive history, e.g. playing with a small object

Signs and symptoms
- Coughing (incomplete obstruction).
- Abnormal breathing sounds, e.g. stridor.
- Absence of breathing sounds and no cough (complete obstruction).
- Struggling for breath, e.g. abnormal chest wall movements.
- The child may be holding their neck or becoming cyanosed.
- The child may be drooling, making gurgling sounds, or attempting to cough.
- If of an appropriate age the child may tell you that they are choking.
- Apnoea.
- Colour change, pallor to mucous membranes, cyanosis.
- The child may be unconscious.

ALERT: Airway obstruction could be caused by soft tissue swelling (e.g. severe allergic reaction). This should be identified for specific emergency management.

Immediate management and treatment
- Should ensure the safety of the child and the rescuer
- Will be based on basic paediatric life support
- Will depend on the severity of the obstruction
- Will depend on the age/size of the child
- Skilled help and resuscitation equipment should be summoned

Management (Resuscitation Council (UK) 2010)

Child who is coughing and conscious
- Encourage the child to cough
- Observe the child carefully for any deterioration.
  The child who is conscious but coughing is ineffective:
- Place the child in a head down position – this allows gravity to assist in dislodging any foreign body and helping it to fall away from the airway/mouth. This can be achieved by holding an infant face down along your arm, ensuring the infant's head is supported, a toddler face down over your knee, or in larger children bending them forward ensuring they are supported.
- Give 5 back blows: these should be directed to the middle of the child's back in between the shoulder blades; the heel of the hand should be used. They do need to be hard in nature.

- If the foreign body is dispelled from the mouth then stop, place the child in the recovery position, assess airway and breathing, and administer oxygen if required.
- If it is not dispelled after 5 back blows then give 5 thrusts:
  - Abdominal thrusts are administered differently depending on the age of the child.
  - In an infant (under 1 year) the thrusts are administered in a similar manner to chest compressions using the same landmark. The infant needs to be turned onto their back with their head down, along the health professional's arm, for example, and 5 chest thrusts administered. They need to be harder in nature and slower than chest compressions.
  - With a child over 1 year, the health professional needs to position themselves behind the child, supporting them, place one fist on the child's abdomen halfway between the umbilicus and xiphisternum, place the other hand on top and exert forceful pressure in an inwards and upwards motion up to 5 times.
- If the foreign body is not expelled and the child remains conscious repeat the process of 5 back blows then 5 abdominal thrusts until the foreign body is dispelled or the child's condition changes.

ALERT: In the child over 1 year of age abdominal thrusts (Heimlich manoeuvre) are used. However, in the child under 1, chest thrusts are used to avoid damage to abdominal organs.

Unconscious child
- Stay with the child
- Summon emergency help
- Place child on a flat, firm surface
- Begin basic life support
  - Open airway
  - If the foreign body is visible one single finger sweep can be used to try to dislodge it.

ALERT: Blind or repeated finger sweeps must NEVER be used. This could result in the foreign body being driven further and more tightly into the airway. Soft tissue damage could also occur.

- Attempt to open airway and deliver 5 rescue breaths. This is achieved in the child under 1 year of age by placing the head of the child in a neutral position and lifting the chin. For a child over 1, tilt head and lift chin. In all cases the soft tissue of the nose should be pinched to achieve a seal.
- With each rescue breath observe for chest wall movement.
- If no movement, adjust head position and proceed.
- If ineffective and no improvement is seen, proceed to full Paediatric Basic Life Support with chest compressions (see Fig. 4.5) (Resuscitation Council (UK), 2010).

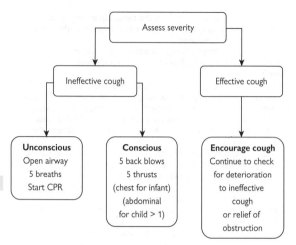

Fig. 4.5 Basic Life Support with chest compressions
(Adapted from the Resuscitation Council (UK) (2010) Basic Life Support management algorithm;
www.resus.org.uk/pages/pchkalgo.pdf)

Background information
- Choking can occur at any age, but pre-school children are most vulnerable.
- Children of this age have a narrow airway, more easily blocked.
- They tend to explore small objects by placing them in their mouth.
- They may have a relatively ineffective/immature swallowing mechanism.
- Parents should be advised to avoid small toys that could be placed in the mouth for their preschool aged children.
- Small, hard items of food should be avoided for the under-fives, e.g. peanuts.

Differential diagnosis
- A child may have a similar presentation with epiglottitis, but there is unlikely to be as much coughing and the child may have been complaining of a sore throat previously.
- It is imperative to obtain a quick, but accurate, history of what the child was doing prior to the choking episode beginning, and to ascertain whether this was witnessed.

Complications
- If the child manages to expel the foreign body with coughing the complications may be minimal.

- However, with any choking episode that presents to the ED a period of observation post choking may be required to ensure the child's oxygen saturations are satisfactory and that the child remains well.
- It has been reported that occasionally abdominal thrusts may cause injury: this should not deter the health professional from performing them, but it may be advisable for the child to be thoroughly examined after abdominal thrusts.
- Occasionally, the foreign body may have caused injury to the throat or airway, so an ENT review should be considered.
- Hypoxia resulting in brain injury or death can occur if the airway obstruction cannot be removed.

Further reading

Resuscitation Council (UK) (2007). Paediatric Immediate Life Support (1st edn). Resuscitation Council (UK): London.

Resuscitation Council (UK) (2010). Paediatric Basic Life Support and Paediatric Advanced Life Support. Available at: www.resus.org.uk/pages/pbls.pdf.

For health promotion advice to give to parents attending the ED see: Child Accident Prevention Trust (2008) Choking Accidents Fact-sheet [online]. Available at: http://www.capt.org.uk/pdfs/factsheet%20choking.pdf [Accessed 12/01/2009].

☠️ Management of drowning in children

Introduction

Drowning is 'the process of experiencing respiratory impairment from submersion/immersion in liquid' (World Congress 2002). Due to the confusion of differing worldwide definitions, 'near drowning' is no longer an official term; however, if used it is said to have occurred if there has been any recovery (however transient) after the submersion.

Signs and symptoms

- Immediate body response to drowning is apnoea and bradycardia.
- Lasting 20 seconds to 5 minutes
  - hypoxia and acidosis
  - causes tachycardia and an increase in blood pressure.
- At some point breathing will recommence involuntarily and cause laryngeal spasm when the inhaled water touches the glottis.
- Eventually subsides and the fluid is aspirated into the lungs.
- Hypoxia is extremely severe by this time, loss of consciousness will have occurred, bradycardia and dysrhythmias may be apparent, and death is imminent.

Immediate management

- Initiate basic life support (Resuscitation Council (UK) 2010).
- Cervical spine immobilization. NB: cervical spinal injury must be assumed until excluded if circumstances are unknown!
- After recovery, close observation is essential due to the possibility of deterioration with respiratory compromise, necessitating intubation and ventilation.

History

- Exposure to contaminated water should be noted and treatment initiated accordingly.
- The initial response for drowning should be to treat the hypoxia, hypothermia and associated injuries.

Examination

- The child should be thoroughly examined from head to toe to ascertain any injury occuring prior to or because of the drowning.
- Chest X-ray changes may occur at a later date due to microbial infection.

Investigations

- Blood glucose
- Blood gas analysis (preferably arterial) and blood lactate
- Urea and electrolytes
- Coagulation status
- Blood and sputum cultures
- Chest X-ray
- Lateral cervical spine X-ray or CT scan if deemed necessary

Treatment

If basic life support is unsuccessful:

- Secure the airway as soon as possible. NB: the stomach may be full of water which will increase the risk of aspiration!
- Insertion of an oro/nasogastric tube if necessary to empty stomach.
- Obtain a core temperature as soon as possible and prevent further hypothermia.
- Monitoring of the vital signs is essential.
- If hypothermia is present, resuscitation should continue until a core temperature of 32°C is reached, unless this cannot be acheived despite attempts.
- Initiate rewarming if necessary according to APLS guidelines.

External rewarming

- Remove cold, wet clothing
- Supply warm blankets
- Infrared radiant lamp
- Heating blanket
- Warm air system

Core rewarming

- Warm intravenous fluids to 39°C to prevent further heat loss
- Warm ventilator gases to 42°C to prevent further heat loss
- Gastric or bladder lavage with normal saline at 42°C
- Peritoneal lavage with potassium-free dialysate at 42°C (use 20mL/kg cycled every 15 minutes)
- Pleural or pericardial lavage
- Endovascular warming
- Extracorporeal blood warming
- Raise temperature by approximately 1°C an hour to reduce haemodynamic instability (there is controversy as to whether maintaining mild hypothermia could have a beneficial effect on neurological outcome)

Complications/prognosis

- If the first breath occurs within the first 3 minutes of cardiopulmonary resuscitation then the prognosis is generally good.
- The majority of children who have been submerged for longer than 8 minutes stand little chance of being neurologically intact.
- The brain is the most vulnerable organ, and if cardiac problems have occurred during submersion then cerebral impairment is highly likely.
- Fever is common in the first 24 hours after resuscitation, but is not necessarily a sign of infection; this would be more likely after 24 hours. Treatment with broad spectrum antibiotics is advisable after blood cultures have been taken.
- Due to posthypoxic brain injury, raised intracranial pressure may become apparent, but aggressive treatment of this has not shown any improvement of the outcome.
- If the patient is hypothermic before the drowning, prognosis may be slightly better.

- If the arterial blood pH remains less than 7.0 and PO_2 remains less than 8.0 kPa despite treatment, prognosis is poor.
- Only after all the prognostic indicators have been considered should resuscitation cease.

Further reading

Mackway-Jones K, Molyneux E, Phillips B, Wieteskas S (2008). Advanced paediatric life support. (4th edn) Oxford: Blackwell Publishing

http://www.who.int/violence_injury_prevention/other_injury/drowning/en/

Resuscitation Council (UK) (2010) Paediatric Basic Life Support.and Paediatric Advanced Life Support. Available at: www.resus.org.uk/pages/pbls.pdf.

World Congress (2002). http://www.cslsa.org/events/archiveattachments/spr03minutes/attachmentG2.pdf

Circulatory problems

☠ Shock

Shock results from an acute failure of circulatory function. Inadequate amounts of nutrients and oxygen are delivered to the body tissues, and there is inadequate removal of tissue waste products. The most common causes of shock in the paediatric patient are hypovolaemia (from any cause), septicaemia, and the effects of trauma.

Shock can develop rapidly in children, because the loss of relatively small amounts of fluid can comprise a high percentage of their intravascular volume.

Early recognition of shock is essential. The outcome of decompensated shock is in general very poor.

Shock may be described as either compensated or uncompensated.

- Compensated shock is when vital organ function is maintained by intrinsic mechanisms, and the child's ability to compensate is effective. Early signs are subtle and include:
  - Irritability, agitation or confusion
  - Increased heart rate
  - Decreased capillary return
  - Normal blood pressure
  - Narrowing pulse pressure
  - Thirst
  - Pallor
  - Decreased urinary output
- Uncompensated shock is when the compensatory mechanisms start to fail and the circulatory system is no longer efficient. The signs may include:
  - Tachypnoea
  - Tachycardia
  - Falling blood pressure
  - Moderate metabolic acidosis
  - Oliguria
  - Very slow capillary return
  - Decreased skin turgor
  - Decreased cerebral state

There are many types of shock, four of which will be discussed here. These are:
- Cardiogenic shock
- Septic shock
- Distributive shock
- Hypovolaemic shock.

Cardiogenic shock

Cardiogenic shock can be defined as shock resulting from a decline in cardiac output secondary to serious heart disease.

Possible causes:
- Arrhythmias
- Cardiomyopathy

- Heart failure
- Myocardial infarction
- Myocardial contusion
- Valvular disease

Septic shock

Septic shock is associated with sepsis. Sepsis is associated with the presence of pathogenic organisms in the blood or tissue.

Possible causes:
- Septicaemia
- Abdominal infection/pelvic infection following trauma or surgery.

Distributive shock

Distributive shock is caused by a profound decrease in systemic vascular tone. The most common aetiology of distributive shock is sepsis due to infection.

Possible causes:
- Anaphylaxis
- Spinal chord injury/shock
- Head injury
- Early stages of sepsis
- Drug intoxication

Hypovolaemic shock

This is the most common form of shock in children and is caused by a reduction in the volume of blood.

Possible causes:
- Haemorrhage
- Dehydration
- Vomiting
- Diarrhoea
- Ketoacidosis
- Ascites
- Pancreatitis
- Intestinal obstruction
- Burns
- Peritonitis
- Volvulus

A child's body can tolerate a loss of 20–25% in circulating volume prior to a drop in blood pressure and cardiac output.

In hypovolaemic shock the body attempts to maintain circulation despite the deficit.

Fluids used in shock

Fluids are given in resuscitation to restore circulating volume and ensure that vital organs are adequately perfused. This is essential to allow the exchange of oxygen and carbon dioxide, and for normal metabolic conditions to be maintained.

Cardiac arrest and hypovolaemia

If hypovolaemia is suspected, infuse intravenous or intraosseous fluids rapidly. In the initial stages of resuscitation there are no clear advantages in using colloids, so use isotonic saline solutions. Avoid glucose-based solutions, as these will be redistributed rapidly away from the intravascular space and will cause hyponatraemia and hyperglycaemia, which may worsen neurological outcome after cardiac arrest.

Further reading

Morton R, Phillips B (1994). Signs of early circulatory failure. In: Accidents and Emergencies in Children. Oxford University Press, Oxford, p. 37

Resuscitation Council UK (2010) Resuscitation Guidelines. Resuscitation Council (UK), London

① Fluid and electrolyte balance

Fluid and electrolyte balance are essential requirements for optimal cellular function. The kidneys are responsible for controlling the body's fluid and electrolyte balance and excretion of metabolic waste. In healthy individuals, they regulate the volume and composition of body fluids by selectively conserving fluids and electrolytes in times of need, and excreting the excess fluids and electrolytes surplus to the body's requirements.

The content and distribution of total body water changes with age (see Table 5.1).

Infants have a high content of body water and a large surface area to body mass ratio, which makes any imbalance potentially more rapid and serious.

The body fluids are split into two main compartments, the intracellular fluid (ICF) and the extracellular fluid (ECF) compartments. The ECF is then further divided into the intravascular (plasma), interstitial (fluid surrounding the tissues), and transcellular (cerebrospinal fluid, sinovial, pleural, peritoneal) compartments. Three quarters of the water distribution in the ECF is located in the interstitial and transcellular spaces and one quarter in the plasma.

It is important to remember that age-related changes affect both body water content and distribution.

Fluid loss at any age consists mainly of urine, insensible losses (skin and respiratory tract), sweat, vomit, and stool. Fluid balance is normally maintained through activities of daily living: adequate fluid intake, nutrition and warmth. The mechanisms to maintain homeostasis are highly sophisticated, and are finely balanced by many complex systems of movement of fluids and electrolytes between the vascular space and the body tissues. This involves osmosis and diffusion, with a complex process of oncotic and hydrostatic forces moving fluid around the body compartments.

Fluid and electrolyte imbalances in the newborn are often due to poor feeding. In children, gastroenteritis, characterized by a sudden onset of diarrhoea and vomiting (D&V), is a more common cause. Imbalances can occur at any age; however, the younger age groups are far more susceptible due to the immaturity of their kidney function (see Table 5.2).

Table 5.3 illustrates the recommended amounts of feeds for infants. Generally, the older child can tolerate a degree of dehydration from diarrhoea and vomiting without requiring medical intervention; however, they are at risk of kidney failure if they become severely dehydrated.

More commonly, dehydration and electrolyte imbalance in this age group is caused by vomiting from alcohol or substance abuse; this is a growing problem in adolescents. Most symptoms resolve spontaneously, but a significant number require some form of advice or treatment in a hospital setting.

Table 5.1 Normal body water content

Age group	Approx body water content
Premature infants	90%
Newborn infants	70–80%
12–24 months	64%
Adolescents and adults	60%

Table 5.2 Classification of dehydration and observations

1. Normal well child with D&V. No clinical signs of dehydration	2. Clinically dehydrated	3. Clinically dehydrated & shocked
Temperature	Temperature	Temperature
Pulse	Pulse	Pulse
Respiratory	Respiratory	Respiratory
Weight	BP	BP
Observe stools	Weight & height/length	Weight & height/length
	Observe stools & send sample	Send stool for M&C, virology, E. coli 0157
	Monitor skin temperature and blood glucose levels	Monitor skin temperature and blood glucose levels; blood sample for U&E & FBC
	If there is blood in the stools send a specimen for E. coli 0157; bloods should also be taken for U&E	Urine electrolytes
	Fluid balance chart including stools as fluid output (weigh nappies in babies), measure urine output in the older child and make a note of the number of times they pass stools in 24 hours.	Fluid balance chart including stools as fluid output (weigh nappies in babies), measure urine output in the older child and make a note of the number of times they pass stools in 24 hours

Table 5.3 Infant feeds (average requirements/kg/day)

Newborn	30mL
2 days	60mL
3 days	90mL
4 days	120mL
5 days	150mL
6 days to 9 months	150mL
> 9 months	120mL

Langmack (2007)

The potential life threatening complication of prolonged D&V results from the loss of electrolytes and water. The National Patient Safety Agency (2007) recommends that children should receive 0.45% sodium replacement as opposed to the traditional rehydration fluid 0.18% sodium chloride and glucose (dextrose saline) to prevent the development of hyponatraemia (see Table 5.4). Hyponatraemia is potentially a very serious complication of rehydration and careful consideration should be taken when deciding what fluid replacement is appropriate (see Table 5.5). Remember that plasma sodium in dehydrated children can appear high; this is usually because they are water depleted. Conversely, low plasma sodium can be a sign of acute renal failure; this occurs as the body is being rehydrated and becomes water overloaded resulting from the kidneys being unable to excrete fluid.

Table 5.4 Infusion therapy

IV replacement	0.9% NaCl/ Hartmann's	
Hypovolaemia		
Daily IV requirement	Weight (kg)	IV fluid
	3–10	100mL/kg
	11–30	100 mL/kg + 50mL/kg for each additional kg > 10kg
	>30	1500mL plus 20mL/kg for each additional kg>30kg

(Willock 2000)

Table 5.5 Management

Action	Rational
Assessment of level of dehydration	Infants and preterm babies are particularly vulnerable partly due to their large percentage of ECF, their immature compensatory mechanisms and high metabolic rate during the first few months of life.

Table 5.5 Management (*Continued*)

Action	Rational
Observations (Table 5.2)	Dehydration can cause shock and impaired renal function.
	Accurate recording of fluid balance is an essential requirement to decide the course of management. This includes documenting and measurement of all episodes of stools and urine passed. Babies' nappies can be weighed before and after they have been used to accurately calculate their fluid output (stools and urine) and episodes of vomiting must be measured (if possible) and recorded for accurate balance.
	Blood in a child's stools is red flag for a serious cause of D&V. Bloods should be taken in these children for U&E and FBC for possible haemolytic uraemic syndrome (HUS)
Fluid and electrolyte maintenance	
An infant's daily requirement of feeds should be calculated according to the infant's expected body weight. (Table 5.3)	
1. Oral rehydration solution (ORS) is recommended for infants and children if tolerated. Fruit juice should be avoided.	This will restore the fluid and electrolyte balance with minimal intervention
2. Children with clinical dehydration	NGT is an efficient way to deliver fluids in babies.
Start with ORS at 50–100mL/kg. It may be necessary to pass an NGT to commence slow safe hydration. If this is not tolerated it may be necessary to start IV hydration.	
3. Intravenous fluids may be required if oral fluids are not tolerated. A bolus may be required followed by maintenance fluids (Table 5.4).	If the child's serum sodium is very low or very high, correction should be gradual to avoid large fluid shifts and cerebral oedema.
Maintenance of fluid balance	Prevention of fluid overload.
Once adequately rehydrated the fluid requirement should be calculated using the previous day's output plus insensible losses (Table 5.5).	

Table 5.6 Example fluid requirements in 24 hour period

Weight 10 kg			Total
Fluid input			
Calculation fluid/kg	100mL/10kg		1000mL
Insensible losses	300mL/m² (300/0.5=150)		150mL
Total fluid requirement	mL/kg + Insensible losses	1000+150mL	1150mL
Output			
Urine and stool output	Fluid intake – insensible loss		Approx 850– 1000 mL

The example in Table 5.6 can be used for all age groups using a simple 5 calculation as follows:

100mL/kg for the first 10kg body weight + an additional 50mL/kg for the next 10kg of body weight + 15mL/kg for each additional kilogramme (see Table 5.7).

Table 5.7 Calculating daily fluid requirement

Child's weight 28kg	Fluid required in mL/kg	mL of fluid
First 10kg	100x10	1000
Second 10kg	50x10	500
Each additional kg	15x8	120
Total fluid required for 28kg child	1000+500+120	1620mL hours in 24 hours

Further reading

Metheny NM (2000) Fluid and electrolyte balance in infants and children. In: Fluid and electrolyte balance. Philadelphia: Lippincott. pp. 392–408

National Patient Safety Agency (2007). Patient safety alert 22: reducing the risk of hyponatraemia when administering intravenous infusions to children. Issued 28th March 2007. www.npsa.nhs.uk (accessed 23 September 2008).

Langmack G (2007) Gastrointestinal problems. In Glasper A, McEwing G, Richardson J, ed. The Oxford Handbook of Children's and Young People's Nursing. Oxford University Press, pp. 390–1

Willock J, Jewkes F (2000) Making sense of fluid balance in children. *Paediatric Nursing* 12:37–42

☼ Haemorrhage

Haemorrhage is one of the more common causes of hypovolaemic shock in children. Serious injury is the primary cause, although other conditions such as clotting disorders, poisoning and malignancy can also be responsible.

Immediate identification of exsanguinating haemorrhage is a key part of the primary survey when assessing the seriously injured child. Early intervention can improve outcome and prevent circulatory failure and subsequent cardiac arrest.

Primary survey
- **A**irway with cervical spine control
- **B**reathing with ventilatory support
- **C**irculation with haemorrhage control
- **D**isability with prevention of secondary insult
- **E**xposure with temperature control.

The assessment and immediate treatment of haemorrhage occur within the primary survey. Concurrent with the circulatory assessment is a rapid assessment for signs of external haemorrhage. Pressure is applied to control obvious bleeding.

It is important to note that while external blood loss in neonates and small infants may appear low, it can amount to a significant proportion of their total circulating volume. Any blood loss in such patients should be regarded as serious.

Assessment of circulation
- Heart rate
- Capillary refill time (CRT)
- Respiratory rate
- Mental state
- Systolic blood pressure

Symptoms and signs
- Anxiety and restlessness
- Marked tachycardia
- CRT over 2 seconds (can be delayed due to body temperature and site of testing)
- Tachypnoea unrelated to thoracic problem
- Altered conscious level unrelated to head injury
- Falling blood pressure*
- Relative bradycardia*
- Cardiac arrest (Pulseless Electrical Activity (PEA))*
- * Severe or preterminal signs

Immediate action
- Facial oxygen at 15L/min via nonrebreathing mask.
- Apply pressure to any obvious external haemorrhage.
- Insert two large intravenous cannulae.
- Intra-osseous cannulation (if IV unsuccessful after 90 seconds).

- IV fluid bolus: two 10mL/kg crystalloid boluses. Assess response between each bolus.
- If no improvement get a surgica.l opinion.
- IV fluid bolus: two 10mL/kg crystalloid boluses. Assess response between each bolus.
- Blood is used when further IV fluid bolus is required.

Massive haemothorax

This is a life threatening haemorrhage which should be identified and treated during the primary survey. Blood collects in the pleural space and impinges on the child's ability to ventilate. The thorax can contain a significant proportion of circulating blood volume.

Signs

- Shock
- Hypoxia despite facial oxygen
- Decreased area entry and dullness to percussion on the affected side.
- Decreased chest expansion on the affected side

Treatment

- High-flow oxygen (15L/min) via a non-rebreathing mask
- Immediate volume replacement
- Chest drain insertion

Volume replacement must be commenced prior to chest drain insertion—one of the few cases where a circulatory problem is addressed before a breathing one. This is because the potentially massive, sudden shift of circulating volume which may result from drainage needs to be pre-empted.

Secondary survey

This is a quick top to toe survey which aims to identify significant injuries. External haemorrhage is uncommon and control is applied during the primary survey. Signs of internal haemorrhage can be more subtle. This is commonly due to an injury of the chest, abdomen and pelvis. In children the liver, spleen and bladder lie intra-abdominally and therefore are more vulnerable in blunt trauma to the abdomen. In addition, the chest wall is very compliant and flexible. Pulmonary contusions are possible without overlying rib fracture. The presence of a rib fracture indicates a significant degree of force, and serious underlying injury should be expected. Blood loss from a closed femoral fracture is significant, but limited by tamponade. Open long bone fractures may result in considerable blood loss, which can be life-threatening.

Signs

- Bruising, swelling and abrasions
- Lacerations and deformity
- Crepitus/surgical emphysema
- Abdominal tenderness, distension or masses
- Palpate for abnormal mobility of the pelvis
- Unexplained haemodynamic unstability

Further management

Once immediate life threatening conditions are identified and treated, the secondary survey is completed and further emergency treatment instituted. A final review and reassessment is carried out, and stabilization achieved prior to transfer to a definitive care facility.

Further reading

Advanced Life Support Group (2004) Advanced Paediatric Life Support: the practical approach. Fourth edition. Oxford: Blackwell.

☠ Managing the child or young person with toxic shock syndrome

Although toxic shock syndrome (TSS) is a rare condition, it is potentially life threatening and should be managed as an emergency. TSS occurs through pathological infection by *Staphylococcus aureus* bacteria. The syndrome was first described in 1978 and was associated with the use of tampons in menstruating females; however, it is also associated with skin or soft tissue infections, abscesses, cellulitis, boils, and lesions caused by burns, insect bites, and infected wound sites.

Immediate identification
- Fever greater than 38.9 degrees Celsius.
- Hypotension (it must be remembered that hypotension is a late sign of circulatory failure in young children).
- A nonpurpuric red rash which is widespread and will later peel particularly around the fingers and toes (desquamation).
- Complaints of muscle aching and pain.
- Abdominal pain.
- Diarrhoea.
- Vomiting.
- Irritability.

Further diagnostic indicators
- Drowsiness with no focal neurological signs.
- Inflammation of the conjunctivae or other mucosal surface.
- Biochemical evidence of renal or liver malfunction.
- Negative culture of organisms from blood cerebral spinal fluid or throat except for *Staphylococcus aureus*.
- Negative serology for measles, leptospirosis, or the tick borne disorder Rocky Mountain spotted fever (Centers for Disease Control and Prevention 2008).

Immediate action and management
- As with any life-threatening condition, the child's airway, breathing and circulation should be assessed in accordance with basic paediatric life support.
  - Close monitoring of vital signs.
- Rapid recognition, diagnosis and hospitalization is essential (Lillitos et al 2007).
- Careful history taking should include past medical and surgical history, possible infection exposure, travel, vocation, hobbies, vaccination history, menstrual status and medication history.
- Identify and decontaminate site of toxin production, e.g. drain or debride lesion, remove foreign body material.
- Investigations will include blood test, swabs, radiographs and echocardiographs (to rule out cardiac causes of shock).
- Supportive therapy, administration of intravenous antibiotics such as flucloxacillin, erythromycin, or clindamycin, and intravenous fluid to maintain blood pressure.

- Maintenance of strict fluid balance documentation.
- These children may need to be transferred to and cared for in a paediatric intensive care unit (Lillitos et al 2007).

Medical and nursing personnel caring for these children and young people should be proficient in basic and advanced paediatric resuscitation skills in accordance with the Resuscitation Council guidelines.

Conditions that resemble TSS

- Severe group A streptococcal infection (scarlet fever, necrotizing fasciitis, and toxic shock-like syndromes). Streptococcal toxic shock-like syndrome may be indistinguishable from TSS. Extensive soft tissue destruction and exudative pharyngitis would suggest streptococcal aetiology.
- Kawasaki syndrome (rare in children over 4 years old).
- Staphylococcal scalded skin syndrome (rare above the age of 5).
- Rocky Mountain spotted fever.
- Leptospirosis.
- Meningococcaemia.
- Gram-negative sepsis.
- Exanthematous viral syndromes (e.g. rubeola, adenoviral infection, certain enteroviral infections).
- Severe allergic drug reaction (www.TSSIS.com).

Further background to staphylococcal toxic shock syndrome

- Pathogenesis of toxic shock syndrome begins with colonization or infection by a strain of *Staphylococcus aureus* capable of producing a TSS toxin, sometimes referred to as a superantigen (Lillitos et al 2007). Production of toxin then takes place followed by toxin absorption.
- Toxic shock syndrome is more likely to be found in children or young people, as most adults have developed specific immunity by their 20s.

Further reading

Centers for Disease Control and Prevention (2008). Toxic Shock Syndrome. http://www.cdc.gov/. (Last accessed August 2008)
Lillitos P, Harford D, Michie C (2007) Toxic Shock Syndrome. *Emergency Nurse*. 15:28–33.
TSSIS. http://www.toxicshock.com

☠ Meningococcal disease

Meningococcal meningitis and meningococcal septicaemia are systemic infections caused by the Gram-negative diplococcus *Neisseria meningitidis*. This bacterium has many different serotypes: A, B, C, W135 and Y. Groups B and C are the most common in the UK, although group C is declining with the advent of the MenC vaccine in 1999.

Meningococcal disease remains a significant cause of mortality in children in the UK. The incidence of meningococcal disease is highest in children under 5 years, with a peak in children under 1 year of age and a second smaller peak in young people aged 15–19 years.

- Meningococci can be found naturally in the throat or nose, with approximately 10% of the population being carriers, rising to 25% in young people aged 15–19 years.
- The majority of cases of meningococcal disease occur sporadically, with <5% of cases occurring in clusters.
  The reason why the disease occurs is not fully understood. However:
- Overcrowding and smoking increase the risk of the disease.
- Travel to the Indian subcontinent, Middle East, and sub-Saharan Africa has in recent years increased the incidence of Group A and W135 cases in UK.
- Increased incidence in winter.
- Transmission is via nasopharyngeal droplets.
- The incubation period is 2–10 days.

Children can present with meningitis alone, septicaemia alone or both. Meningococcal septicaemia is the more serious. Meningococcal disease continues to be a significant cause of mortality and morbidity in children in the UK. Early recognition and aggressive early treatment improve outcome. In meningococcal septicaemia, death occurs due to cardiovascular failure whereas in meningococcal meningitis death occurs as a consequence of CNS damage.

Signs and symptoms

Frequently, mild nonspecific signs and symptoms are followed by severe illness, and in >50% cases a rash appears.

Symptoms of septicaemia

- Rash: may be very diverse being sparse or profuse, and vary from tiny petechial spots to large purpuric lesions which look different according to skin type. In early disease approximately a third of all rashes can be blanching.
- Fever
- Aches: children usually experience muscle and joint aches, making them feel restless and uncomfortable.
- Myalgia and especially leg pain.
- Weakness.
- Gastro-intestinal symptoms, including abdominal pain, vomiting and diarrhoea.

Symptoms of meningitis
- Fever
- Headache
- Vomiting
- Irritability/drowsiness/confusion
- Seizures
- Photophobia
- Neck stiffness
- Infants may also have a bulging fontanelle

Young children can be very hard to assess and parents' anxieties about their child should always be taken seriously. All febrile children should be thoroughly assessed no matter how well they look. Young people often present late and the disease can be very advanced.

Nursing management
- Initial assessment includes patency of the airway, and adequacy of breathing and circulation in line with APLS guidelines (2010). Resuscitation should start where indicated and should follow the Early Management of Meningococcal Disease algorithm (Pollard et al 1999).
- Give oxygen to all patients even if oxygen saturations are normal to optimize tissue oxygenation.
- Assess circulation, including heart rate, capillary refill time, core-peripheral temperature, demarcation of circulatory insufficiency and systolic blood pressure.
- Secure venous/intraosseous access. Rapid fluid resuscitation should be commenced, boluses of 20mL/kg administered over 5–10 minutes should be given and response evaluated. The nurse's role in the administration, monitoring and evaluation of efficacy of fluid administration cannot be overstated.
- Assessment of conscious level – AVPU scale, pupil size and reaction, GCS.
- Must assess and document temperature, heart rate, respiratory rate, blood pressure, capillary refill time (CRT), oxygen saturation measurement, assessment of conscious level, pupil size and reaction, and rash including whether it blanches, extent, speed of development, whether it is petechial or purpuric.
- Assessment is essential to determine whether shock or signs of raised intracranial pressure are present.
- Early signs of shock include: tachycardia; tachypnoea; oxygen saturation <95% in air; cool peripheries; CRT >3 seconds or core/peripheral temperature gap of >3 degrees; pallor; mottling; reduced urine output <1mL/kg/hour; drowsiness, agitation, confusion. A low BP is a preterminal sign.
- Signs of raised ICP include: decreasing or fluctuating level of consciousness; unequal, dilated or abnormally reactive pupils; seizures; abnormal posturing; Cushing's triad (low pulse, elevated BP, abnormal respiratory rate and pattern).
- Take bloods for full blood count, urea and electrolytes, glucose, calcium, magnesium, phosphate, clotting studies, cross match, culture,

venous blood gas (to assess base excess) and meningococcal PCR. May also need to take throat swab.
- Blood glucose must be monitored and hypoglycaemia corrected.
- Administer definitive treatment, IV antibiotics cefotaxime or ceftriaxone.
- Glasgow Meningococcal Septicaemia Prognostic Score (GMSPS) is a useful scoring tool to assess the severity of disease (Table 5.8). The higher the score the more severe the disease. Must be repeated on a regular basis.

Table 5.8 Glasgow Meningococcal Septicaemia Prognostic Score

Observation	Score
Systolic BP >75mmHg in children <4 years	3
Systolic BP > 85mmHg in children ≥4 years	
Core-peripheral temperature difference >3 degrees	3
Modified GCS <8 or a deterioration of 3 points or more in 1 hour	3
Parental opinion that the child's condition has deteriorated in last hour	2
Absence of meningism	2
Extending purpuric rash or widespread purpura	1
Base deficit > 8	1
Total score	Maximum 15

- Meningococcal disease is a notifiable disease; the Department of Health must be notified and prophylaxis provided for close contacts.
- Provide psychological support for the family; help them to cope with their child suffering from a highly critical illness.

Further reading

Pathan, N., Faust, S.N., Levin, M. (2003) Pathophysiology of meningococcal meningitis and septicaemia. *Archives of Diseases in Childhood.* 88:601–7.
Meningitis Research Foundation. http://www.meningitis.org/
Meningitis Trust. http://www.meningitisuk.org/
Isabel–a clinical decision support system. http://www.isabelhealthcare.com/home/default
Pollard, AJ et al (1999) Early Management algorithm. Dept Paediatrics, Imperial College at St Mary's Hospital. *Arch Dis Child* 80:290.
APLS guidelines (2010) – http://www.resus.org.uk/pages/pals.pdf

☠ Cardiac tamponade and pulseless electrical activity (PEA)

Cardiac tamponade is a life-threatening condition. Penetrating or blunt trauma to the chest directly injures the heart or major vessels, causing bleeding, which fills the pericardial sac and compromises ventricular filling. The progressive reduction in cardiac output eventually leads to complete circulatory failure. The electrical activity of the heart and, therefore, the ECG remains normal, a condition known as pulseless electrical activity (PEA).

Though uncommon, cardiac tamponade is one of the key conditions to be identified in the primary survey of the seriously injured child.

Primary survey
- **A**irway with cervical spine control
- **B**reathing with ventilatory support
- **C**irculation with haemorrhage control
- **D**isability with prevention of secondary insult
- **E**xposure with temperature control.

Cardiac tamponade may also be seen in cardiac patients after pacing wires have been removed, and in those with electrolyte imbalances.

Key signs
- Shock:
  - Anxiety and restlessness
  - Marked tachycardia
  - Relative bradycardia
  - CRT over 2 seconds (can be delayed due to body temperature)
  - Tachypnoea unrelated to thoracic problem
  - Altered conscious level unrelated to head injury
  - Falling blood pressure is a pre-terminal sign
- Muffled heart sounds
- Distended neck veins
- An impalpable pulse with a normal cardiac electrical rhythm (PEA)

Diagnosis of cardiac tamponade is difficult and some of the key signs are not clearly identifiable. Muffled heart sounds are especially difficult to identify during resuscitation, due to the inherent level of background noise in this situation. Distended neck veins may not be present if there is concurrent hypovolaemia. Other causes of inadequate circulation, such as tension pneumothorax and hypovolaemia, are identified and treated first by following the ABC approach. In patients where circulatory inadequacy remains, treatment for cardiac tamponade should be considered quickly, especially in patients with PEA, as this is a pre-asystolic state.

Treatment of cardiac tamponade
Immediate action
- High flow oxygen
- Intravenous access and fluid replacement
- Emergency needle pericardiocentesis
- Consult cardiothoracic or paediatric surgeon for definitive treatment (usually thoracotomy)

Aspirate from pericardiocentesis may be small in volume, but can improve cardiac output significantly. Conversely, a large volume of aspirate may indicate aspiration from the ventricle. Pericardial drainage may need to be repeated if signs of tamponade recur.

Treatment of PEA

PEA is a momentary pause on the way to cardiac arrest; therefore treatment of this condition is identical to that of asystole.

Immediate action
- Ventilate with high flow oxygen
- Perform CPR
- Administer IV/IO adrenaline 10mcg/kg
- Continue CPR
- Identify and treat causes
  - Hypoxia
  - Hypovolaemia
  - Hypothermia
  - Hypo/hyperkalaemia and hypocalcaemia
  - Tension pneumothorax
  - Cardiac tamponade
  - Toxins
  - Thromboembolism

Further management

Once immediate life threatening conditions are identified and treated the secondary survey is completed and further emergency treatment instituted. A final review and reassessment is carried out, and stabilization achieved prior to transfer to a definitive care facility.

Further reading

Advanced Life Support Group (2004) *Advanced Paediatric Life Support: the practical approach.* Fourth edition. Oxford: Blackwell.

☠ Management of electrocution in children

There are a number of important factors to consider when assessing children who have been electrocuted.

Immediate action centres on the child's resuscitation. This is best achieved by following current guidelines from the Resuscitation Council (UK) and the Advanced Paediatric Life Support group.

⚠**Electricity will try to find the earth by the quickest route.**

Current type
Alternating current (AC) is more dangerous, especially at lower voltages, than direct current (DC), and can result in ventricular fibrillation. Additionally, AC causes violent muscle contractions. These contractions make many victims unable to let go after contact with the circuit.

Current pathways
Electrical current will follow the pathway of least resistance to the ground. Any current that crosses the heart or brain is the most dangerous.

Resistance
Immersion in water or having wet skin can decrease resistance sharply, resulting in increased electrical current being delivered to tissue, but fewer surface burns.

Lightning follows the same laws of physics as all other types of electricity, but the burns associated with other forms are often missing. Lightning normally induces cardiac arrest, and neurological problems may occur in patients who survive lightning strikes.

Injury pattern
Cardiac
Cardiac dysrhythmias are a major concern from electrocution. These will be apparent from the time of the injury. Other concerns are ventricular fibrillation, requiring immediate resuscitation of the child.

Burns
There are potentially four types of burn injury resulting from electrocution.
- **Direct injury** from the contact with the electrical source.
- **Flash burn** from the electricity source
- **Arc burn,** usually from high voltage electricity
- **Flame burn** caused by clothing catching fire during the electrocution

Trauma can be caused by the intense and often violent muscle spasms the child displays when being electrocuted. In addition, the child may have fallen from some height such as from an electric pylon.

Direct injury electrocution is common with younger children who poke things into electrical sockets or touch live wires. This can leave the child with serious full thickness burn injury at the contact point, and there may also be an exit point burn. Also worth considering is the damage to the tissue between entry and exit point, which may lead to compartment syndrome developing (Davies 2003).

Immediate action

- Isolate child from the source of the electricity without endangering yourself.
- Rapid assessment of airway, breathing, circulation and disability following APLS and Resuscitation Council guidelines is needed and start resuscitation if needed.
- Give pain relief early, preferably opiod based medications, and cover burns to prevent infection.

Cardiac

- If on arrival the child is in normal sinus rhythm then cardiac monitoring is not usually required.

Burns

- Be aware that burns in and around the child's airway may become complicated if the airway swells, so get an anaesthetist early. This is especially so if the child is hoarse, wheezing, dribbling, has a stridor, or soot particles in the airway.
- Cool the burn with cool water, but be careful not to make the child hypothermic.
- Treat the pain before assessing burns in any great depth with opioids such as morphine.
- A simple dressing of cling film is all that is needed if the child is being referred to a burns unit. Otherwise follow local protocols for burns dressings in your department or discuss with the local burns unit.
- Fluid resuscitation should follow your local burns centre guidelines as well as APLS guidelines for shock and burns management.
- Consider nonaccidental causes and take appropriate action.

Trauma assessment

- Always be suspicious of other injury when electricity is involved. This includes cervical spine injury, other broken bones and internal injury. Consider the electrical current pathway from entry to exit and the body organs it may have damaged on route.
- Have a high index of suspicion for serious internal injury at all times. Complete a trauma assessment (see APLS guidelines).

Further reading

Gausche-Hill M, Fuchs S, Yamamoto L (eds) (2006) APLS. The Pediatric Emergency Medicine Resource (revised 4th edn). Boston: Jones and Bartlett

Davies F (2003) Minor Trauma in Children, A Pocket Guide. London: Arnold

:☠: Gunshot injuries

Immediate identification

Entrance wounds

Note wound size is determined by:
- Speed of bullet (velocity): faster bullets have more energy, making bigger holes and causing more damage internally.
- Size of the bullet.
- Scorching or powder stippling, from gunshot made close to the skin.

Exit wounds
- Usually larger
- Have ragged edges

Note:
- Not all patients will present with an exit wound
- Projectile may still be lodged in the body
- Size of the wound is not indicative of the degree of injuries sustained

Immediate action
- Prior warning from ambulance staff is often given
- Initial assessment – ABCDE principles of trauma management (Resuscitation Council UK, www.resus.org.uk)
- Gain IV access
- Assess conscious level
- Assess degree of pain
- Assess track of bullet and potential tissues/organs affected

Assessment should include

History
Either the patient or those accompanying will need to be asked:
- What sort of weapon was used? For example, an airgun, handgun, shotgun or rifle.
- What range was it fired at?
- What kind of bullet was fired?

Effects/damage caused
- Laceration or crushing as the bullet tears and displaces the tissues
- Compression injuries as shock waves emanate through the tissues
- Gouged track as the bullet creates a cavity in the tissue it passes through
- Tissues surrounding the bullet's track also affected, e.g. bone fragmentation
- Fractured bone splinters can act as secondary missiles

Potential complications
- Pneumothorax
- Hypovolaemic shock
- Infection: this can localize in an abscess if left untreated initially

Investigations

Patient may require assessment to establish extent of injuries by:

- Orthopaedics, to stabilize and manage fractures
- Surgery, also for excision of necrotic tissue

Treatment considerations

- Airway/breathing: consider pneumothorax and need for ventilation
- Circulation: control bleeding; this will have started prehospital
  - Manage hypovolaemia and shock
- Disability: assess level of consciousness, and maintain comfortable position for the conscious casualty
  If the patient is conscious:
- Age appropriate explanations of what is happening and constant reassurance will be required
- Provide effective analgesia
- Ascertain tetanus status

Additional considerations

A crucial part of the nurse's role in the ED will be:

Preservation of evidence

A possible criminal investigation may be undertaken by the police, so:

- Assist in the preservation of forensic evidence.
- Follow locally based protocols concerning patient's clothing and belongings, e.g. document and bag them.
- In particular, be aware of the need not to cut clothing through the entry and/or exit sites.

Emotional support

- Communication
- Parents, family and friends may have difficulties coming to terms with the situation, with heightened emotions and frustrations due to the uncertainty of prognosis, severity of injury, unexpected nature and anxieties.

Reporting of gunshots to the police

- Safety is of paramount importance.
- For all gunshot injuries the police will need to be notified. This is usually the responsibility of the treating medical practitioner.
- Police often arrive with the patient, having accompanied them in the ambulance. On arrival, consideration will need to be given to whether the patient is still armed, so liaison with the police is crucial.
- The General Medical Council (GMC) advises that for gunshot wounds, doctors report to the police all patients on their arrival at hospital.
- The Nursing and Midwifery Council (NMC) advises the following statement in the Code of Professional Conduct (2008):
  - You must disclose information if you believe someone may be at risk of harm, in line with the law of the country in which you are practising.
  - If you are at all concerned that you are not equipped to deal with the situation then you must liaise with senior colleagues.

Media involvement
• Adhere to local trust policy
• Maintain patient confidentiality
• Police can be extremely useful in managing media involvement

Background information
• Rare in paediatrics, male adolescents at greatest risk
• Greatest risk: 16–30 age group
• Highest incidence: metropolitan areas of large cities, although becoming more widespread
• Number of firearm mortalities is decreasing, but the number of injuries is increasing
• General public's perception is there has been a proliferation of gun related injuries
• Not all gunshot injuries are linked to criminal activity
• Children and young people can have access to firearms through sport or in the home resulting in suicide attempts and unintentional injuries

Further reading

Cotton, BA, Nance, ML (2004) Penetrating trauma in children. *Seminars in Pediatric Surgery* 13:87–97

General Medical Council (2003) Reporting Gun Shot Wounds. Guidance for Doctors in Accident and Emergency Departments. GMC guidance available at: http://www.gmc-uk.org/guidance/current/library/reporting_gunshot_wounds.asp

☠ **Knife injuries**

Immediate identification
- Bleeding from laceration/stab wound
- Can be severe bleeding if artery is damaged
- Commonly knives, also screwdrivers, scissors, pencils, etc.

Immediate management
- Adopt the principles of an ABC approach to trauma management
- Assess the airway, breathing and circulation
- Assess for hypovolaemia
- Possible blood products transfusion
- Fluid resuscitation and balance
- Stem bleeding if possible
- Assess conscious level
- Assess degree of pain
- Assess wound
- Gain IV access
- Provide effective analgesia

Examination
- Knife wounds may appear insignificant, but can have devastating consequences.
- If the patient attends with the knife still in situ then it should not be removed as vital structures can potentially be damaged as the knife is withdrawn.

Management/treatment
- Ascertain the history of the incident
- In the majority of instances the victim will know their attacker
- Commonly associated with quarrels, loss of temper, revenge, and self harm
- In all situations, consider the patient's tetanus status

Superficial wound
- Thorough cleansing
- Irrigation of the wound (if needed)
- Closure of wound as appropriate with sutures, steristrips, glue, etc.

Penetrating wound
- Requires surgical assessment
- Exploration in theatre where thorough cleansing and surgical repair of damaged structures can occur

Background information
- Ages: adolescents/young adults are at greatest risk
- Males are at greatest risk
- Most injuries are superficial
- Most injuries are the result of accidents
- There is public perception that knife injuries are increasing
- Stab wounds can be made with minimal force
- Crucial factor is the sharpness of the tip of the object

- Greatest force is required to penetrate clothing and skin, and once through, remarkably little force is required to follow through to create a deep knife wound.
- A faster stabbing action makes it easier to penetrate skin.

Incised wounds
- Sharp cut-like injuries, made by knives or broken glass, etc.
- Slit-like incision
- Edges of the wound will vary according to the nature of the cutting edge of the object

Slash wounds
- Wounds where the length is greater than the depth
- Generally not life threatening unless in exceptional circumstances the wound involves a major blood vessel.

Pulp wounds
- Pulp laceration – pulp of the finger is sliced off – wound generally bleeds copiously and the affected arm needs to be elevated. This may also require the use of an alginate dressing to stem bleeding.

Further considerations

Disclosure of information
- Currently there is no requirement for health care professionals to report knife injuries to the police.
- The Nursing and Midwifery Council Code of Conduct (2008) states that information must be 'disclosed if you believe someone may be at risk of harm, in line with the law of the country in which you are practising'.
- The General Medical Council is presently revising guidance for medical staff, which may also have ramifications for nurses.
- Disclosure without consent should only be in exceptional circumstances in collaboration with other health care professionals and/or senior staff.
- Keep a clear and accurate record, as an aggrieved individual can take civil action.
- The difficulty with knife injuries is that they can and frequently do occur unintentionally, and therefore there needs to be a degree of flexibility to enable health care professionals to act in the best interests of patients.

Preservation of evidence
Possible criminal investigation may be undertaken by the police, so:
- Assist in the preservation of forensic evidence.
- Follow locally based protocols regarding patient's clothing and belongings such as documenting and bagging.
- In particular be aware of the need not to cut clothing through the entry and/or exit sites.

Further reading
Christensen, MC, Nielsen, TG, Ridley, S, Lecky, FE, Morris, S (2008) Outcomes and costs of penetrating trauma injury in England and Wales. *Injury* 39:1013–1025
Trauma Audit Research Network (2008) data available at: www.tarn.ac.uk

223

Gastrointestinal problems

:O: Damage from ingestion

Background

Children, from the age of just a few months, will explore to make sense of their world, and this exploration frequently involves putting things into their mouths. Children may ingest either foreign bodies or liquids. In contrast to adults, ingestion is usually accidental, and significant injury is therefore far less common.

Foreign bodies

Children often swallow radio-opaque objects such as coins, toy parts, pins, screws, or button batteries. In most instances (99%), swallowed objects pass harmlessly through the digestive tract and are expelled within the faeces. Problems occur due to either:
- Impaction
- Systemic reaction to toxic products

Impaction

Impaction usually occurs in the oesophagus, with the thoracic inlet being the most common site, accounting for 70% of cases. The remaining 30% occur equally at the mid-oesophageal region or the lower end of the oesophagus where it joins the stomach. Pointed objects, however, may impact at any level. Symptoms may be minimal, but could include pain, irritability, vomiting, bleeding, or obstruction. Occasionally parents may simply report food refusal or weight loss. Migration through to adjacent structures is a rare but serious and potentially life-threatening complication. Once the object has passed into the stomach it will usually continue harmlessly through the gut to be expelled in the stool.

In an asymptomatic child, use of a metal detector or chest X-ray to confirm that the object is below the level of the diaphragm may be sufficient. Once in the stomach, most objects will pass without a problem. It is not necessary to advise parents to inspect the stool!

Hazardous objects, or those found to be within the oesophagus, may be imaged again after 12 hours to ensure they are moving. The opinion of a paediatric surgeon may be required if the object is not passing or the child is symptomatic.

Button batteries

These may be particularly hazardous, as the seal may be digested by gastric acid exposing the toxic contents. They should be managed as a hazardous object, but bear in mind that they may not be detected by a metal detector. If they are found in the oesophagus, are below the diaphragm but not moving, or the child has become symptomatic, refer urgently to a paediatric surgeon for removal.

Liquid ingestion

Modern households are full of potentially toxic liquid products ranging from cleaning products to medicines.

Fortunately, children do not swallow large quantities of unpleasant substances, and even the accidental ingestion of tastier products such as paracetamol syrups tends to be less that initially thought, as the child usually spills some of it.

The key to management is determining exactly what may have been ingested and the National Poisons Information Service can provide advice regarding specific products.

Caustic and corrosive products may be either acid or alkali and cause tissue injury by chemical reaction.

Alkaline products
- Rapid and severe injury occurs within minutes of contact
- Tissues that first come into contact are most severely damaged
- Tissue oedema initially occurs, which may cause stridor
- Over 2–4 weeks, scar tissue forms that can lead to stricture formation but this is uncommon

Acid products
- Cause injury by coagulation necrosis and eschar formation
- The stomach is the most commonly affected organ
- 3–4 days later the eschar sloughs and granulation occurs
- Over 2–4 weeks a scar forms, which contracts and can cause obstruction
- Perforation or haemorrhage may occur

History and examination
Despite the potential for serious damage to occur, many children remain asymptomatic.

Symptoms may include:
- Vomiting
- Drooling
- Dysphagia
- Refusal to swallow
- Irritability
- Stridor or respiratory distress
- Haematemesis

Treatment
- Resuscitation is the first priority
- Dilution using small amounts of water or milk may be helpful
- Acute oesophagoscopy may help to identify burns, but is unlikely to alter the management as there is no effective treatment
- Depending on the substance ingested, give activated charcoal

Cautions
- With all inadvertent ingestions, it is important to explore the social circumstances surrounding the event. There may be concerns regarding household safety or child supervision.
- Forced ingestion may occur as a manifestation of child abuse.

- Older children may ingest substances or objects as part of a psychiatric illness.
- Children with pre-existing GI tract abnormalities are more likely to have complications.

Further reading

http://emedicine.medscape.com

Cameron et al, editors. (2006) Textbook of Paediatric Emergency Medicine. Churchill Livingstone Elsevier.

Toxbase. UK: National Poisons Information Service. Available from:http//www.toxbase.org

① Abdominal pain

A large variety of disorders can present as abdominal pain in children. The most common medical cause is gastroenteritis and the most common surgical cause is appendicitis (see Table 6.1 for more causes). Abdominal pain is often accompanied by vomiting, and is a frequent reason for parents to seek emergency medical advice. In surgical conditions, pain usually precedes vomiting, whereas the opposite tends to occur in medical conditions. Infants and young children are frequently unable to localize their pain, and may present with referred pain in the abdomen, e.g. from pneumonia or as the result of a metabolic cause such as diabetic ketoacidosis. Abdominal pain is often a recurrent problem so history is an important element.

Initial assessment
- Overall appearance of child: is the child pale, clammy, flushed? Look for facial expressions, e.g. grimacing. In babies and toddlers observe whether the child is drawing their knees up to their abdomen. Visually assess the child's abdomen for distension.
- Assess pain using the FACES, CRIES, FLACC, QUESTT scales. Administer appropriate analgesia for child's weight (loading dose if child has not already had a dose in the same day). Babies should be stripped to be weighed.
- Observations: pulse, respiration rate, oxygen saturations, temperature, blood glucose, capillary refill time, Glasgow Coma Score, capillary refill time. Also look for signs of rashes.

Table 6.1 Some common causes of abdominal pain

Medical causes	Surgical causes	Gynaecological causes
Gastroenteritis	Appendicitis	Ectopic pregnancy
Mesenteric adenitis	Meckel's diverticulum	Ovarian cyst
Inflammatory bowel disease	Intestinal obstruction	Pelvic inflammatory disease
Urinary tract infections	Intussusception	Endometriosis
Constipation	Trauma	Dysmenorrhoea
Diabetic ketoacidosis	Testicular torsion	
Henoch Schonlein Purpura (HSP)	Incarcerated hernia	
Lower lobe pneumonia	Peritonitis	
Volvulus	Hirschsprung's disease	
Infantile colic		
Pneumonia		

- Keep all children nil by mouth until assessed by a doctor, as the child may need to have surgery.

Further investigations

- Urinalysis: ensure that babies have been having wet nappies and that older children have not been complaining of pain, burning, stinging, or frequency on passing urine. Always perform a urine dipstick test. If any positive results send sample for microscopy, culture and sensitivity (MC&S).
- In female patients, if sexually active perform pregnancy test (BHCG– beta human chorionic gonadotropin). The sensitivity of this must be recognized and appropriate consent obtained.
- Blood tests +/− cannula: full blood count (FBC), urea and electrolytes (U&E), amylase, blood glucose. Consider the need for topical anaesthetics, e.g. Ametop® gel/EMLA® cream or ethyl chloride (cold spray). Also consider the use of distraction therapy.
- Imaging: chest X-ray, abdominal X-ray or abdominal ultrasound scan may be required.
- Stool sample: a stool sample may be required in children with diarrhoea.

Further reading

Kumar P, Clark M (Eds) (1998). Clinical Medicine. 4th Edition. Edinburgh: W.B. Saunders.
Longmore M, Wilkinson I, Torok E. (2001) Oxford Handbook of Clinical Medicine (5th edn). Oxford: Oxford University Press.

☼ Management of intussusception

Intussusception is when a part of the bowel slides back inside another part of the bowel. This most commonly occurs where the terminal ileum slides back into the caecum. Enlarged lymphatic tissue in the bowel walls may be a causative factor.

Immediate identification
- History of severe colic
- Episodes of screaming linked to pallor; may appear well in between
- Age usually 3 months to 2 years (may occur up to school age child)
- May have had history of viral illness or gastroenteritis
- Drawing up of legs
- Vomiting
- Lethargy
- Redcurrant jelly stools (75% of cases; this is a late sign)
- Visible peristalsis over distended abdomen
- Very sick infant; signs of shock and dehydration

ALERT: Correct dehydration and hypovolaemic shock.

Immediate action
- Will depend upon extent of resuscitation needed.
- Will depend on whether perforation has occurred.

Immediate nursing care
- Reassure child/family.
- Explain and give support throughout procedures.
- Obtain and record observations; heart rate, respiratory rate, blood pressure, temperature.
- Assess pain, score using an appropriate pain score tool.
- Administer analgesia as prescribed and assess its effectiveness.
- Note when the child last ate and drank.

Management
- Palpation of abdomen.
- Abdominal ultrasound scan or X-ray to confirm diagnosis.
- Nonsurgical reduction via barium enema if history less than 24 hours.
- Surgical correction: may require resection of part of the bowel if necrosis evident.

Nursing management
- Correct dehydration
- Monitor fluid balance
- Nil by mouth
- Intravenous cannulation will be required
- Monitor cannula site
- Prepare for surgery
- Reassure child/parents
- Pain assessment, analgesia

- Monitor vital signs
- Prognosis good if diagnosed promptly
- Risk of death if diagnosis missed

Further reading

Candy D, Davies G, Ross E (2006). Clinical Paediatrics and Child Health (Chapter 11), Saunders (ed). Edinburgh: Elsevier.
http://www.ich.ucl.ac.uk/gosh_families/information_sheets/intussusception/intussusception_ families.html

:☼: **Appendicitis**

Appendicitis is the inflammation of the vermiform appendix, which is situated at the end of the large intestine, in the right iliac fossa (RIF). The surgical removal of the inflamed appendix is the most common surgical emergency in paediatric practice (Humes and Simpson 2006). Appendicitis is commonly seen in children aged 10 years and above, but can affect children of any age.

Recognition of appendicitis

The most common signs and symptoms include:
- Central abdominal pain which radiates to the lower right side into the iliac fossa
- Vomiting or nausea
- Loss of appetite
- Pyrexia
- Flushed skin, especially the face
- Rebound tenderness and guarding of the area when palpated
- Pain in the RIF when coughing
- History of abdominal pain for less than 48 hours
- Pain on movement

Nursing requirements on admission

- Obtain and record observations; heart rate, respiratory rate, blood pressure (all of which may be elevated due to pain, anxiety, temperature and infection), temperature.
- Obtain a pain score, using the most age-relevant pain score tool. Administer analgesia as prescribed and assess its effectiveness.
- Provide urine sample collection equipment and collect sample. Urinalysis will be required to eliminate the possibility of a urinary tract infection (UTI) and a pregnancy test may also be requested by the surgical team in girls of child-bearing age. (NOTE: verbal consent from the patient will be required in some Trusts/Health Boards, depending on local policy.)
- Note when the child last ate and drank.

NOTE: Keep the child nil-by-mouth (NBM) until the surgeons have performed their examination (in preparation of possible surgery).
- Apply local anaesthetic cream (Ametop® or EMLA®) for blood tests and cannulation. Remember that some children may become more anxious or upset when blood tests are mentioned. Careful explanation and reassurance may be required about how the cream works. Distraction techniques may also be helpful.
- Prepare equipment for venepuncture/cannulation and assist as necessary.
- The child may require intravenous antibiotics (IVABs) or intravenous fluids (IVI) should be administered and subsequent care following this procedure should be provided.
- Prepare child for surgery, complete relevant paperwork, and involve play specialists if available.
- Liaise with surgical team about child's condition and any changes.

Management

There is no definitive diagnostic test for appendicitis (Humes and Simpson 2006) (sometimes an ultrasound scan is performed to eliminate other abdominal surgical conditions), but the diagnosis is often a clinical one following examination by the surgical team.

Blood tests may be taken:
- C-reactive protein (CRP)
- Full blood count (FBC)

These tests help to identify any infection in the blood; the white cell count (WCC) and CRP will both be raised if infection is identified.

The main treatment for appendicitis is the removal of the appendix via a surgical appendectomy, via a small incision in the abdomen or via keyhole surgery.

Pain relief

Analgesia should always be administered as per surgical instructions. An age-appropriate pain score tool should be used and pain scores should be reassessed following any administration of analgesia, to evaluate its effectiveness.

The child who is nil by mouth will not be able to have analgesia orally and it may be necessary to administer the analgesia intravenously or per rectum (PR). The administration of PR medication may be new to the child and family; explanation of why this route is necessary should be provided, and their consent gained before administration. This consent should be documented in the child's notes.

It is important to keep the child and family updated and ensure their understanding of the situation. Any problems identified or any concerns raised by them should be addressed.

Further reading

Davenport M (1996) ABC of General Surgery in Children: Acute Abdominal Pain in Children. *British Medical Journal* 312:498–501

Humes DJ, Simpson J (2006) Acute Appendicitis. *British Medical Journal* 333:530–534

:✪: Gastroenteritis

Gastroenteritis is an inflammation of the gastrointestinal (GI) tract caused by infection (virus, bacteria or protozoa). Patients present with a sudden onset of diarrhoea with/without vomiting. Gastroenteritis is a transient disorder, although fluid loss can be severe, especially in children under 1 year old. Most children with gastroenteritis can be managed at home with support and advice from healthcare professionals. Diarrhoea usually lasts for 5–7 days, ceasing within 2 weeks. Vomiting usually lasts for 1–2 days, ceasing within 3 days.

Incidence

- Common: infants and young children may experience more than one episode in a year. Gastroenteritis is the most likely reason for children presenting with sudden onset diarrhoea. The peak age for infection is between 6 months and 2 years of age; the most likely cause is viral infection (about 70% of cases) and the commonest modes of infection are the faecal-oral or respiratory routes.

Causes

- Viral (stools rarely bloody):
  - Rotaviruses
  - Noroviruses
  - Enteric adenoviruses
  - Caliciviruses
  - Astroviruses
  - Enteroviruses
  - Cytomegalovirus
- Bacterial (may be bloody):
  - *Salmonella*
  - *Campylobacteri jejuni*
  - *Escherichia coli*
  - *Shigella*
- Protozoa (<10% of cases):
  - *Cryptosporidium*
  - *Giardia lamblia*
  - *Entamoeba histolytica*

Signs and symptoms

- Sudden onset diarrhoea
- Vomiting
- Fever (high if due to bacterial infection)
- Dehydration

Immediate management

Isolate source and apply universal precautions used to prevent cross infection.

Assess hydration status using the National Institute of Health and Clinical Excellence (NICE 2009) assessment tool (see also Table 6.2). Identifying a red flag indicates need for immediate action.

- If no clinical dehydration, prevent dehydration, encourage fluid intake, and use low osmolarity solution (ORS–oral rehydration solution) if at increased risk of dehydration

Table 6.2 Increasing severity of dehydration

	No clinically detectable dehydration	Clinical dehydration	Clinical shock
Symptoms (remote and face-to-face assessments)	Appears well	*Appears to be unwell or deteriorating	–
	Alert and responsive	*Altered responsiveness (for example, irritable, lethargic)	Decreased level of consciousness
	Normal urine output	Decreased urine output	–
	Skin colour unchanged	Skin colour unchanged	Pale or mottled skin
	Warm extremities	Warm extremities	Cold extremities
Signs (face-to-face assessments)	Alert and responsive	*Altered responsiveness (for example, irritable, lethargic)	Decreased level of consciousness
	Skin colour unchanged	Skin colour unchanged	Pale or mottled skin
	Warm extremities	Warm extremities	Cold extremities
	Eyes not sunken	*Sunken eyes	–
	Moist mucous membranes (except after a drink)	Dry mucous membranes (except for 'mouth breather')	–
	Normal heart rate	*Tachycardia	Tachycardia
	Normal breathing pattern	*Tachypnoea	Tachypnoea
	Normal peripheral pulses	Normal peripheral pulses	Weak peripheral pulses
	Normal capillary refill time	Normal capillary refill time	Prolonged capillary refill time
	Normal skin turgor	*Reduced skin turgor	–
	Normal blood pressure	Normal blood pressure	Hypotension (decompensated shock)

*Red flag

- If clinically dehydrated, use oral rehydration therapy
- If clinically shock suspected or confirmed, give immediate intravenous therapy (IVT) for shock until resolved.

History
- Onset and duration of illness to date
- Recent contact with people with gastroenteritis, travel abroad or to known source of infection
- Nature and frequency of stools and vomit
- Fluid intake and urine output
- Use of antibiotics or drugs that may cause diarrhoea

Examination and investigations
- Record vital signs
- Exclude other potential causes if high fever, prolonged symptoms or indicators of a surgical cause
- Obtain blood biochemistry if intravenous therapy is required or there are signs/symptoms of hypernatraemia
- Assess blood acid-base status and chlorine concentration if shock is suspected or confirmed
- Obtain stool specimens for virology and bacterial culture if an outbreak is suspected, if the child has bloody diarrhoea or a history of recent foreign travel, or is young or immunocompromised and has a high fever

Treatment
- Post-rehydration
  - Encourage milk feeds (breast or other) and fluid intake
  - Consider use of ORS after each large watery stool in high risk children
  - Start ORT if dehydration recurs
- Nutrition
  - During rehydration:
    - continue breastfeeding,
    - do not give solids,
    - do not give fruit juices or carbonated drinks
    - use ORS solutions as oral fluids
    - consider supplementing with usual fluids if ORS solution being refused (not applicable to high risk children, e.g. tachypnoeic, tachycardic, sunken eyes, altered responsiveness)
  - After rehydration:
    - give full strength milk
    - reintroduce solid food
    - avoid fruit juices and carbonated drinks until diarrhoea has stopped

(Nice 2009)

Children at increased risk of dehydration
Complications
- Dehydration
- Metabolic acidosis
- Electrolyte imbalance

- Carbohydrate intolerance
- Reinfection
- Development of food intolerance
- Haemolytic uraemic syndrome
- Iatrogenic complications
- Death

Further reading

Elliot E.J. (2007). Acute gastroenteritis in children. *British Medical Journal* 334:35–40.

Hartling, L., Belkmare, S., Wiebe, N., Russell, K.F., Klassen, T.P., Craig, W.R. (2006) Oral versus intravenous rehydration for treating dehydration due to gastroenteritis in children. *Cochrane Database of Systematic Reviews* 1469493x.

National Institute of Health and Clinical Excellence (2009). Diarrhoea and vomiting in children under 5 (CG84). Diarrhoea and vomiting caused by gastroenteritis: diagnosis, assessment and management in children younger than 5 years. http://www.nice.org.uk/nicemedia/pdf/CG47NICEGuideline.pdf

☼: Abdominal trauma

The principles of family centred care and the psychological care of the child who has been involved in trauma should be considered throughout.

Causes

- Road traffic accident (RTA): direct impact, crush injuries, acceleration injuries.
- Accidents, such as falls from heights, objects impaled, blunt trauma, direct impact with object, crush injury.
- Children are more susceptible to accidental injury due to their risk-taking behaviour.
- Assault: direct blow, knife, gunshot, accelerated impact.
- Consider non-accidental injury where indicated by history, mechanism of injury, delay in seeking treatment or inaccuracies in account of how injuries occurred.
  Consider and assess for abdominal trauma when the following present:
- Children can have abdominal injuries that are not immediately obvious. More of the impacting energy exerted from an injury can be transferred internally, damaging internal organs, without external evidence of injury (www.resus.org.uk).
- History of mechanism of injury indicates possible abdominal injury, e.g. direct impact of object with abdomen.
- Multiple injuries due to trauma (See p. 104).
- Chest and/or pelvic injuries.
- No available history, but symptoms suggestive of trauma, e.g. injured child brought in unaccompanied.
- Visual clues, e.g. contusions/bruising, lacerations to abdomen, haematuria, blood in faeces, rectal bleeding, and blood in vomit.
- Moderate/severe pain in abdomen.
- Shoulder tip pain (referred pain).
- Guarding.
- Tachycardia.
- Signs of shock
  - Reduced peripheral pulses
  - Increased capillary refill time
  - Hypotension
  - Unconscious/reduced conscious level
- Abdominal distension/increasing girth size (not relieved by gastric tube decompression).

Abdominal trauma may be obvious and acute, masked by more serious injuries, or insidious and vague.
  Organs that may be involved:

- Spleen
- Liver
- Bowel
- Kidneys

Management

Primary survey

- As described on pages 72 and 76, assessment and management of ABCDE (www.resus.org.uk) will be the priority. Airway management should be combined with cervical spine immobilization, when clinical signs or mechanism of injury indicate possible spinal injury. Obvious abdominal trauma should not detract from the systematic ABCDE assessment. Other problems may require more immediate treatment.
- Problems identified during the primary survey should be treated as they are found.
- 'Treat first what kills first.'

Secondary survey

- In less serious abdominal injury and in the presence of more serious problems, abdominal trauma may not be diagnosed and managed until secondary survey has taken place, when a top-to-toe examination is undertaken.
- Emergency treatment.
- This should be prioritized and managed in order of severity of problems identified.
- Airway and breathing problems managed first, if required.
- Treatment for circulatory problems, including fluid resuscitation intervention and blood transfusion.
- Obvious bleeding can be managed by applying pressure to a profuse bleeding abdominal wound with sterile gauze.
- Assessment and regular re-assessment of observations, including respiratory, circulatory and neurological assessments.
- Pain assessment and management. Relieving moderate/severe pain may assist with diagnosis in a conscious child, as they are likely to be more co-operative.
- Investigations, including abdominal ultrasound scan/X-ray/CT scan. Bloods for group and cross match.
- Preparation for emergency surgery and obtain consent (Section 2).

Definitive care

- Definitive care will depend on the expertise on-site, such as paediatric surgeons and provision of on-site paediatric HDU/PICU facilities.
- Child requiring emergency surgery:
  - Surgery may take place on-site, if appropriately trained paediatric surgeons available. Otherwise transfer to regional unit with appropriately trained paediatric surgeons will be necessary.
- Child requiring HDU/PICU care:
  - Intubation/ventilation/stabilization and preparation for safe transfer/ retrieval to on-site or regional HDU/PICU.
  - Contact on-site or regional HDU/PICU centre for bed availability/to allow for preparation of staff, equipment and environment.
  - Arrange for retrieval or transfer with appropriately trained practitioners.

- Child not requiring paediatric surgeon/HDU or PICU:
  - Transfer to children's ward.

Further reading

Browning J G, Wilkinson A G, Beattie T. (2008) Imaging paediatric blunt trauma in the emergency department: ultrasound versus computed tomography. *Emergency Medicine Journal* 25:645–648

Stylianos S, Ford H R. (2008) Outcomes in pediatric trauma care. *Seminars in Pediatric Surgery* 17:110–115

Skin and connective tissue problems

ⓘ Gluing wounds

Introduction

Wound glue has been used to close superficial wounds on faces and scalps for over 15 years, and is an established method for closing appropriately sized wounds.

Application

- Clean wound thoroughly; if the wound is in the scalp ensure that the patient's hair is not in the wound before closure.
- Achieve haemostasis.
- Hold the wound edges together ensuring good opposition.
- Place the glue along the wound edges, either by using the spot welding method or in one continuous thin line.
- Hold the wound edges together for 30–60 seconds.
- Ensure that good closure has been achieved.

Advice on discharge

- Keep wound clean and dry for 5 days.
- Avoid picking at or touching wound.
- The glue will form a scab and will flake off after 5–10 days.
- If bleeding reoccurs seek medical advice.

Tips for gluing wounds

- Do not apply glue directly into the wound.
- Avoid using an excessive amount of glue, thin layers are most effective.
- Avoid gluing yourself to the patient.

Further reading

Elmasahne FN, Matbouli SA, Zuberi MS (1995). Use of tissue adhesive in the closure of small incisions and lacerations. *J. Ped. Surg.* 30:837–8

Quinn JV, Drzewiecki A, Li MM, et al. (1993) A randomized controlled trial comparing a tissue adhesive with suturing in the repair of pediatric facial lacerations. *Ann. Emerg. Med.* 22:1130–5

Wang MY, Levy ML, Mittler MA, Liu CY, Johnston S, McComb JG (1999). A Prospective Analysis of the Use of Octylcyanoacrylate Tissue Adhesive for Wound Closure in Pediatric Neurosurgery. *Pediatr Neurosurg* 30:186–188

! Facial lacerations

Introduction

It is common for children to present to emergency departments with facial lacerations. Soft tissue trauma is much more common than fracture, particularly in younger children whose facial skeletons are resistant to injury. Therefore emergency practitioners must be skilled and confident at assessing and managing this type of injury.

Incidence and causes

Facial lacerations are frequently seen in younger children, especially those who have not long been walking, as they are unsteady on their feet, unaware of danger, and their heads and faces are at the right height to collide with items of low furniture. Hence, many facial lacerations are over the forehead, around the eyebrows or on the chin.

⚠ A facial laceration in a nonmobile child should be treated with extreme caution. There may be a child safeguarding issue.

Immediate management

Points to remember

- Facial lacerations bleed profusely as a result of the rich blood supply to the face.
- This bleeding can be a source of great distress to parents/carers who also worry about the cosmetic outcome.
- This blood supply facilitates healing, and, while parents should be informed that it is difficult to predict the level of scarring, they can be reassured that the vast majority of these wounds heal very well.

Wound closure

- The majority of lacerations to the face are suitable for closure with wound closure strips or skin glue after wound cleansing (see page on wound closure).
- As the aesthetic outcome is of vital importance, it is often helpful to approximate the edges of the wound with wound closure strips, which can be adjusted until the best result is achieved, rather than starting with skin glue.
- Some children have a tendency to fiddle with wounds and to pick at strips; other wounds may be liable to being dribbled on. In these cases a combination of wound closure strips and glue can be useful.
- It is imperative that children are appropriately prepared through distraction (use starlight distraction box) for the procedure and then kept as still as possible so that the best cosmetic result can be achieved.
- Beware of using tissue glue near to children's eyes. To prevent accidental instillation into the eye if the child wriggles, protect the eye with a patch of gauze.
- Only a small minority of facial lacerations require suturing. This will usually need to be done under conscious sedation or general anaesthetic as children do not tolerate it well. It should be carried out by an expert.

Special wounds

Eyebrow lacerations

Lacerations through the eyebrow require particular care to avoid developing a distortion in the line of the eyebrow, which would be especially noticeable. In general, horizontal lacerations within the eyebrow respond well to careful closure with tissue adhesive. Those that dissect the eyebrow vertically should be referred to the maxillofacial or plastic surgery team (according to local procedure) for specialist closure. If in doubt, ask for specialist help.

Ear and nose lacerations

Lacerations involving ear or nasal cartilage must always be referred onwards to the maxillofacial or plastic surgery team.

Eyelid lacerations

Eyelid lacerations must always be referred to ophthalmology.

Wounds in and around the mouth

Lip lacerations

Lacerations to the lip usually heal well with conservative management. Those that are gaping or continue to bleed may need to be sutured.

Important! Lacerations that cross the vermillion border need to be sutured to achieve perfect alignment. An obvious step in the line of the lip border will be cosmetically undesirable. These must always be referred to a plastic surgery service.

Mouth and tongue lacerations

Lacerations of the mouth and tongue usually heal well and quickly with conservative management. Only those where haemorrhage is uncontrollable, where the wound is gaping, or where there is a partially severed segment of the tongue will require suturing.

Full thickness lacerations

Full thickness lacerations, i.e. those that extend from inside the mouth to the skin surface, need suturing to avoid adverse cosmetic outcomes or formation of a sinus. This requires expert help from a senior consultant or a plastic surgeon.

Torn frenulum

Laceration of the frenulum (torn frenulum) does not usually require treatment beyond initial haemorrhage management with pressure.

Warning! Torn frenulum can be a non-accidental injury, but is not considered to be pathognomonic of abuse. If in doubt follow child safeguarding policy.

The majority of facial lacerations are straightforward to manage. By having knowledge of special wounds and considerations, the practitioner can avoid the potential pitfalls.

Further reading

http://cks.library.nhs.uk/lacerations
Davies FCW, Robson WJ, Smith A (2003) Minor Trauma in Children. London: Arnold.

⊙ Lacerations, cuts and contusions

Introduction

Definition of cuts

A separation in the skin where none of the skin is missing. They are caused by sharp objects, e.g. knife, glass. A deep cut may reveal underlying structures such as tendons, fat, muscle or bone.

Definition of laceration

An irregular tearing or ripping of the skin, often involving underlying tissues. They are caused by blunt force trauma, falls, or crush injuries.

Identification of a laceration

- Ragged or torn edges
- Crushing and bruising
- Hairs driven in to tissues
- Nerves, fibres and vessels may cross the depths of the wound.

The force at which these wounds are caused can often breach through all layers of the skin, damaging surrounding tissue and underlying blood vessels; therefore it is possible for lacerations and cuts to bleed profusely. Lacerations are often regarded as the more serious of wounds as the injury has penetrated beyond the protective layer of the body, introducing the possibility of infection.

Classification of wounds

- Superficial: damaging only the epidermis, have normal skin colouring
- Partial thickness: damaging through epidermis and dermis, will look pale pink.
- Full thickness: reaches the subcutaneous fatty tissue, and may go through to muscle or bone. These wounds may expose yellow fat islands, tendons, or nerves.

Immediate management of haemorrhaging wound

- Minor haemorrhage: apply direct pressure for 10 minutes then dress wound with saline soaked gauze (to prevent adherence) and bandage until wound can be explored further under controlled conditions.
- Uncontrollable major haemorrhage: ensure the child is lying down, as there may have been a significant blood loss prior to arrival at hospital. Apply direct pressure and elevate the affected area above the level of the heart. Secure expert help immediately, particularly if an arterial bleed is suspected. Record a set of vital signs.

Nursing management

- Ask when, where, and how wound was sustained.
- Identify any weakness, numbness, or reduced movement to the area.
- Assess depth of wound.
- Foreign bodies: an X-ray may be needed if the wound is deep.
- In the case of dirty wounds, ensure that immunization status is ascertained. Most children in the UK receive immunizations for tetanus at 2, 3 and 4 months with a booster at 5 and 15 years. This means that they will be guarded against tetanus for 10 years from the last booster.

If this time frame has been exceeded and the wound is dirty, then antitetanus immunoglobulin is advised. Otherwise, a further booster will be needed.

- Is the wound painful? Is analgesia required? Use a pain assessment tool to ensure the most appropriate analgesia is given.
- Remove any rings from extremities to prevent tourniquet effect if limb swollen.
- Consider timing of the injury. Wounds more than 12 hours old may be better left to heal by secondary intention.
- Clean wound as thoroughly as possible using tap water or normal saline. In case of extremely dirty wounds an antiseptic, e.g. povidone-iodine, may be indicated. This can be painful, so entonox should be used if child is old enough. If the wound is to be sutured under general anaesthetic then careful consideration should be given to leaving the wound cleansing until this stage, and covering the wound with povidone-iodine soaked gauze in the meantime.
- Consider method of wound closure, such as glue, steristrips or suturing. Whilst the former are the preferred choice and can be easily managed using distraction techniques, the latter may be necessary in large deep wounds or wounds under tension (see wound closure section).

Contusions

Definition

Also known as bruising. They are caused by capillaries under the surface of the skin rupturing and bleeding as a result of a blunt object striking the skin. There is not an opening to the wound, so the blood has nowhere to go and causes a purple discolouration of the skin with localized swelling. Contusions are often tender to touch.

Causes

- Falls or bumping into something.
- Medicine or medical treatments (such as chemotherapy).
- Allergic reactions and viral infections.
- Babies are sometimes bruised during the birthing process.
- Certain illnesses and diseases can cause bruising.
- Unexplained bruises in children may be the result of child abuse.

Nursing management

- Elevation of the affected part.
- Application of ice packs (not directly on to the skin) for 24 hours, leaving them on for 20 minute intervals.

Always consider safeguarding issues when assessing lacerations, cuts and contusions. Do the injuries fit with the story or mechanism? Is there an issue of safety and supervision at home? Is the wound/contusion a result of self harm or nonaccidental injury?

Further reading

Wardrope J, Edhouse JA (1999). The Management of Wounds and Burns. Oxford: Oxford University Press.
Benbow M (2005). Evidence-Based Wound Management. London: Whurr

① Cellulitis

Introduction

An acute spreading infection of the skin involving the dermis and subcutaneous tissue, cellulitis has an indistinctive edge and advancing border that can be a serious sign. If treated promptly and appropriately, most children recover completely.

Background information

- Any area of the body can be affected and given classification accordingly (e.g. orbital, periorbital).
- Most likely causative organisms are beta-haemolytic streptococci (80%) or *Staphylococcus aureus*.
- In infants under 3 months, the most likely organism is Group B streptococcus.
- Facial cellulitis in children under 2 years caused by *Haemophilus influenza type B* is now rare since introduction of vaccination (check immunization status).
- Perianal cellulitis is a condition found mainly in young children, and is caused by Group A streptococcus. It is characterized by painful bright red skin around the anus, and painful bowel movements that may be accompanied by blood in the stools.
- Periorbital cellulitis is usually caused by upper respiratory pathogens such as Group B streptococcus, *Moraxella catarrhalis* and non-typeable *Haemophilus influenzae*.

Incidence/causes

Cellulitis is a relatively common infection usually caused by a break in the skin from trauma (burns, bites, lacerations) or skin disorder (eczema), but it may be more seriously spread through bacteraemia or underlying osteomyelitis.

Signs and symptoms

- Initial flu-like symptoms such as fever and shivering lasting a few hours, followed by pain, redness, heat and swelling of affected area.
- The child may be systemically unwell with fever, vomiting, rigors and general malaise.
- Infection typically unilateral, although facial cellulitis is usually symmetrical, spreading from around the nose to the cheeks.
- Red streaks of lymphangitis spreading away from area of cellulitis.
- Localized lymphadenopathy.

Immediate management

⚠ Consider need for admission and intravenous antibiotic treatment in severe and rapidly worsening infection, uncertain diagnosis (e.g. possible necrotizing fasciitis), systemically unwell child, vomiting child. Maintain a low threshold for admission if:

- Suspected orbital or periorbital cellulitis
- Facial cellulitis in a child
- Immunocompromised

- Diabetes mellitus
- Neonate or child under 1 year
- Failure to respond to initial treatment
- Significant comorbidity
- Parental concern or inability to cope.

History

- History suggestive of skin abrasion, trauma or pre-existing skin condition allowing portal of entry for infection (e.g. lacerations, puncture wounds, bites, dermatitis, tinea infection).

Investigations

Diagnosis is based on findings and clinical history. Depending on clinical condition and area involved consider:

- Swabs for culture and sensitivity when obvious broken skin
- Full blood count, erythrocyte sedimentation rate and C-reactive protein
- Blood cultures if cellulitis severe or not responding to treatment
- Lumbar puncture in infants and children with features of sepsis
- CT head to assess orbital or periorbital cellulitis
- Radiological investigation if foreign body, underlying osteomyelitis, or necrotizing fasciitis suspected.

Nursing management

- Manage children without systemic symptoms and with mild to moderate infection in primary care.
- Prescribe and administer antibiotics according to local policy and the child's age/weight, usually for 7 days:
  - Flucloxacillin: first line in uncomplicated cellulitis
  - Erythromycin: if child allergic to penicillin
  - Clarithromycin: if child intolerant of erythromycin.
  - Co-amoxiclav: if facial cellulitis (seek advice from local microbiologist if allergic to penicillin).
- If exposure to fresh or salt water has occurred at site of infection, seek advice from a microbiologist, as doxycycline should not be used in children under 12 years and ciprofloxacin should be avoided in children and growing adolescents.
- Reduce pain and fever.
  - Administer paracetamol or ibuprofen
  - Rest infected area and elevate if possible to reduce swelling and pain
- Manage underlying condition (e.g. tinea infection, foreign bodies, dermatitis, etc.)
- Advise use of emollients until infection resolves to keep skin well hydrated.

Discharge/follow up

- Review within 48 hours.
- Draw around erythematous area with marker pen to assess whether cellulitis is improving or worsening.

- Advise to return immediately if symptoms rapidly worsening or oral antibiotics not tolerated.
- Consider admission if not responding to treatment.
- Stress the importance of completing the course of antibiotics and continuing antibiotics for longer than 7 days if symptoms not fully resolved.
- Refer diabetic patients to nurse specialist to ensure optimal glycaemic control.
- Give preventative advice such as wearing appropriate footwear to reduce injury to skin, and the importance of wound cleansing and care.
- Review immunization status, particularly for tetanus and *Haemophilus influenzae* type B (Hib).

Prognosis/complications

Daily improvement should be seen with appropriate antibiotic therapy.

ALERT: Serious and life threatening complications may result from spread of infection via lymphatics or blood.

- Septicaemia/bacteraemia
- Abscess formation (orbital cellulitis may progress to cerebral, orbital or subperiosteal abscess)
- Meningitis or cavernous sinus thrombosis (spread from orbital cellulitis)
- Toxin mediated disease (toxic shock syndrome or scalded skin syndrome)

Further reading

Al-Nammari S, Roberton B, Ferguson C (2007). Towards evidence based emergency medicine: best BETs from the Manchester Royal Infirmary. Should a child with preseptal periorbital cellulitis be treated with intravenous or oral antibiotics? *Emergency Medical Journal* 24:28–29

Brilliant LC (2000) Perianal Streptococcal Dermatitis. *American Family Physician* 61:391–3. Available at: http://www.aafp.org/afp/20000115/391.html

For table of likely micro-organisms implicated in specific presentations of cellulitis go to: http://www.prodigy.nhs.uk/cellulitis/evidence/references#-219601

NHS Clinical Knowledge Summaries (2005) Cellulitis National Library for Health. http://www.prodigy.nhs.uk/cellulitis#219569001

⑦ Impetigo

Introduction
Impetigo is a highly contagious bacterial infection of the superficial layers of the epidermis. It is usually managed by the GP, but may be seen in an emergency department. Care must be taken to observe cross-infection policies as applied to individual departments.

Background information
- Primary impetigo is classified as direct bacterial invasion of healthy skin.
- Secondary impetigo follows underlying skin disease such as eczema, scabies or trauma to the skin.
- Nonbullous impetigo is the most common form (70% of cases), with vesicles or pustules that quickly rupture leaving a yellow-brown crust.
- Bullous impetigo is usually due to toxin-producing *Staphylococcus aureus* and is characterized by large, fluid filled blister formation.

Incidence/causes
Common in children, impetigo is caused by *Staphylococcus aureus* (90% of non-bullous impetigo) or *Streptococcus pyogenes*. Peak incidence occurs at 2–6 years of age. Spread rapidly by direct contact from school, nursery, and family, and more prevalent in overcrowded conditions.

Signs and symptoms
- Thin walled vesicular lesions which rapidly erupt to leave superficial skin erosions covered in honey-coloured crusts.
- Lesions may be itchy or painful in bullous impetigo, but are often asymptomatic in non-bullous.
- In severe impetigo there may be systemic illness with fever and malaise.
- History
  - Lesions typically appear within 4–10 days of exposure to known contact (school, nursery, sibling).
  - Underlying skin disease or trauma such as eczema, scabies, insect bites, chickenpox, burns, abrasions, herpes simplex.

Investigations
Diagnosis is based on findings and clinical history; treatment is rarely based on results of skin swabs, which are unreliable in differentiating infection from colonization. Send swabs for culture if:
- Infection is extensive or severe
- Treatment with oral antibiotics fails
- Infection is recurring.

⚠ Swab for nasal carriage of meticillin-resistant *Staphylococcus aureus* (MRSA) if patient has been exposed to a known contact:
  - Swab the lesion
  - Follow local protocols
  - Contact the Centers for Disease Control and Prevention if there is a local outbreak

Immediate and nursing management

- Topical fusidic acid for small localized lesions, following local antibiotic guidance.
- Topical mupirocin as second-line therapy when fusidic acid not tolerated or ineffective.
- Flucloxacillin oral for extensive disease, lesions not responding to topical treatment, lymphadenopathy or systemic illness.
- Erythromycin as alternative oral antibiotic.
- Soften crusts by soaking in warm water prior to applying topical treatments.
- Cover sores with loose clothing or gauze bandage to prevent spread of infection.
- Keep child off school/nursery and away from newborn babies until sores have stopped blistering/crusting, or 48 hours after treatment with antibiotics.

Discharge/follow up

- Hygiene advice to reduce risk of spread of infection and recurrence.
- Frequent hand washing, keep fingernails short, avoid scratching, avoid sharing towels, flannels, clothing and bathwater until lesions cleared.
- Follow up not necessary if lesions have healed with treatment.
- Referral indicated if impetigo is severe or extensive, recurring frequently or is unresponsive to oral treatment.

Prognosis/complications

Usually resolves within 2 weeks even without treatment and heals without scarring. Complications rare but can include lymphadenitis, cellulitis, and post-streptococcal glomerulonephritis, in less than 1% of cases.

Further reading

HPA and Association of Medical Microbiologists (2008) Management of Infection: Guidance for Primary Care for Consultation and Local Adaption. Health Protection Agency http://www.hpa. org.uk/web/HPAwebFile/HPAweb_C/1194947340160. Accessed 17/12/08

Sladden MJ, Johnston GA (2004). Common skin infections in children. *British Medical Journal* 329:95–99

NHS Clinical Knowledge Summaries (2005) Impetigo National Library for Health. http://cks.library. nhs.uk/impetigo#-225401. Accessed 17/12/08

☠ Management of eczema herpeticum (Kaposi varicelliform) in children

Introduction
Eczema herpeticum is a severe primary herpes infection that occurs in individuals with eczema.

⚠ This is a dermatological emergency with potentially fatal complications in its severest forms (Buxton 1998). Treatment with antiviral medication should take place before confirmatory swab results return (NICE 2007), so reliance upon clinical identification is a key element.

Background information
- Eczematous skin has a disturbed barrier function that predisposes to bacterial and viral infections.
- Children with eczema should avoid contact if at all possible with people who have active cold sores.
- Primary infection of a child with atopic eczema with herpes simplex is often the worst episode. Subsequent herpetic infections (the affected person often carries the virus for life) are often less traumatic, and the parents are likely to seek medical attention earlier if they recognize the condition.
- Subsequent infections often respond to early use of aciclovir cream alone, without the need to use oral/IV medication. Some practitioners would give a prescription for aciclovir cream for parents to hold in readiness for such an event.

Differential diagnoses
- Chicken pox.
- Eczema herpeticum may occur also on a background of the rare condition of Darrier's disease.
- Erythema multiforme can occur as a rare reaction to herpes simplex and is characterized by lesions that look 'target' like. Erythema multiforme mainly appears on the hands, forearms and lower legs.

Signs, symptoms and history
- Child has a previous background history of eczema.
- Parents or carers say that the skin has changed very rapidly, perhaps overnight or within a day, and is not the usual eczema appearance the child normally manifests (a reliable indicator).
- The delicate top of the vesicles often breaks down very quickly, so ask parents what the skin looked like when they first noticed the problem.
- Suggestive history: contact with someone who has a cold sore (herpes simplex), or if the child has recently had a cold sore themselves.
- The child presents with small pustules/vesicles with a prior history of eczema.
- Lesions begin at the same time and progress all together with similar appearance (linear progression of monomorphic lesions):
  - Begin as small vesicles, grow to small pustules with a delicate top (easily broken to reveal clear fluid)

- • After 24 hours or so, the broken pustules break down to form erosions or small 'ulcers'
  - • Ulcers often coalesce into larger areas of raw looking erosions that give a 'raw-meat looking' appearance to the affected skin
  - • Erosions may take on a golden crusty appearance if secondary colonization with *Staphylococcus aureus* occurs.
- Lesions are very painful.
- Child has an elevated temperature (unusual with atopic eczema on its own).
- Child will often look very unwell.
- The affected area is often localized and confined to the areas most affected by eczema, but it can be widespread with chicken pox-like vesicles, filled with clear fluid in the early stages and crusting later.

Immediate management

- Assessment of severity, site of skin affected, and stage of development to determine appropriate antiviral therapy route (IV or oral aciclovir).
- Immediate referral to a medical officer with dermatology experience, if available.

Nursing management

- Oral/IV aciclovir (depending on clinical picture of severity) will reduce the severity and duration of the course of the infection. In widespread eczema herpeticum or the immunocompromised child, urgent administration of aciclovir can be lifesaving.
- Antibiotics to control secondary infection (oral or IV depending on severity). NB: secondary infection is usually staphylococcal, so the drug of choice is flucloxacillin, usually used at the higher dose regimen for skin infections.
- Appropriate regular pain relief.
- Barrier nurse, and isolate from the immunocompromised on the ward.
- Use gloves and gown for initial handling if herpes is suspected.
- Lukewarm compresses of potassium permanganate can be used to give symptomatic relief and dry weeping sores (potassium permanganate at a concentration of 1:10,000 should look the colour of a dark 'rosé wine' colour. Dilutions made up to this concentration can be applied for 10–15 minutes at a time). It may help to dry oozing skin and bring some pain relief. The child and parent should be advised that it will stain the skin brown for a week or so.

Complications

⚠ Skin involvement that includes the eye or the skin near the eye would require a child to be seen by an eye specialist on the same day as presentation (NICE 2007).

Further reading

Buxton P (1998) ABC of Dermatology (3rd edn). London: BMJ Publishing Group.
Harper J, Oranje A, Prose N, (eds) (2000) Textbook of paediatric dermatology. Oxford: Blackwell Science.
NICE (2007) Guidelines Atopic Dermatitis in Children. http://www.nice.org.uk/CG57

☠ Emergency management of burns and scalds

Introduction
The key priority when faced with a burn is to stop the burning and arrest any further tissue damage.

In tandem with this, it is a priority to deal with the pain that the child will be experiencing and to provide information to the parents/family.

Signs and symptoms
- First degree burns have redness, pain, minor swelling, but no blisters.
- Second degree burns produce blisters, which sometimes burst, give severe pain and show redness.
- Third degree burns are dry, waxy, white, leathery brown or charred. Because of nerve damage there may be little pain, and the area may feel numb.

Immediate management
As for all children coming to accident and emergency, the management of the child should start with an assessment of their airway, breathing and circulation (ABC). The next consideration should be appropriate analgesia.

Airway
If the child has been in a house fire, then there is a possibility that he/she has inhaled hot gases and has sustained an airway burn injury.

Examine the airway: if there is suspicion of an airway burn, e.g. a burn around the mouth and nose or the presence of soot in mucus, then anaesthetic assessment is required as a matter of urgency.

Early intubation may be indicated to offset the problems associated with oedema.

Breathing
Check the child's respiratory rate and observe the work of breathing.

Is breathing smooth or laboured or noisy? If the latter, then again alert the anaesthetic team.

Circulation
At least two unburned areas should be identified that are suitable for the insertion of an intravenous cannula.

Fluid loss is a major problem in someone who has been burned, so fluid must be replaced rapidly.

Who do I need to call?
- The child will need a more thorough assessment from the thermal injury management team on call.
- The burn ward/unit will need to be alerted about the child's impending admission if the burn is major (>10%).

History

On presentation there are several key facts that the nurse needs to know in order to effectively manage the child who has been burned or scalded. These should be ascertained by history taking and examination.

- When did the burn happen?
  This is important to know as any actions that subsequently occur need to be calculated from the time the injury took place and not the time of arrival (there could be a significant delay between the time the burn occurred and the child's admission).

Examination

Assess type of burn
- Burns are caused by a variety of elements and some require specific actions.
- You need to know what caused the burn and seek additional information.
  The types of burns encountered are:
  - Scalds
  - Flame burns
  - Chemical burns
  - Electrical burns
  - Contact burns
  - Radiation burns

Assess burned area
- The total body surface area (TBSA) burned is important to determine to see if you're dealing with a minor or major burn/scald. This can be achieved quickly using the Wallace Rule of Nines (there is an adapted Wallace Rule of Nines for babies and young children), but can be more accurately assessed using a Lund and Browder chart. It is important to remember that the burn itself is being assessed, so surrounding areas of erythema (redness) should be excluded.
- TBSA >10% = Major burn
- TBSA <10% = Minor burn

Assess the depth of the burn
- Burns vary in depth according to the layers of skin involved/penetrated in the injury and are commonly classified as:
  - Partial thickness: superficial or involving the epidermis only and will be pink/red in appearance
  - Full thickness: the burn extends down through the dermis into the fascia and underlying muscle and will be white or leathery/charred in appearance

Nursing management

Assess whether fluid resuscitation is required
- If the burn exceeds 10% TBSA then it should be regarded as a major burn and fluid resuscitation should begin.
  - Fluid resuscitation is calculated using the Parkland formula that estimates the amount of fluid required over the 24 hours after a burn. Half of the fluid is given in the first 8 hours and the remainder is given in the subsequent 16 hours.

- Do not neglect the child's normal fluid requirements, which must also be given.
- Oral feeding should be encouraged as soon as possible to offset further gastrointestinal complications, provided the child is not fasting for a procedure.
- Closely observe the child's urine output as this is an indicator of the effectiveness of the fluid resuscitation.
- The child should be catheterized and urine output should be maintained above 1 mL/kg/hour.

Assess the child's pain
- ALL burns are painful whether minor or major and adequate pain relief should be prescribed and administered.

Assess the need for a dressing
- At this early stage minimal dressings will be required, so that the wound may be easily accessed for assessment by medical staff.
  - It is important to remember that the dressing used should be of a non/low adherence material.
  - Ensure that the child does not become hypothermic because of prolonged exposure.
  - Do not apply any topical agents until the burn has been thoroughly assessed by the burn team. Topical agents applied too soon can obscure the burn's appearance.
  - Remember that following a burn the child will be susceptible to infection, so precautions should be observed.

Care of the family
- Don't forget that the family will need reassurance and a continuous flow of information about what is going on.
- Include the family in decision making and encourage a family-centred approach to care.
- Burns and scalds in children are distressing, life-changing and life-threatening events that affect the whole family.

Further reading

Herndon D. (2002). Total Burn Care (2nd edn). London: Saunders
http://www2.warwick.ac.uk/fac/med/research/hsri/emergencycare/prehospitalcare/
    jrcalcstakeholderwebsite/guidelines/burns_and_scalds_in_children_2006.pdf

☠ Snake bites

Introduction

- Snake bites occur when a snake bites the skin, and if the snake is poisonous it can result in a medical emergency.
- When contact is made, hollow fangs in the upper jaw discharge snake venom into the tissues.
- Snake venom is a combination of many different proteins and enzymes. Most are harmless but some of these proteins are toxic to humans.

Incidence/causes

- The UK's only indigenous poisonous snake is the adder. UK poisons centres are contacted on average for 100 human cases each year. In approximately 70% of patients, envenoming is minimal or localized, causing pain, swelling and inflammation of the bitten area.
- The adder is common and most bites will occur in the summer months from people walking through long grass.
- There are also exotic snakes in the UK held legally by zoos, research establishments, and licensed private individuals. Some are kept illegally as 'macho pets' and there will be occasions when the owners will seek medical attention for a bite.

It is unusual, but envenoming can be life-threatening, particularly in children. See Fig. 7.1 for the management of a potentially venomous bite.

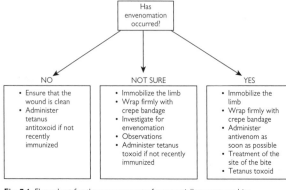

Fig. 7.1 Flow chart for the management of a potentially venomous bite

Signs and symptoms
- The symptoms are generally rapid in onset, and the diagnosis of envenomation is straightforward. The symptoms may be as a direct result of the bite or an allergic reaction to the toxin.
- Symptoms usually manifest themselves within 1 hour of the snake bite, and antivenoms are not often available at the site of the incident. By the time the individual has reached a medical centre it will be evident if envenomation has occurred.

Clinical features
- Immediate sharp pain.
- Tingling sensation and local swelling.
- Spreading pain, tenderness, inflammation, and enlarged, tender lymph nodes.
- Anaphylactoid symptoms may occur within 5 minutes or may be delayed for several hours. These include nausea, vomiting, sweating, fever, vasoconstriction, tachycardia, loss of consciousness, shock, oedema.
- Hypotension.
- Bleeding from the gums and nose into the lungs, gastrointestinal and genitourinary tract.
- Acute renal failure (more common in children).
(APLS 2005)

Immediate management
- Assessment of ABC (refer to recognition of a seriously ill child), and in addition be aware of the following:
  - Airway: may be compromised due to depressed level of consciousness, bulbar palsy, paralysis and airway oedema. Clearance of secretions is commonly required. Assessment of the airway must be frequent.
  - Breathing: venoms may cause paralysis and patients may require ventilatory support.
  - Circulation: shock may be present due to massive leakage of fluid into the tissues, cardiac arrhythmia and bleeding secondary to coagulopathy.
  - Disability: assess the patient's level of consciousness.
  - Exposure: full exposure required to locate the site of the bite.
(APLS 2005)

History
- Details of the snake: with captive snakes this may be known exactly. Others are identified according to size, colour, patterning and other characteristics (e.g. a 'rattle').
- Ascertain time of the bite and onset of pain.
- Routine history of allergies and medications.

Examination
- Observe for angioedema and shock
- Note confusion/drowsiness
- Monitor vital signs
- Observe the wound for tissue destruction, oedema, blisters and erythema
- Examine for systemic effects such as changes in skin sensation, hypotension, bleeding and lymphadenopathy

Investigations
- Blood tests:
  - FBC
  - U&Es
  - Clotting studies
  - Fibrinogen
  - Crossmatch
  - Blood gas is indicated.
- Other investigations:
  - Chest X-ray if indicated
  - Wound X-ray for retained teeth/fangs.

Nursing management and treatment
- Limit the uptake of the venom into the circulatory system (application of a crepe bandage, firmly applied and immobilization of the limb using a splint).
- If appropriate and available administer the antivenom. In general, the child will receive the same dose of antiserum as an adult, as it is based on the amount required to neutralize the toxin as opposed to the weight of the patient.
- Provide supportive care to systems affected by the toxin.
- Pain management: titrated intravenous opiates may be required.
- Treat the site of the bite and observe for the development of compartment syndrome.
- If venom is sprayed into the eyes they must be thoroughly irrigated as soon as possible.
- The patient should be monitored for at least 24 hours post envenomation.

Complications
- Local wound complications
- Compartment syndrome
- Cardiovascular and haematological complications
- Respiratory complications
- Renal failure
- Neuromuscular blockade

Prognosis

- Fatalities are rare; the last reported fatality in the UK was over 30 years ago.

Further reading

Harborne DJ (1993) Emergency treatment of adder bites: case reports and literature review. *Archives of Emergency Medicine*. 10:239–43

Warrell DA (2005) Treatment of bites by adders and exotic venomous snakes. *British Medical Journal*. 33:1244–7

Advanced Paediatric Life Support Group (APLS) (2005) Advanced Paediatric Life Support: The Practical Approach, 4th Edition. BMJ Publishing Group, London.

① Animal bites

Introduction
Approximately 1% of all visits to Emergency Departments are as a result of animal bites. Up to 50% of these attendances are school age children, between the age of 5 and 14 years.

Due to the potential emotional, psychological and physical consequences, bites require careful management aimed at both the short and long term recovery of the child.

Incidence/causes
- The majority of bites are inflicted by dogs which account for up to 80–90% of all bites.
- Cats account for between 5 and 10%.
- Human bites and others such as rodents, and in rare instances wild animals or exotic pets, account for the rest. NB: human bites are a child safeguarding issue, and it will require a forensic dentist to differentiate an adult from a child bite.
- Boys are bitten by dogs more than girls, and girls are bitten or scratched by cats more often than boys.
- Fatalities, although rare, usually involve infants and preschool children.
- Dog bites are usually the result of children teasing or unknowingly threatening an animal. In the majority of cases, the dog is known to the child and is very often the family pet. Younger children tend to be bitten more often in the home. There is some evidence to suggest that, with the rise in popularity of more 'aggressive' breeds of dog, unprovoked incidents are on the increase. However, this has to be treated with caution due to the intense media coverage in such instances.
- School age children are usually bitten or scratched on the hand, arm or leg. The incidence of bites to the head, face and neck increases in children under the age of 5.
- Cat bites are more likely to result in puncture wounds as opposed to lacerations and contusions from dog bites. The incidence of infection is generally higher as a result of a cat bite.
- Bites to hands are generally more susceptible to infection than other areas.
- The bite of a large dog can exert forces of up to 450 pounds per square inch, which can result in significant crush and laceration injuries often with large areas of devitalized tissue, or in severe cases damage to underlying organs.
- Fatalities are usually as a result of significant haemorrhage.

Immediate management
The priority in all cases should be the assessment of airway, breathing, circulation and disability (ABCD) (APLS 2005).

Refer to p. 68, Recognizing a seriously ill child, to identify and address potential life threatening injuries. This is especially important in children who have been bitten by a large, powerful animal.

History

It is useful to identify the type, breed, and size of animal involved, the time the incident occurred, and the duration of the attack. Other factors, such as the mechanism of the injury, should be considered, for example:

- Did the animal bite and let go?
- Did it bite and shake?
- Did the animal drag or move the child?

These are all important observations in ascertaining the potential severity of injuries.

The circumstances leading to the injury should be identified, for example:

- What caused the animal to bite the child?
- Where did the incident occur?
- Who owns the animal and who was present at the time?

These observations may be important later when considering any potential safeguarding issues, and the child's future safety and wellbeing.

At this point it may also be useful to identify what first aid the child has received, and if the child has any other medical conditions.

Examination

- The location and number of bites should be noted and recorded as this will give an indication as to the potential seriousness of the injury and the potential complications that may occur.
- The wounds inflicted should be described, i.e. is the wound a scratch, laceration, puncture, etc.?
- Any bruising, deformity, or deficit in function, and the amount of blood loss should also be noted. Again, other associated injuries should be recorded and treated. It may be useful to measure and record the size of any laceration or tissue/blood loss.

Nursing management

During the assessment phase, the wound should be irrigated and then covered with saline soaked gauze to prevent the tissues drying, which can lead to a delay in the healing process. Referral to appropriate specialties should have taken place if the bite is substantial, or in an area that may require surgical intervention such as the face, hand, or genital area.

Treatment

- Pain assessment should be carried out using a recognized age-appropriate assessment tool.
- Appropriate analgesics (clinically and allergy permitting) may include one or a combination of analgesic methods including local anaesthetics, entonox, and distraction techniques.
- Animal bites require good wound cleansing to minimize the risks of infection.
- Irrigate the wound with a 30 mL syringe and 19 g needle (use a blunt needle to minimize injury) with normal saline or water (dependent on clean source). Optimal pressure should be between 5 and 15 psi.
- NB: Too much pressure may redistribute bacteria into other tissues. (Gardner & Franz 2008)

- The use of antiseptic solutions in irrigation is controversial, with evidence suggesting that it discourages wound healing.
- Re-examine wound to ensure that internal structures are not damaged, remove any devitalized tissue, and check for foreign bodies (e.g. teeth). (NB: care should be taken to ensure that this minimizes any potential damage to wound healing or appearance of the wound.)

Wound care

Wound closure following an animal bite will depend upon the type of wound and location. Facial/scalp bites, where a good cosmetic result is essential, will need to be closed. Faces tend to heal well due to a good blood supply compared to hands, which have increased risk of infection. Other areas may be left for either delayed primary repair or healing by secondary intention.

Due to the increased risk of infection, a nonadhesive povidone/iodine dressing such as Inadine® can be applied, provided that there are no contraindications.

Care should be taken if large areas are covered with this dressing or if being used in infants under 6 months old, due to the absorption of iodine.

Complications/prognosis

NB: Check local hospital and departmental policy before giving antibiotics.

Common antibiotics for the treatment of animal bites include:
- Co-amoxiclav and amoxicillin
- Doxycycline or metronidazole (if allergic to penicillin; not to be used in pregnancy)
- Cefradine and metronidazole (if pregnant and penicillin-allergic)
- Wound swabs are required only if wound appears infected, and should be taken for both aerobic and anaerobic organisms. Tetanus status should be checked and as per Department of Health policy (1996).
- Rabies should be considered if the bite was sustained in a country where the disease is endemic, or in high risk bites such as those from bats. Advice should be sought from clinical virologists and the Health Protection Agency (Drug and Therapeutics Bulletin 2004).
- Children who have sustained animal bites may need follow up for delayed primary suturing, and/or wound checks. This may need to be carried out in the emergency department, specialist clinic, or by the practice nurse usually after 48 hours (check local policy). Events such as severe animal bites may cause psychological trauma to the patient, which should not be underestimated. Patients should be advised to seek support from their local GP/health visitor.
- Education on how to prevent further incidences should be offered. Websites such as the RSPCA and DEFRA sites may be useful sources of information.

Further reading

Gardner and Franz (2008) Wound bioburden. In: Baranoski S, Ayello EA (eds) Wound care essentials (2nd edn). London: Lippincott Williams and Wilkins, pp. 108–109

Kannikeswaran N, Kamat D (2008). Mammalian Bites (Online). *Clinical Pediatrics* available at http://clp.sage.com.

Morgan M (2005). Hospital management of animal and human bites. *Journal of Hospital Infection.* 61:1–10..

www.defra.gov.uk

www.rspca.co.uk

Advanced Life Support Group (2005) Advanced Paediatric Life Support. 4th Edition. BMJ Publishing Group, London

Department of Health (1996). http://cks.library.nhs.uk/bites_human_and_animal/mangement/detailed_answers/managing_an_animal_bite#-287861

Drug and Therapeutics Bulletin (2004) **42** (9) pp. 67–71.

⑦ Suturing wounds

When suturing children's wounds, careful consideration must be made as to whether the wound really requires suturing. Modern, more appropriate wound closure measures have been developed, in order to reduce scarring, pain and anxiety both for the child and their parents. However, one must not avoid suturing an appropriate wound simply because other methods are easier. The object of suturing a wound is to oppose the skin, aiming for slight eversion of the wound edges. Before suturing a child, they need to be prepared both physically and mentally for the procedure (refer to communicating through play, p. 14); this should involve an explanation of the procedure and of the risks associated with the procedure.

- Prepare a clean field by opening a suturing pack over a clean dressing/suturing trolley.
- Infiltrate around the wound with local/topical anaesthetic (1% lidocaine, or lidocaine, adrenaline and tetracaine gel, do not use adrenaline on wounds involving digits, genitalia, or mucous membranes).
- Decide on the appropriate suture material (see Table 7.1).

Table 7.1 Suture materials

Wound site	Which material and size	When to remove
Face	5/0 or 6/0 nonabsorbable	3–5 days
Scalp	3/0 nonabsorbable	7 days
Hand	5/0 or 4/0 nonabsorbable	7–10 days
Small wounds	4/0 nonabsorbable	7 days
Large wounds	4/0	10–12 days
Over joints	4/0	10–12 days

- The wound must be thoroughly cleaned with normal saline and all debris irrigated out of the wound. This is best achieved using a 10 mL syringe.
- The wound must be closed using the appropriate sutures as per the techniques shown in Fig. 7.2.

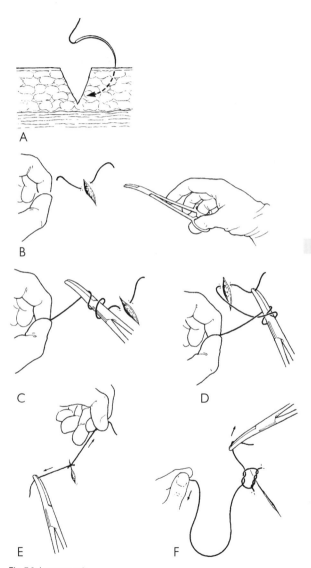

Fig. 7.2 Instrument tie
Oxford Handbook of Emergency Medicine 3e, Wyatt et al, (2006), p.406-407, with permission from Oxford University Press

Key points for suturing
- Do not be afraid to remove sutures, especially the first one applied.
- Do not close dirty wounds.
- Fully explore wounds; if not confident or competent to know what you are examining, seek more senior help.
- Do not close wounds under too much tension.
- Do not overtighten suture knots.
- Always ask for help when unsure.

Further reading

Sano, Kazufumi MD, Yoshizu, Takae MD, et al. (2005) Easy-Removal "Ribbon-Knot Suturing" For Pediatric Wound Care. *Plastic and Reconstructive Surgery*. 116:694–695

Bonadio WA, Carney M, Gustafson D (1994) Efficacy of nurses suturing pediatric dermal lacerations in an emergency department. *Ann Emerg Med*. 24:1144–6.

Musculoskeletal problems

⑦ Overview of fractures and dislocations

Introduction
- Most children's fractures follow simple fracture patterns and are caused by low-velocity trauma.
- A child's bones are less brittle than an adult's, and often deform to produce buckle or greenstick fractures.
- Children's ligaments are stronger than their bones, so sprains and dislocations are unusual, and growth plate fractures more common.
- As the child gets older and skeletal maturity occurs (approximately age 14 in girls and 16 in boys), an adult injury pattern emerges.
- Bone injuries in young children may be associated with nonaccidental injury, especially in children under 1 year in age.

Definitions
- Fracture: a fracture is a loss of continuity of the margins of a bone. A break is the same as a fracture, but the terms are frequently misunderstood.
- Dislocation: complete separation of the surfaces of a joint.
- Subluxation: a partial shift of the surfaces of the joint, where some contact remains.

Types of fractures common in children
- Plastic deformation: bowing of a long bone.
- Buckle fracture: a compression-type injury. Sometimes referred to as a torus fracture. A small outward buckle can be seen in the cortex.
- Greenstick fracture: occurs when a bone is bent, and one side (the side under tension) starts to fracture. The fracture line does not pass entirely through the bone.
- Complete fracture: a fracture that passes completely through a bone.
- Growth plate fracture: a fracture that involves the growth plate. Growth plate fractures are usually described using the Salter-Harris classification (Fig. 8.1a).
  • Type I – the fracture line passes through the growth plate, separating the epiphysis completely from the metaphysis.
  • Type II – the fracture line travels through much of the growth plate before passing through the metaphysis and detaching a triangular metaphyseal fragment. This is the most common injury.
  • Type III – the fracture line passes along the growth plate for a variable distance before entering the joint through a fracture of the epiphysis. These are very rare.
  • Type IV – the fracture line passes from the joint surface across the epiphysis, growth plate and into the metaphysis.
  • Type V – these are crush injuries of the growth plate. There is often very little to see on the X-ray at first, but deformity appears months or years later because bone growth has stopped. These are rare.

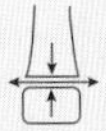	Type I: Injuries occur when the fracture line is along the plane of the growth plate. Pain on weight bearing will be the main symptom
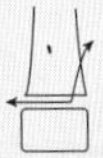	Type II: Injuries occur when the fracture is along the plane of the growth plate but extends into the metaphysis (the growing portion of a long bone) on one side
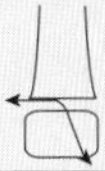	Type III: Injuries occur when the fracture line is along the plane of the growth plate, but extends into the epiphysis (bone end) on one side
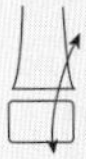	Type IV: Injuries occur where the fracture extends from the epiphysis through the growth plate into the metaphysis
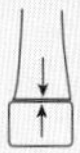	Type V: Injures involve a crush injury to the growth plate. This may not be obvious on X-ray but the clinical signs will suggest a serious injury

Fig. 8.1a Salter-Harris classification of fractures
Oxford Handbook of Children's and Young People's Nursing, Glasper et al., (2006), p.475, with permission from Oxford University Press

Other classifications of fractures

(see Fig 8.1b)

- Closed: the skin over the facture site is intact.
- Open: the skin over the fracture site has been broken, and this skin break communicates with the fracture. This may occur either from the inside out (when a sharp bone splinter at the fracture site pierces the skin) or from the outside in (when the force that fractures the bone also breaks the skin). These fractures were previously referred to as compound fractures.
- Pathological: the fracture occurs through a bone abnormality, e.g. neoplasm or bone cyst. There may be minimal force required to cause the fracture.
- Comminuted: the fracture causes the bone to fragment into many pieces. This is rare in children.
- Displaced fractures: fractures may move in one of three ways:
  - Shift: the bone ends may shift with respect to one another at the fracture site
  - Angulate: the bone may angulate at the fracture site
  - Rotate: the long axes of bones may rotate at the fracture site

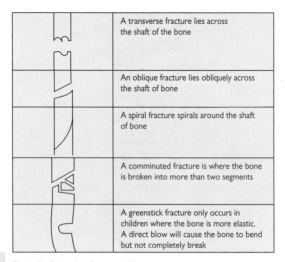

	A transverse fracture lies across the shaft of the bone
	An oblique fracture lies obliquely across the shaft of bone
	A spiral fracture spirals around the shaft of bone
	A comminuted fracture is where the bone is broken into more than two segments
	A greenstick fracture only occurs in children where the bone is more elastic. A direct blow will cause the bone to bend but not completely break

Fig. 8.1b Other classifications of fractures
Oxford Handbook of Children's and Young People's Nursing, Glasper et al., (2006), p.474, with permission from Oxford University Press

Signs and symptoms
- Mechanism of injury:
  - Direct forces (e.g. kicked on side of lower leg playing football) are likely to cause a fracture at the site of the injury, and a degree of soft tissue injury overlying it.
  - Indirect forces (e.g. fall onto outstretched hand) may cause a fracture further up the limb where the forces are dissipated, e.g. in the wrist, elbow, or clavicle.
- Tenderness
- Swelling/bruising: not always obvious, can often be 'felt' rather than seen.
- Loss of function: can usually be observed by watching the child. Do not ask the child to attempt to move an obviously fractured limb.
- Deformity: compare with uninjured side if not immediately obvious.
- Crepitus: do not try to elicit crepitus, but it may be felt if supporting an injured limb.

Immediate management
- Wounds: photograph wounds, then cover with a sterile dressing.
- Critical skin is an area of blanching over the fracture/dislocation site where the skin is stretched and its circulation is compromised. Report immediately as the injury will need to be reduced as a priority.

- Check distal pulses, skin temperature and sensation—looking for neurovascular damage.
- Immobilize/support the affected part. This may require a splint, or may simply require a sling.
- Elevate the limb to reduce pain and swelling.
- Analgesia should be provided following an appropriate pain assessment. In all but minor greenstick or buckle fractures an opiate may be required, e.g. diamorphine intranasally or morphine IV. Entonox is useful as an adjunct or while alternative analgesics are being prepared. A femoral nerve block may also be considered.
- X-ray: a minimum of two views should be taken, and in long bone injuries the X-ray should show the whole of the bone and the joints above and below it.

Further management
- Most fractures in children are undisplaced and a short period in a cast restores normal function.
- Some fractures with only a small amount of angulation do not need reduction, as normal growth will allow remodelling of the fracture to occur over time.
- Most children with displaced fractures or dislocations will require a general anaesthetic for reduction of the injury.
- Most fractures and dislocations can be reduced using a closed method. Some may need open reduction and internal fixation to achieve stability.
- Some dislocations may be reduced relatively easily with entonox, e.g. dislocations of the patella, and some may be reduced with local anaesthetic, e.g. dislocations of fingers.
- The majority of fractures and dislocations will require some form of immobilization/support after reduction, until healing occurs.

Further reading
Ring D, Waters PM, (1996) Management of fractures and dislocations of the elbow in children. *Acta Orthop Belg* 62(Suppl 1):58–65

① Applying splints

Introduction

Splints are used to treat a variety of injuries and conditions. The principles of family centred care, and psychological care of the child who has been involved in trauma and attended the Emergency Department, should be considered throughout.

When to apply a splint

- Limb injuries, such as fractures, dislocations, sprains.
- To immobilize a damaged limb, for example for osteomyelitis.
- To immobilize a limb/prevent further damage due to movement.
- To correct/maintain alignment/position.
- For pain relief, particularly when moving the child, for example transfer to X-ray or ward.
- To reduce muscle spasm.

Types of splints (most common)

- Thomas splint, which may be used as a resting splint or have traction applied to it.
- Box splint (padded, plastic covered splint), used as a resting splint.

Immediate care

- As described on pages 72 and 76, assessment and management of ABCDE (www.resus.org.uk) will be the priority, as the child may have other, more urgent problems.
- Once immediate life threatening problems have been ruled out or managed, the child's limb can be splinted.
- Application of the splint:
  - Explain procedure to parents and give age appropriate explanations to the child.
  - Gain consent from child and/or parents for procedure.
  - Identify the correct splint for the type and location of injury, e.g. a Thomas splint is commonly used for a fractured femur.
  - Ensure all relevant equipment is located and prepared, e.g. appropriately sized splint for the child.
  - Ensure a competent practitioner is available to apply the splint and an adequate number of practitioners are able to assist with the application.
  - Manual traction of the limb will need to be applied while applying the skin extensions for a Thomas splint, to ensure correct position.
  - Application of a splint to an injured limb is a painful procedure. The child should receive adequate pain relief in preparation for splint.
  - The child may have already received pain relief for the injury. For example, once the absence of other injuries such as head injury has been established pain should be managed. This should include intranasal diamorphine or intravenous morphine, and oral analgesia such as paracetamol and/or a nonsteroidal anti-inflammatory drug (NSAID) (www.nice.org.uk).
  - However, further analgesia for procedural pain, such as when the splint is applied, may be required. Entonox is one of the

recommended methods of pain relief for prevention of procedural pain. Regional anaesthesia (femoral nerve block) may also be considered if there is a practitioner with the relevant expertise.
- Throughout the application of the splint the child's pain should be assessed and managed.
- Following application, the child should be made comfortable and the limb should be in an acceptable alignment (depending on whether definitive or temporary intervention).
- Assess for neurovascular compromise due to the initial injury and from the application of the splint. Neurovascular observations include assessment of pulse, level of swelling, colour, warmth, movement and sensation of the affected limb, distal to the fracture/injury.
- It is important that neurovascular observations are carried out for early detection and treatment of compartment syndrome (see p. 286)
- Child may be admitted to the children's ward, or be prepared for immediate surgery depending on extent of the injuries.

Further reading

British Association for Emergency Medicine (2004) Guideline for the management of pain in children. London: BAEM

Wright E (2007). Evaluating a paediatric neurovascular assessment tool. *Journal of Orthopaedic Nursing*. 11:20–29

① Applying casts

Introduction

A cast is a rigid 'shell' which must be well fitting to support the architecture of the body and underlying soft tissue of a limb, or other part of the child's body. A cast provides external protection and maintains correct anatomical alignment, to prevent any further damage and to allow healing to take place. A cast may be used to support broken bones, dislocations, and soft tissue damage to ligaments and tendons.

Purpose of casting

- Restore bone alignment
- Rest and protect a limb or joint
- Restore function
- Limit movement
- Reduce pain, muscle spasm and swelling
- Prevent/limit further damage to neurovasculature and soft tissue
- Prevent complications such as malunion

Immediate management: application

- Application should be according to local policy or guidelines. Prior to application explain the procedure to the child or young person if alert and responsive.
- Involve parents/carers or guardians or trusted adult; consent should be obtained.
- Analgesia and/or sedation may be required prior to application; use distraction and/or play as appropriate.
- Ensure that there are adequate numbers of suitably qualified staff available to ensure safe application, as some casts may require more than two members of staff.
- A freshly applied cast should be treated gently until fully dry. A cast can be made from plaster or from fibreglass/polyester materials; the age of the child or young person and their injury or condition may determine the best type of material to use. Plaster casts are cheaper, and are composed of a cotton bandage impregnated with plaster of Paris, which hardens when it has been made wet. Plaster casts are absorbent and porous, allowing a limb or the immobilized part of the body to breathe. They can be more easily moulded to make a snug fit, and split easily to accommodate swelling. Fibreglass/polyester casts are more waterproof, and are lightweight but strong. The cast cannot be moulded easily in the same way as the plaster cast, but bathing and movement are easier in these casts.
- Do not rest the freshly applied cast on a hard surface as it may become dented or distorted, which may interfere with the functional ability of the cast.
- The child or young person is usually discharged home after a cast is applied in the emergency department or clinic. Parents/carers MUST be issued with instructions on drying, checking for complications and use of aids or crutches and pain relief.

⚠️Never use direct heat on a cast, and never slide anything down inside the cast to relieve itching.

Complications
- Swelling
- Pain
- Discolouration (darker or lighter than other extremity or digits)
- Digit or extremity becomes cool

Assessment

⚠️The 5 P's of ischaemia should be reported immediately; they include: pain, especially associated with passive movements, pallor, pulselessness, paraesthesia and paralysis.

⚠️Compartment syndrome: this constitutes an emergency situation, when post traumatic swelling may gradually compromise the circulation within a closed fascial compartment. This can cause ischaemia and death of the muscle contributing to compartment syndrome (see pp 286–7).

Features of a good cast
- Well fitting
- Has a smooth interior
- Does not cause constriction
- Is light in weight

Limitations of casts
- Applying a cast is difficult if a dressing would be unreachable during treatment, although a window can be left in the cast for observation of a wound and dressing change.
- Plaster casts can be heavy, thus restricting movement especially for young children,
- Removal or bivalving of the cast, although painless, may involve the use of the circular saw, which can be noisy and distressing for children during this procedure. Child play specialists can help by providing distraction or guided imagery.
- If plaster casts become wet they will break down, reducing their effectiveness, and the underlying skin may become macerated.
- Insertion of implements to scratch under the cast risks injury to the skin, which may cause an infection, or in some instances the implement cannot be retrieved and becomes lodged inside the cast.

Complications
- The skin under the cast can become dry and scaly.
- In hot weather, a staphylococcal infection of the hair and sweat glands can lead to severe and painful dermatitis.

Further reading

Royal College of Nursing (RCN) (2007) Benchmarks for Children's Orthopaedic Nursing Care: RCN Guidance. London. RCN
http://www.orthoseek.com
http://www.orthoters.co.uk

! **Application of skin traction in emergency situations**

Introduction

Traction applied via skin extensions is no longer the orthopaedic surgeon's treatment of choice for leg fractures. This is due to recent rapid advancement in surgical techniques and the desire to get children home as quickly as possible.

Incidence

Traction is the application of a pulling force to a part of the body.
Skin traction is still used as a short term treatment for:
- Some fractures prior to other treatments such as casting or internal fixation/external fixation
- Contractures of muscles
- Muscle spasms.
Other uses include:
- Resting a diseased or painful joint as in 'irritable hip'
- Reduction of a dislocated joint

Gallows traction is used to immobilize a femoral fracture in an infant until swelling subsides, prior to application of a hip spica. (NB: this is appropriate for very young children less than 16 kg in weight. Some authorities specify 12 kg; it is therefore important to check the specified maximum weight against local policy before placing a child in Gallows traction.)
- The procedure may cause distress and/or discomfort. A careful explanation should be given to the child and parent and administer prescribed analgesia/entonox where appropriate.
- Ensure the child's skin is clean to prevent possible pressure sores and/ or skin infection. Adhesive skin traction is usually essential for fractures and therefore older children may need to be shaved.
- Privacy and dignity should be maintained throughout the proceedure.
- Nonadhesive traction is ideal in short term situations such as 'irritable hip' or when the child is to be removed from the traction for periods of physiotherapy or other interventions.

Management (Fig 8.2)

In addition to the extension kit you may need other equipment such as:
- Traction bars/frame (Balkan beams)
- Pulleys
- Extra cord
- Prescribed number of weights
- Container for weights.

Applying simple skin traction requires two people, at least one of whom should be experienced in traction applications.
- Ascertain the need for either an adhesive or nonadhesive traction kit or appropriate bandages.
- Prepare the bed with appropriate Balkan beam bed frame and pulleys, and weights as prescribed. Some hospitals have special beds and cots with orthopaedic frames already attached.

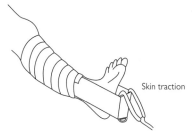
Skin traction

Fig. 8.2 Skin traction.
Oxford Handbook of Children's and Young People's Nursing, Glasper et al., (2006), p.505, with permission from Oxford University Press

- Provide appropriate information to the child and family members using a variety of methods. Involve a play specialist to provide distraction/preprocedural play when required.
- Ascertain the integrity of the skin. Check allergy status of the child with parent/guardian.
- Measure the traction extensions against the unaffected limb to avoid causing pain, making sure that you have left enough space to allow the child to plantar flex the foot without restriction when the spreader bar is inserted. Cut off the excess material with scissors.
- Apply bandage (not too tightly) starting just above the malleoli. Leave the knee free.
- Take the traction cords at the spreader and pass through the pulley at the end of the bed and attach securely to the prescribed weights.
- Elevate the foot of the bed to provide the counter traction, ensuring that the child does not slide down the bed too much.
- Ensure neurovascular observations are recorded to detect potential neurovascular impairment (compartment syndrome).

Always carry out neurovascular assessment to prevent a child in traction from developing a potential lifelong disability. Andrews (1990) describes the 5 P's of neurovascular assessment. These are:
- Pain
- Pallor
- Paraesthesia
- Pulselessness
- Paralysis

The first two points are early indicators, the final three are late signs of damage. Seek an urgent medical opinion if these early signs are apparent.

Further reading

Davis PD (1999) Principles of traction. *Journal of Orthopaedic Nursing*. 3:222–237.
Andrews LW (1990). Neurovascular assessment. *Advanced Clinical Care*. 6:5–7.
Buechsenschuetz K E, Mehlman C T, Shaw K J, Crawford A H, Immerman E B (2002). NHS Economic Evaluation Database (NHS EED). Femoral shaft fractures in children: traction and casting versus elastic stable intramedullary nailing. *Journal of Trauma* 53(5): 914–21.

① Bone infections

Introduction
Acute osteomyelitis is a potentially serious infection of the bone and marrow usually caused by pus-forming bacteria, and should be considered in any child who presents with fever and a limp and is generally unwell.

Classification criteria
Acute osteomyelitis is defined as a history of relevant symptoms of less than 14 days, and subacute osteomyelitis as a history of 14 days or more.

Incidence and ratio
Osteomyelitis can occur at any age, but is most frequent between the ages of 5 and 13 years. Recent evidence suggests a change in the epidemiology of acute and subacute osteomyelitis, which has some geographical variability. Any bacteria can cause osteomyelitis, but there appears to be a relationship between the age of the child and the bacteria responsible.
- 2:100 000 population
- The incidence is greater in boys than girls

Acute osteomyelitis: common causative organisms
- Gram +ve bacteria
  - *Staphylococcus aureus*
  - *Streptococcus pyogenes*
  - *Streptococcus pneumoniae*
- Gram −ve bacteria
  - *Haemophilus influenzae* type B
  - *E. coli*
  - *Pseudomonas aeruginosa*
  - *Proteus mirabilis*
- Gram −ve osteomyelitis is seen in children with sickle cell anaemia, and an infected umbilical stump may be the precursor to an acute episode in an infant.
- More rarely, fungi, viruses, or parasites may cause osteomyelitis, and tuberculosis should also be a consideration.

Pathophysiology
Infective emboli from the main infected source break away and travel to the small end of the arteries in the bone metaphysis, where the infective process becomes established. Due to the unique blood supply in childhood, acute osteomyelitis frequently affects the metaphyseal region of long bones, which is close to the growth plate or epiphysis, and a joint. The infective process initiates local bone destruction and abscess formation, which gradually exerts more pressure on the rigid structure of the bone. The pressure lifts and strips the periosteum; as the infection spreads underneath the periosteum this causes thrombosis of vessels and exacerbates bony necrosis. Eventually, the abscess will rupture into the subperiosteal space. In some instances the infection may cause a walled-off abscess, rather than an infiltrating infection. Occasionally, there are multiple foci, for example in disseminated staphylococcal or *H. influenzae* infection.

Osteomyelitis can be acquired from exogenous or haematogenous sources.

- Exogenous osteomyelitis is acquired by direct invasion of the bone from an external source such as the result of a penetrating wound, open fracture, contamination during surgery, or secondary invasion from overlying abscess or burns.
- Haematogenous osteomyelitis (via the blood stream) is commonly caused by organisms from pre-existing foci such as carbuncles, furuncles, skin abrasions, impetigo, respiratory tract infections, acute otitis media, tonsillitis, abscessed teeth, infected burns, or pyelonephritis. Other contributory factors may include immunosuppression, poor physical condition and malnourishment.
- Whilst the most common infecting organism has been reported to be *Staphylococcus aureus* in 80% of cases, more recent evidence from the USA would suggest that the spectrum is changing and in one third of cases no causative organism can be isolated. Fastidious organisms such as *Kingella kingae* may be responsible for a considerable proportion of cases of haematogenous osteomyelitis with a negative routine culture.

Signs and symptoms
- Severe pain
- History of recent infection, trauma, surgery or burns
- Reluctance to move affected limb (pseudoparesis) and decreased range of movements, which may include difficulty in sitting up if there is spinal involvement
- Warmth, erythema and localized swelling
- Reduced movement of neighbouring joint(s)
- Toxaemia and generally unwell
- Pyrexia
- Malaise and nausea

Differential diagnosis
- Septic arthritis
- Irritable hip
- Cellulitis
- Still's disease
- Sickle cell crisis
- Gaucher's disease

Immediate management
- Prompt and rigorous IV antibiotic therapy is commenced as soon as possible after initial blood culture. The choice of drug is influenced by the child's age and the likely causative organisms. The dosage must be high enough to ensure high blood and tissue levels, which penetrate bone and joint cavities. The drug regime is changed once the causative organism has been isolated.
- Current drug regimes following local protocol.
- After the initial clinical response, antibiotics are switched to the oral route and continued for a total of 6 weeks.

- Serial measurement of inflammatory markers such as C-reactive protein or sedimentation rate may be useful for monitoring treatment progress, coupled with clinical improvement in the child's condition.
- Failure to respond suggests a resistant organism or abscess formation.
- For infants who have not been immunized with the HiB vaccine, the drug of choice is a cephalosporin.
- Surgical treatment is performed if the condition fails to respond rapidly to antibiotic therapy.

Clinical investigations

- Full blood count: marked leukocytosis, elevated erythrocyte sedimentation rate (ESR).
- Blood culture. This will be positive in the early phase, and it is important diagnostically to establish causative organisms prior to commencing a definitive IV antibiotic regime.
- X-rays have limited diagnostic value as they are often negative (or show normal), and only reveal soft tissue swelling, as it takes between 7 and 10 days for subperiosteal new bone formation to occur.
- Bone scan.
- Ultrasound.

Nursing management

- Pain relief
- Rest and immobilization of the affected limb (backslab may be considered)
- 4-hourly monitoring of temperature and vital signs
- Monitoring fluid intake and output
- Child may be nauseous and/or vomiting
- Monitoring of IV site and cannula

Complications

- Septicaemia
- Chronic osteomyelitis
- Metastatic infection
- Septic arthritis
- Altered bone growth and growth-plate arrest
- Non-union of fractures
- Disability and deformity

Further reading

Chamley CA, Carson P, Randall D, Sandwell M (2005). Developmental Anatomy and Physiology of Children: A Practical Approach. London: Elsevier.
Royal College of Nursing (2007). Benchmarks for Children's Orthopaedic Nursing Care: RCN Guidance. London: RCN.
http://www.orthoseek.com/
http://www.orthoteers.co.uk

:☠: **Compartment syndrome**

Introduction
- Acute compartment syndrome occurs when swelling occurs within a closed fascial space.
- Because the swelling is contained, the pressure within the closed compartment rises.
- The rise in pressure reduces capillary perfusion below the level necessary for tissue perfusion.
- This results in muscle and nerve ischaemia, which will lead to muscle infarction and nerve damage if not treated promptly.

ALERT: Acute compartment syndrome is a limb-threatening emergency that requires prompt treatment

Causes
- Can occur with orthopaedic injuries, vascular injuries and soft tissue injuries.
- Commonest fractures associated with compartment syndrome are those of the tibial shaft and the shaft of the radius and ulna.
- Comminuted fractures are more prone to compartment syndrome.
- Can occur with open fractures.
- In children crush injuries to the foot may lead to foot compartment syndrome.

Signs and symptoms
- Pain out of proportion to the injury and that requires frequent strong analgesia.
- Pain that is made worse by passive stretching of the distal joints.
- A tense, swollen limb.
- Paraesthesia (pins and needles, loss of 2 point discrimination).
- Skin colour, temperature, capillary refill and distal pulses are all unreliable indicators of compartment syndrome.
- Pallor, loss of pulses and paralysis are very late, ominous signs.
- Children with associated head or spinal injuries (or those who are very young) may be unable to identify/verbalize the above signs, so a high index of suspicion must be maintained.
- Andrews (1990) describes the 5 P's of neurovascular assessment:
  - Pain (early indicator of damage)
  - Pallor
  - Paraesthesia
  - Pulselessness (late sign of damage)
  - Paralysis.

Document neurovascular assessment findings; this facilitates ongoing evaluation.

Immediate management
- Split any casts around the limb, including all padding, right down to the skin.
- Reduce/release traction on the limb.

- Release compressive bandaging.
- Obtain urgent orthopaedic assessment.
- Start regular monitoring of the child and the affected limb (every 15–30 minutes).
- Physical measurement of intracompartment pressure is available in most centres, and will be specifically helpful in young children or those whose conscious level is impaired.

⚠When compartment syndrome is suspected, do not elevate the limb. This has no effect on reducing the intracompartment pressure and may reduce arterial inflow, adversely affecting perfusion pressure.

Treatment
- Urgent fasciotomy may be required, so the child and parents should be prepared for the possibility of emergency surgery.

Complications
- Permanent injury to nerves and muscles resulting in impaired function, e.g. Volkmann's ischaemic contracture
- Rhabdomyolysis and renal failure
- Loss of the limb
- Death
- Cosmetic deformity from fasciotomy

Further reading
Paula R (2008). Compartment Syndrome, Extremity. http://emedicine.medscape.com/article/828456-overview. Accessed 24 December 2008

Shadgan B, Menon M, O'Brien PJ, Reid WD (2008) Diagnostic techniques in acute compartment syndrome of the leg. *J Orthop Trauma* 22:581–7

Andrews LW (1990) Neurovascular assessment. *Advanced Clinical Care* 6:5–7.

☹ Spinal injuries in children

Introduction
Spinal injuries are relatively uncommon in children, but they do occur, and their management, especially immediately following the injury, is crucial to prevent secondary damage to the spinal cord and spinal column.

Causes
Spinal injuries in children and young people commonly involve the upper part of the cervical spine; this is due to the neck muscles being weaker and not coping with any sudden movement of the child's heavy head, for example, following a severe acceleration-deceleration injury. Causes of spinal injury include:
- Falls (especially if child lands direct onto both feet or has fallen from three-times their own height or higher)
- Collisions (especially road traffic collisions/accidents)
- Sports injuries (e.g. diving, rugby, horse riding and trampolining)
- Non-accidental injury

The history and mechanism of injury must always be considered in relation to a spinal injury; any suspected injury or possible injury should be treated as such and the child should be immobilized

Signs and symptoms
- Weakness of limbs
- Numbness of limbs
- Pain in limbs
- Spinal pain
- Physical evidence of head and/or spinal trauma
- Altered consciousness level

Immediate management
Spinal immobilization
- The hospital play specialist can be invaluable in distracting distressed children.
- If cervical spine injury is suspected, the airway should be opened (if necessary) using a jaw thrust; do not use a chin lift/head tilt.
- Neutral in-line cervical spine immobilization should be commenced immediately post-injury and maintained until other methods of immobilization (cervical collars/head blocks/tapes/spinal board) have been placed in position.
- Children may require extra padding positioned around them when on spinal board to prevent movement of the body and head.
- Strapping should not be too tight as this causes discomfort, decreases circulation and compromises chest expansion and therefore breathing.
- Cervical collars alone are not adequate for immobilization; however, in paediatric practice, where the child is uncooperative, this may be the only immobilization method tolerated.
- Smaller children have a larger occiput, and if placed onto a board the head may be flexed forward; consider using a small amount of padding under the shoulders to return child's head to a neutral position.

Nursing management

- High flow oxygen delivery via nonrebreathe bag, to prevent hypoxia.
- Keep the child warm.
- Observe for vomit, blood or foreign body in the mouth; if present give gentle suction. A health care professional should be present at all times in case of vomiting and subsequent risk of aspiration.
- Commence observations: temperature, heart rate, respiratory rate, oxygen saturations and blood pressure.
- Neurological status: observe for any changes in consciousness level using paediatric approved scoring system.
- Administer pain relief.
- Explain to the family what is happening and what investigations are going to be performed (age appropriate explanations). Remember, the child may have been admitted into a busy Emergency Department (ED), the trauma team and paediatric registrar should be in attendance, and there may be other related activity around the child. The child will be immobilized and will not be able to see anything around them, and may be scared.

Examination, investigations and treatment

NB: the child should remain in cervical spine immobilization (if possible) until he/she has been examined by a senior ED doctor.

There are two types of spinal injury:
- Primary: occurs at the moment of impact
- Secondary: due to swelling, ischaemia and bony fragments being dislodged.

To enable the doctor to examine the child (and also to remove the child from the ambulance spinal board) the child will require 'log-rolling':
- For a smaller child, 3 people are required
- For an older child, 4 people are required
- Immobilization of the cervical spine is required throughout
- An experienced member of staff will hold the child's head, and they have control: every member of the team should be aware of their directions during log-rolling (the leader should ensure everyone is aware of this before commencing the log-roll).
- The doctor will physically examine the child's neck and back; the child (if appropriate) will tell them if they have any pain on examination.
- Once log-rolled for examination the blocks and tapes should be re-positioned.

The NICE guidelines for Head Injury (NICE 2007) recommend the following investigations:
- Plain X-rays are initial choice of investigation (two views for children under the age of 10)
- CT scan, dependent on child's age: children under the age of 10 should have a CT scan considered if they show signs of severe head injury (GCS ≤8), if there is a strong suspicion of injury despite normal plain X-ray film, or if the plain films are inadequate.

Treatment may include spinal surgery, neurological surgery and possible transfer to a specialist centre or Paediatric Intensive Care Unit for further care.

Complications/prognosis
- Increase in secretions (requiring suction to maintain airway patency)
- Muscle weakness
- Shock
- Haemorrhage
- Urinary retention
- Pressure sores from being immobilized

Complications are reduced and prognosis is enhanced with good care and management during all stages—prehospital, acute care and rehabilitation.

Further reading
Sheerin F (2005) Spinal cord injury: causation and pathophysiology. *Emergency Nurse* 12(9). February (author has produced three articles in this series: March 2005, issue 10, and December 2004, issue 8)

JR CALC (2004) Clinical Practice Guidelines – UK Ambulance Service (www.nelh.nhs.uk/emergency) (for prehospital care)

NICE (2007) Head Injury. NICE Clinical Guideline 56. London: NICE

Sensory problems

⑦ Management of eye problems

Introduction

There are only two types of eye injury and one type of eye infection that are considered paediatric ophthalmic emergencies:

- chemical injury
- trauma (penetrating/perforating)
- orbital cellulitis.

NB: eye injuries should whereever possible be managed by an experienced practitioner.

Also included under eye injuries are:

- blunt trauma (and how different structures are affected)
- abrasions (corneal and conjunctival)
- foreign bodies, including subtarsal (under upper eyelid)
- exposure to glue, typing correction fluid, etc.

Infections and inflammatory problems are listed in order of eye structure (after orbital cellulitis):

- lids
- conjunctiva
- cornea, including contact lens-related
- inflammation of iris

Immediate management

In the management of any eye problem the first two things to be done are:

- history taking
- testing and recording of visual acuity by Snellen chart, Kay Picture Test, or Sheridan–Gardiner cards.

After the eye examination itself you will be able to decide on:

- how to write down your findings
- what to report/handover to the ophthalmolgy team
- the appropriate treatment/action to take.

Be aware of nonaccidental injuries/possible signs of child abuse. If suspected, follow local child protection (CP) guidelines, e.g.:

- refer to paediatrician
- alert CP team.

Anatomy and physiology

See Fig. 9.1.

History taking

Where possible, ask the child as well as the parent what has happened.

- What happened?
- When did it happen?
- Where did it happen?
- Was any force involved?
- Has anything been done to the eye already?
- Any previous eye problems or operations?

Visual acuity assessment

An assessment of vision is a fundamental part of an ocular examination; it is undertaken regardless of whether vision is mentioned as part of the

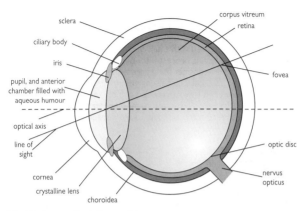

Fig. 9.1 Cross sectional diagram of the eye

chief complaint, as it measures the function of the eye and gives some idea of the patient's disability. It may also have considerable medicolegal implications in young people, as in the case of ocular damage at school/work or after an assault.

* Once a child can talk and recognize simple pictures, you can probably check their vision using a Kay Picture Test (Fig. 9.2) or Sheridan–Gardiner cards when available.
* Once a child can recognize letters you can use a single letter Snellen chart.

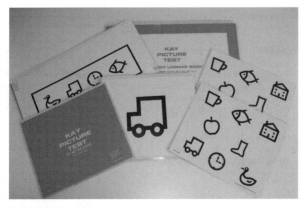

Fig. 9.2 Kay Picture Test

- Once a child is confident with letters, they should manage the normal Snellen chart, but you might have to point to the lower letters individually if they become confused.
- Cooperation is increased with small children if an element of play is introduced to the testing process—try to make it a game!
- If the child is in pain, consider using a local anaesthetic drop such as proxymetacaine 0.5% before checking vision.
- If vision is below 6/9 it is worth trying a pinhole test. Place a pinhole occluder over the child's nose, get them to hold it in place if they can, and ask them to read the chart again to see if vision improves (see Fig. 9.3).

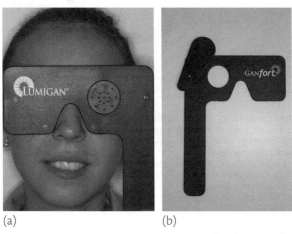

(a)   (b)

Fig. 9.3a and b Using a pinhole occulder

Helpful hints for examining children's eyes
- Show them the torch light and let them play with it if appropriate.
- Explain what you are going to do and what you are going to use, e.g. ophthalmoscope, portable slit lamp.
- Use of engaging toys can be a great method of getting small children to look where you need them to; ask parents or an assistant to hold them for you.

How to record your findings
- It is easiest to follow a logical sequence each time; see Table 9.1 for an example grid for reporting sequential examination.

Table 9.1 Example grid for reporting a sequential examination

Right		Left
	Lids	
	Conjunctiva	
	Cornea	
	Anterior chamber	
	Pupils	

Reporting your findings

The ophthalmologist will want to know the patient's vision, and what you have seen when you examined the eye. Even if you do not know what the specific diagnosis is, if you can clearly describe what you are seeing in relation to the structures of the eye, the ophthalmologist will be more likely to understand what you are telling them. Make sure you tell them about any history of force with the injury.

Further reading

Fraser S, Asaria R, Kon C (2001) Eye Know How. London: BMJ Books.
Simcock P, Fallows J (2001) Patient pictures: clinical drawings for your patients: ophthalmology. Abingdon: Health Press.

☼: Eye injuries

Introduction

Eye injuries during childhood can be serious and can cause loss of vision. The causes of eye injuries are varied. Throughout this section the correct terminology for drops and ointment will be used: Oc = ointment and G = drops.

NB: eye injuries should wherever possible be managed by an experienced practitioner.

Chemical injuries to the eye

- Chemical injuries to the eye (burns): alkaline substances cause more serious damage to the eye than acidic or thermal injuries.
- Common causes include spray cleaners, perfumes/deodorants, nail polishes, and washing detergent capsules (NB: these are very alkaline).

Immediate management

- Ask what chemical was involved and check pH in both eyes if possible; normal pH is 7.5.
- Irrigate for 10–20 minutes with normal saline:
  - warm the saline (unless a thermal burn)
  - place child/adolescent in reclining chair (or on parent's lap) or wrap child in blanket on a couch
  - rest patient's head on (affected) side with receiver to catch irrigated fluid
  - use an apron/towels under affected side to keep patient dry
  - run a little normal saline onto face, under affected eye, to get patient used to the temperature
  - get child to look up and run solution into bottom lid
  - get child to look down, then evert upper eyelid:
    - gently pull upper lid lashes away from the globe
    - using a glass rod or fingertip, press down gently just above the upper lid crease while lifting lid up and back
    - this exposes the underside of lid; irrigate under the lid and irrigate the eyeball from above
  - ask the child to look up and blink to get lid back in position
  - ask child/adolescent to look left, right, up, and down while you irrigate.
- Wait 5 minutes then recheck pH
- Irrigate with further normal saline if pH not within normal limits
- While waiting between irrigating and rechecking pH take full history by asking:
  - what happened and how, and what chemical was involved
  - when did it happen
  - which eye is affected
  - irrigated already/action already taken prior to arrival
  - check and record visual acuity (VA)
- Refer immediately to ophthalmology

Superglue or cyanoacrylate injuries to the eye

Introduction
These glues are commonly sold under the trade name of Superglue, and are widely and freely available.

Immediate management
The glue may just stick lashes together, and if not causing pain treat with liberal amounts of chloramphenicol ointment and frequent warm wet compresses to encourage glue to come free.

If causing pain, the hardened glue may be rubbing the cornea and child should be referred immediately to an ophthalmologist.

Tear gas/pepper spray injuries to the eye (irritation should only last 15 minutes)

Introduction
Pepper sprays made from capsaicin (hot chilli pepper), used for self defence, are illegal in the United Kingdom; however, such sprays are freely available for purchase on the internet.

Immediate management
- DO NOT irrigate.
- Blow air into eyes (with fan/cool hairdryer) but keep yourself away from direction of flow of air.
- Examine the eye as outlined above after the instillation of fluorescein sodium 2% eyedrops.
- Prophylactic chloramphenicol 0.5% once daily for 5 days.

Trauma: penetrating/perforating injury to the eye

Introduction
Penetrating injuries to the eye may occur in children for a variety reasons.

Immediate management
- Determine the history of the event and attempt to ascertain the force or speed of injury, e.g. hitting stones with a hammer, helping/watching in a workshop.
- Record visual acuity (VA).
- With pen torch, examine eye. Determine whether any parts look abnormal (compare with other eye), in particular whether the cornea looks damaged, the pupil appears an abnormal shape, or the depth of the anterior chamber between the cornea and the iris looks shallow. Suspect penetration/perforation injury if any of these signs appear, or if strongly suggested from history.
- Lie the child down and cover eye with shield (taped on), NOT pad/patch (Fig. 9.4).
- Send to Eye Casualty/Ophthalmology Unit immediately.
- Check tetanus status if tetanus-prone injury.

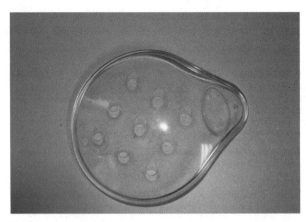

Fig. 9.4 Universal eye shield

Blunt trauma injury to the eye

Introduction

This type of trauma is commonly caused by impact injury during contact sports or fights

Immediate management

Establish history of the event and check visual acuity. If child is unable to open eye, check to see whether the child can tell when a light is shone at the affected eye.

Check tetanus status if appropriate.

Examine eye for injuries from the outside in, structure by structure:

- Orbit: possible fracture
  - Feel along orbital rim.
  - Check eye movements for restriction, pain on upward gaze or double vision.
  - Check for decreased sensation of skin just below the eye compared to the other side.
  - Suspect if eye looks sunken or if there is severe bruising around the eye.
  - Advise not to blow nose.
  - Order X-rays and refer to maxillofacial team and ophthalmology.
- Lids
  - Note bruising and swelling.
  - Check depth of any lacerations and location, especially if involving lid margin and/or tear duct/punctum.
  - Irrigate any burns with cold saline.

- Conjunctiva
  - Subconjunctival haemorrhage (bright red patch of blood under the conjunctiva).
  - Location of any lacerations or abrasions.
  - Draw diagrams.
- Cornea
  - Check for abrasions/lacerations using fluorescein solution.
  - If fluorescein seems to flow away from defect this indicates perforating injury, also indicated by iris tissue protruding through wound.
  - Cover eye with a shield, not a pad, and do not apply pressure on globe.
  - Refer immediately to ophthalmology.
- Iris/anterior chamber
  - Check for hyphaema or blood in anterior chamber covering part of iris detail.
- Pupil
  - Check pupil shape.
  - Pupil peaked (pointed or tear drop shape) indicates possible globe rupture.
  - Enlarged unreactive pupil could be traumatic mydriasis.
  - Check pupil reactions.
- Be aware of knock-on effects to rest of globe
  - On lens (traumatic cataract).
  - Retina (bruising 'commotio' and/or retinal detachment).
  - Check for flashing lights and floaters in vision, or missing areas of vision.
- Give oral analgesia.
- DO NOT DILATE the child's eyes.
- Refer to Eye Casualty/Ophthalmology Unit, telephoning first with history.

Foreign body

Immediate management
- Ascertain history and assess visual acuity
- Get child comfortable, e.g. on parent's lap with parent seated in chair
- Position child in good light and wear magnifying spectacles
- Instil drop of topical anaesthesia (proxymetacaine 0.5%) first then fluorescein 2%, or use a combined drop
- Evert lid (see 'Chemical injuries to the eye')
- If subtarsal foreign body (under the eye lid)
  - Remove foreign body with moistened (by normal/saline) cotton bud (perform subtarsal 'sweep')
  - Examine with blue light for corneal abrasion
  - One dose of Oc chloramphenicol 1%
- If corneal
  - Refer to ophthalmology department

Corneal abrasion

Immediate management
- Instill one dose G fluorescein 2% and G proxymetacaine 0.5%
- Examine with blue light
- Oc chloramphenicol 1% three times daily for 5 days
- Will require regular oral analgesia for the next 24–48 hours as this condition is painful
- Refer to Eye Casualty for review within 2 days
  (The NHS Clinical Knowledge Summaries,
  Corneal Superficial injury guidance)

Cigarette burns

Immediate management
- Local anaesthetic drops to facilitate examination.
- Check history and visual acuity.
- Irrigate eye gently with saline, as there are often fragments of ash in the eye. Use this opportunity to remove child's upper body clothing with child's and parent/guardian's consent; this will enable you to check for other burns or scars on the body, as cigarette burns can be a sign of abuse.
- Examine eye with G fluorescein and any abrasion using procedure outlined above.
- Arrange review with Eye Casualty or Ophthalmology within 48 hours.

Ticks on lids

Immediate management
- Needs removal as close to skin surface as possible with tick remover or fine forceps, without applying pressure to body of tick. Best done by ophthalmology.
- May need to consider advice regarding Lyme disease.

Lice on lashes

Immediate management
- Can be smothered with simple eye ointment or picked off with forceps
- Some medicated treatments may be useable on the lashes and brows
- Bear in mind that pubic lice are more common than head lice on eyelashes and the child should be referred for formal child protection assessment

Laser penlight 'injury'

- Laser pointers are unlikely to cause retinal damage unless shone directly in the eye for several seconds. However, to assess the damage a dilated retinal examination may be required.
- If the child complains of a persistent after-image effect (like the one you see after a photographic flash or after looking directly at a light source), refer to an ophthalmologist for review within 48 hours.

Further reading

Elhers JP, Shah CP (eds) (2008) The Wills Eye Manual: Office and Emergency Room Diagnosis and Treatment of Eye Disease. London: Lippincott Williams & Wilkins.

Webb LA (1995) Eye Emergencies. Oxford: Butterworth Heinemann.

http://www.library.nhs.uk/eyes/SearchResults.aspx?searchText=eye%20injuries&tabID=288

The NHS Clinical Knowledge Summaries, Corneal Superficial injury guidance. http://www.cks.nhs. uk/home.

☼ Eye infections

NB: eye infections should, wherever possible, be managed by an experienced practitioner.

Introduction

There are a range of eye infections that may present during childhood that may require emergency management.

Orbital cellulitis

This is an ocular emergency and can be fatal in a child.

Signs and symptoms
- Swollen lids and swelling around eye, often a deep purple-red.
- Swelling tense to gentle touch.
- Forward protrusion of the eye ball (proptosis).
- Purulent discharge from eye.
- Pyrexia.
- Conjunctival swelling and injection (nonuniform redness).
- Restriction or pain in eye movements.
- Child unwell.
- May have just had conjunctivitis/bad cold/sinusitis.

Immediate management
- Take history and record visual acuity.
- Check temperature.
- Refer urgently to ophthalmology registrar and ENT registrar (warn parents of likely admission to hospital).
- Will need urgent intravenous antibiotics as soon as diagnosis is confirmed by ophthalmologist.

Preseptal cellulitis

This is a complication of cyst, insect bite or sting, or infected spot on eyelid.

Signs and symptoms
- May have inflamed cyst/lump on lid, which does not restrict movement
- May have slightly raised temperature
- May also have conjunctivitis

Immediate management
- Take history and record visual acuity
- Check temperature
- Refer to paediatrician/ophthalmologist for oral antibiotics as per local protocol

Blepharitis

Signs and symptoms
- Red-rimmed eyelid edges, may be sore/itchy, child may rub eyes
- May have frequent conjunctivitis and/or lid cysts

Immediate management

- Instruct parent to clean eyelid edges, first with warm compresses and then cotton buds moistened with diluted baby shampoo (one part shampoo: three parts boiled water).
- G chloramphenicol 0.5% drops 4 times a day for 5 days if concurrent conjunctivitis.
- Advise parent/child that this is a chronic condition and may require referral to an ophthalmology outpatient department via their GP.

Cysts on eyelid

Immediate management

- Advise warm compresses several times a day.
- Advise massage of lid edges/cyst over steam for 10 minutes, 4 times a day.
- Apply Oc chloramphenicol 1% to site twice a day for 2 weeks.
- Refer patient to eye outpatients, via GP, if not resolving in 6 weeks.
- May require incision and curettage by ophthalmologist.
- If conjunctivitis present, apply Oc chloramphenicol 1% 3 times a day for 5 days.

Styes on lids

Immediate management

- May be able to release pustule at base of eyelash by removing this eyelash.
- If not, apply hot steam bathing and compresses as with cysts.
- Oc chloramphenicol ointment 1% 3 times a day for 1–2 weeks.

Conjunctivitis (bacterial)

- Red eye, purulent discharge, child complaining of itching/soreness.

Immediate management

- Treat with G chloramphenicol 0.5% 4 times a day for 5 days, or fusidic acid twice a day for 1 week.
- Give parent and child advice on preventing contagion, e.g. not sharing towels, flannels, etc.

Conjunctivitis (viral)

- Symptoms are red eye, watery discharge, may complain of itching/ soreness/foreign body-sensation (especially if cornea also involved, as in adenoviral conjunctivitis), positive pre-auricular node. Child may have had recent cold/flu.

Immediate management

- G hypromellose (artificial tears) between 4 and 6 times daily for duration of viral infection (usually 7–10 days) to keep eye comfortable.
- G chloramphenicol 0.5% 4 times a day for 5 days if evidence of/ prophylactically for secondary bacterial infection.
- Warn child and parents about spread of virus, and advise on not sharing towels, etc.
- If worsening symptoms (e.g. photophobia) refer to Eye Casualty.

Conjunctivitis (chlamydial)

Remember that chlamydia is a sexually transmitted disease.
Chlamydial conjunctivitis is found in:
- Neonates (newborn babies within first 28 days of life), contracted during descent of birth canal of infected mother
- Sexually active adolescents
- Sexually abused children.

Immediate management
- Suspect if any of the above or if bacterial/viral conjunctivitis excluded/ not responding to treatment.
- Refer to ophthalmology (where swabs will be taken and condition treated, and babies will receive eye ointment and oral erythromycin).
- Advise parents of neonates to attend genito-urinary clinic for testing and treatment.
- Refer to safeguarding team if appropriate.

NB: ophthalmia neonatorum (a purulent conjuctivitis within the first 28 days of life) is a notifiable infectious disease under the Public Health (Control of Diseases) Act 1984.

Acute allergic response/allergic conjunctivitis

Presents as grossly swollen conjunctiva, often only slightly red; may also have swollen lids.

Immediate management
- Irrigate with 100mL (unwarmed) normal saline
- Oral antihistamine without delay
- Antihistamine drops such as Otrivine-Antistin® may be administered

Corneal infections, 'keratitis'

Contact lens-related, patient presents with painful red eye, photophobia and watering, and may have white lesion (ulcer) visible on the corneal surface.

Immediate management
- If white area visible do not stain with fluorescein
- Refer urgently to ophthalmology for treatment
- Advise young person not to use contact lenses for at least 2 weeks

Herpes simplex keratitis (HSK) (cold sores)

Presents as red conjunctiva mainly around iris, and patient may have photosensitivity and history of cold sores elsewhere (e.g. lips/nose) either recently or currently. May or may not have significant pain as HSK desensitizes cornea.

Immediate management
- Dendritic (branch like) ulcer visible on staining with G fluorescein 2%
- Refer to ophthalmology for treatment (with Oc aciclovir 3% 5 times daily)

Iritis (inflammation, not infection)
- Inflammation of iris, often associated with juvenile arthritis (or ankylosing spondylitis in young adults).

- Patient complaining of aching eye, photophobia, visual acuity impaired/ down.

On examination:
- redness is around the cornea/iris, known as circumcorneal or ciliary injection
- pupil may be of different size to other eye, or may be irregular in shape.

Immediate management
- Refer to ophthalmology as soon as possible

Further reading

Elkington A, Khaw R (1988) ABC of Eyes. BMJ Publishing Group
Stollery R, Shaw M, Lee A (2005) Ophthalmic Nursing (3rd edn). Blackwell Science.
www.patient.co.uk/doctor/Orbital-Cellulitis.htm
http://www.library.nhs.uk/eyes/SearchResults.aspx?searchText=eye%20infections&tabID=288
Elhers JP, Shah CP (eds) (2008) The Wills Eye Manual. Wolters Kluwer/Lippincott Williams & Wilkins
Fraser S, Asaria R, Kon C (2001) Eye Know How. BMJ Publishing Group
Simcock P (2001) Patient pictures: clinical drawings for your patients: ophthalmology. MSD
Vaughan DG, Asbury T, Riordan-Eva P (1992) General Ophthalmology (14th edn). Lange Medical Publications
Webb LA (1995) Eye Emergencies. Butterworth Heinemann

⑦ Foreign body in the ear

Introduction
Children may place various objects in their ears, such as toys or beads. This is a relatively common occurrence.

Signs and symptoms
- Change in normal hearing function
- Discharge from the ear
- Pain
- Alteration in balance
- Feeling dizzy

Identification
- May have been witnessed
- Suggestive history, e.g. playing with a small object

Immediate action
- There is no urgency for the foreign body to be removed, unless it is likely to corrode or be harmful, e.g. a battery.

Investigations
- The child may present with ear discharge, and the foreign body is seen when examined using an otoscope.

Nursing management
- Foreign bodies in ears can be difficult to remove. Children will often only allow one attempt at removal, so it is advisable for it to be removed by expert hands. It is usually best done in an ear, nose and throat department.
- Organic material should not be removed by syringing as the water makes the material swell and therefore even more difficult to remove.
- If there is any suspected trauma, infection, or perforation to the tympanic membrane the child may require antibiotic ear drops.
- If the foreign body cannot be removed in clinic, it may need to be done under general anaesthetic. Although usually not an emergency, a foreign body in the ear needs to be removed as soon as possible.
- It is important to ask the child and parent/carer if there has been any change to the child's hearing; if so, audiometric testing would be advisable.
- If the child is in any pain, prescribed analgesia should be given.

Further reading
Bluestone C, Stool S. Cuneyt A, Arjmand E, Casselbrandt M, Donar J, Yellon R (2003) Pediatric Otolaryngology. Fourth Edition. Saunders.
Drake-Lee A (1996). Clinical Otorhinolaryngology. Churchill Livingstone.
http://www.patient.co.uk/doctor/Foreign-bodies-in-the-Ear.htm

⑦ Examination of the ear

History taking

- Identify the child's symptoms and take a careful history.
- Questions will depend on the child's problem.
- Explain each step of any procedure of examination, and ensure that the patient and parent/carer understand and give consent.
- It is important to ascertain the child's level of hearing. If the child is old enough, you could ask the child questions such as whether they have problems hearing at home, or whether they can hear their teacher at school. You can ask the parent or carer what they think about the child's hearing. It is often useful to ask the parent or carer how the child is performing in school, as often teachers pick up a hearing deficit.
- Is there any discharge from the ear canal? Questions to ask include:
  - Does the discharge affect both ears?
  - What is its quantity?
  - What is its colour?
  - Is it sticky?
  - Is it painful or painless?
  - Is it wax?
- Is there any pain? Questions to ask include:
  - Where is it localized?
  - Is it bilateral or unilateral?
  - Is there itching?
  - Is there discharge?
  - If so, did it commence with the pain?
  - Was the pain relieved by the discharge?
  - Is the pain referred?
  - Is there pain and/or swelling behind the pinna?

Examination

- Ensure that the older child is sitting comfortably, and that you maintain privacy.
- A young child may sit on his/her parent/carer's knee for the examination, but if that is not possible, another carer can assist. The best position for the examination is if the child sits sideways on the parent's knee with the ear facing the examiner. The parent/carer should then be advised to place one of their hands gently on the top of the child's head and their other hand on the child's shoulder. This position is comfortable for all concerned, and is reassuring for the child.
- First examine the pinna, outer meatus and adjacent scalp by direct light and check for scars from previous surgery. Examine both pinnae. Look at the size, shape and position of each pinna. A pinna that is small, unusual in shape, or unusually low down on the face could be variations of the norm, but may indicate a congenital disorder/syndrome.
  - Is the ear red and inflamed, and are there signs of trauma or possible infection?
  - Is it deformed due to previous trauma?
  - Is there any damage to the earlobes from earrings or studs?
  - Is there any scaling or cracking of the skin, associated with scaling of the scalp or eyebrow region (possible seborrhoeic eczema).

- Gently pull the pinna upwards and backwards (in infants downwards and backwards) to straighten the meatus. Any localized infection or inflammation will cause this procedure to be quite painful. Common causes of pain might be a boil (furuncle) or a fungal infection in the meatus. Remember that the skin lining in the meatus is very delicate and sensitive.
- Holding the otoscope as you would a pen, with your little finger resting against the patient's face, insert the specula gently into the meatus, using the largest size specula that will fit comfortably in the ear.
- Can you see the eardrum or is it obscured by wax? Earwax is a normal physiological substance that protects the ear canal. The quantity produced varies between individuals. If the earwax obscures the view of the tympanic membrane, the wax should be removed by an experienced practitioner.
- Carefully check the ear canal and the eardrum. The normal eardrum has a pearly grey appearance and you should be able to see the handle of the malleus in the middle ear through the drum. It is often possible to make out the long process of the incus. In a normal drum there is a reflection of light, called a cone of light, extending from the handle to the lower part of the drum, the pars tensa.
- The ear cannot be judged to be completely normal until the entire eardrum has been seen. You may need to ask the patient to move his/her head to see into the roof of the meatus (pars flaccida and pars tensa). The normal appearance of the membrane varies and can only be learned by practice. Practice will lead to recognition of abnormalities.
- Methodically inspect all parts of the meatus and eardrum by varying the angle of the speculum. Carefully check the condition of the external auditory meatus as you withdraw the otoscope.
- Communicate with the child and parent.
- Record findings.

Further reading

Bluestone C, Stool S, Cuneyt A, Arjmand E, Casselbrandt M, Donar J, Yellon R (2003). Pediatric Otolaryngology. Fourth Edition. Saunders
Wormald P, Browning G (1996). Otoscopy - a structured approach. Arnold.

① **Acute otitis media**

Introduction

Otitis media is the generic term for inflammation of the middle ear. Subcategories of otitis media include acute otitis media, otitis media with effusion (glue ear) and chronic suppurative otitis media. Along with the nose and throat, the middle ear is often mildly inflamed when a child has a cold. Otitis media is common in children, because the Eustachian tube is relatively short, making it easy for infections to spread from the nose and throat. In the United Kingdom about 30% of children visit their GP with acute otitis media per year.

Incidence
- White children are more commonly affected than black children.
- Boys are more commonly affected than girls.
- Children with craniofacial abnormalities or Down's syndrome are at greater risk.
- There is an increased risk of children from lower socioeconomic groups being affected by acute otitis media.
- Children who have enlarged tonsils and adenoids have a greater risk of being affected.
- There is a lower incidence of otitis media among breast-fed children.
- Recurrent episodes of acute otitis media or chronic otitis media in young children increase the risk of hearing impairment.

Causes
The most common bacterial causes of acute otitis media are *Streptococcus pneumoniae*, *Haemophilis influenzae*, and *Moraxella catarrhalis*.

Signs and symptoms
- Rapid in onset.
- Often associated with a common cold.
- Child presents with a fever, irritability, crying, and sometimes vomiting and diarrhoea.
- Child may pull at their ears, showing signs of otalgia, and on inspection the tympanic membrane will be red and inflamed.
- The pain is acute, severe, and deep in the ear.
- Often there is an effusion behind the tympanic membrane. If the effusion persists beyond 3 months, it is known as otitis media with effusion.

Immediate management
- When examined the normal appearance of the tympanic membrane is translucent with visible bony landmarks and the cone of reflective light should be identifiable. A few blood vessels may run down the handle of the malleus, but there should not be blood vessels on the tympanic membrane itself. Radial blood vessels are a sign of an effusion in the middle ear.
- If there is an acute otitis media present, one may see a bulging tympanic membrane with loss of visible bony landmarks.

- The diagnosis of acute otitis media is based on changes in the tympanic membrane with regards to colour (red or yellow), opacity, contour, the light reflex, and mobility (if tested).
- If there is a perforation of the tympanic membrane a discharge may be present and otalgia is often relieved as pressure subsides (www.cks. library.nhs.uk).

Differential diagnosis

- Ear pain with discharge could be a sign of a foreign body in situ.
- Eustachian tube dysfunction can cause transient ear pain, but the tympanic membrane is normal.
- Ear pain can be confused with dental pain.

Nursing management

- In about 80% of children the condition resolves without antibiotic treatment in about 3 days.
- In acute otitis media, antibiotics should not be given routinely.
- There are exceptions, however: all children under 6 months, children between 6 months and 2 years if diagnosis certain, if the child has bilateral acute otitis media, or if the child has a systemic illness (www. cks.library.nhs.uk)
- Antibiotics such as amoxicillin may be used for 5 days.
- Analgesia such as paracetamol or ibuprofen may be used to reduce the pain.
- Some children will have a persistent effusion which needs to be monitored on a 3 monthly basis. If this does not resolve and it is affecting the child's hearing and development, insertion of grommets may be indicated.

Complications

- Complications are rare, but they include hearing loss and acute mastoiditis, which may lead to meningitis and/or cerebral abscess. In this case a cortical mastoidectomy and drainage of pus would be indicated.

Further reading

Barnes K (2003). Paediatrics – A Clinical Guide for Nurse Practitioners. Elselvier Science
Bluestone C, Stool S. Cuneyt A, Arjmand E, Casselbrandt M, Donar J, Yellon R (2003). Pediatric Otolaryngology. Fourth Edition. Saunders.
www.nice.org.uk - Surgical management of otitis media with effusion in children
www.cks.library.nhs.uk

① Perforated eardrum

Introduction
- A perforated eardrum means there is a hole in the eardrum, between the middle ear cavity and the external ear canal.
- A perforation in the eardrum can occur spontaneously, following infection, or following an injury.

Signs and symptoms
- Ear ache or discomfort
- Discharge
- Tinnitus

Immediate identification
- A hole in the eardrum can be identified by looking into the ear canal with an otoscope.

Immediate management
- If the child is in pain, prescribed analgesia should be given.
- If the child has a discharging ear, they should see a doctor as they may require antibiotic ear drops.

Nursing management
- Quite often a hole in the eardrum may heal itself.
- Sometimes it does not cause any problems.
- However, a perforation in the eardrum may lead to recurrent ear infections with a discharge from the ear.
- The child and parent should be advised to keep the ear affected dry while washing their hair or swimming.
- There is an operation available to repair the perforation, which is called a 'myringoplasty'. This is usually done when the child is in their teenage years. The older the child is the greater the success of the operation. www.entuk.org.

Complications
- Risk of otitis media.

Further reading
Bluestone C, Stool S. Cuneyt A, Arjmand E, Casselbrandt M, Donar J, Yellon R (2003). Pediatric Otolaryngology. Fourth Edition. Saunders.
Wormald P, Browning G (1996). Otoscopy - a structured approach. Arnold.
www. nhs.uk/Conditions/Perforated-eardrum/Pages/ Symptoms.aspx

⑦ Removal of foreign body from the nose

Introduction

Children may place various objects in their nose such as toys or beads. This is a relatively common occurrence in children between 1 and 4 years old.

Immediate identification

- May have been witnessed.
- Suggestive history, e.g. playing with a small object.

Immediate management

- Ensure that the child can breathe. If the child has any difficulty with breathing at all, you need to seek immediate medical attention.

Symptoms

- In some cases, nobody has witnessed the child putting a foreign body in their nose. However, a child who presents with an ongoing unilateral nasal discharge is likely to have a foreign body in their nostril and should be treated as such until proved otherwise. The discharge may be purulent or bloody.
- If the child has had a foreign body in a nostril for some time, such as sponge, it is likely to smell offensive.

Nursing management

- Although generally not an emergency, a foreign body in the nose needs to be removed as soon as possible.
- Removing such objects needs considerable skill and it is usually best done in an ear, nose, and throat department by a specialist.
- If no foreign body is seen but the history is convincing, an examination under anaesthetic is necessary.

Further reading

Bluestone C, Stool S. Cuneyt A, Arjmand E, Casselbrandt M, Donar J, Yellon R (2003). Pediatric Otolaryngology. Fourth Edition. Saunders.
Drake-Lee A (1996). Clinical Otorhinolaryngology. Churchill Livingstone.
www.gpnotebook.co.uk/simplepage.cfm?ID=825556999

ⓘ **Fractured nose**

Introduction
This is a fracture of the bone over the bridge of the nose and is the commonest facial fracture. This injury is usually caused by blunt trauma such as when the child or young person sustains injury during play, sports, accidents, fights, and falls. It is sometimes difficult to tell whether the nose is broken, and in some cases swelling can make the nose look crooked even when not broken.

Signs and symptoms
- Tenderness when touching the nose
- Swelling of the nose or face
- Bruising of the nose or under the eyes (black eye)
- Deformity of the nose (crooked nose)
- Nosebleed
- When touching the nose, a crunching or crackling sound or sensation like that of rubbing hair between two fingers
- Pain and difficulty breathing out of the nostrils

Immediate management
- Ensure the child is safe
- Ensure the child can breathe adequately
- If the child cannot breathe, follow resuscitation procedures (ABC) and seek immediate medical advice
- Manage any epistaxis accordingly

Examination and investigations
- The diagnosis of a fracture is difficult to make at the time of the injury (unless there is obvious deformity) because of bruising and soft tissue injury. Review by ENT after 5–7 days is recommended to confirm the diagnosis of a fracture for medicolegal reasons and to decide on management (www.entuk.org).
- X-rays are not required to diagnose the fracture. The diagnosis is clinical, observing tenderness and mobility of the nasal bones (www. entuk.org).

Assessment and treatment
- The decision to manipulate a nasal fracture in children is often difficult. If the child has an adequate nasal airway bilaterally and the nose is not too misshapen, often it is better to leave things well alone. The reason for this is the nose changes shape up until the age of 16–17, and the long term results may not be good.
- Manipulation must take place within 14 days following the injury, and the patient and parent must be made aware that the deformity may not be corrected completely. Any residual deformity after manipulation may require more surgery 12 months or more after the injury.

Nursing management/discharge advice

- Place some ice wrapped in a cloth over the nose for about 15 minutes at a time. Repeat several times throughout the day. Commence as soon after the injury as possible and continue for 1–2 days to reduce pain and swelling. Do not apply the ice directly to the skin.
- Take analgesia to reduce pain.
- Be aware of nonaccidental injuries/possible signs of child abuse. If suspected follow local Child Protection (CP) guidelines, e.g.:
  - refer to paediatrician
  - alert CP team

Further reading

Drake-Lee A (1996). Clinical Otorhinolaryngology. Churchill Livingstone.
Wetmore R, Muntx H, McGill T, Potsic W, Healy G, Lusk R (2000). Pediatric Otolaryngology. Thieme.
www.entuk.org

☼ Epistaxis

Introduction

Epistaxis is defined as acute haemorrhage from one or both nostrils, the nasal cavity, or the nasopharynx. This can range from mild oozing to severe blood loss. The rich supply of blood vessels in the nose predisposes it to bleeding. This is exacerbated by removal of crusts from the mucous membrane, infection, trauma, or coagulation disorders.

Causes

- Epistaxis is common in children and is usually caused by damage to blood vessels in the nose caused by small fingers!
- Other possible causes include infections and allergies, or objects (foreign bodies) being inserted in the nose.
- Much more rarely, it may be a sign of a blood coagulation problem.

Immediate prehospital management

- Ensure the safety of the child and carer.
- Reassure child and carer.
- Sit the child upright on a chair, with the head tilted forwards so that the blood does not run back into the throat.
- Identify the Kiesselbach plexus, or the Little area: this is the soft part of the nose, and represents a region in the anteroinferior third of the nasal septum where all three of the chief blood supplies to the internal nose converge. Pinch between the thumb and finger for at least 10 minutes. Squeeze firmly and do not let go until the 10 minutes has elapsed (www.entuk.org)
- Apply crushed ice or a bag of frozen peas wrapped in a towel to the bridge of the nose. This will cause the blood vessels in the nose to constrict and helps slow the bleeding.
- In most cases the bleeding should stop fairly quickly.
- Sometimes it is necessary to pack the nose to stop the bleeding.
- If the child's nose bleeds for more than 20 minutes, take the child to the nearest emergency department.

Nursing management in a health care facility

- A child who has frequent nose bleeds should be referred for further investigations.
- It is important to ask about any past medical history, such as bleeding disorders, which may explain the epistaxis.
- Sometimes, applying ointment regularly to the inside of the nostril will keep the inside of the nose moist, and will prevent the blood vessels cracking and bleeding.
- It may be necessary to cauterize blood vessels in the front of the nose that are giving rise to bleeding. This can be done by an ear, nose and throat specialist in clinic, sometimes under a general anaesthetic.

Points to remember
- Do not tilt the child's head backwards, otherwise they will swallow the blood.
- Do not put cotton wool up the nostrils.
- Advise child not to have any hot drinks for the next 24 hours.
- Advise child not to blow the nose for the next 24 hours.

Further reading

Bluestone C, Stool S, Cuneyt A, Arjmand E, Casselbrandt M, Donar J, Yellon R (2003). Pediatric Otolaryngology. Fourth Edition. Saunders.
Wetmore R, Muntx H, McGill T, Potsic W, Healy G, Lusk R (2000). Pediatric Otolaryngology. Thieme.

Haematology and immunity

① Haemophilia

Introduction

- Haemophilia is a long established disease, which has been linked to many European royal families.
- It is X-linked, which means that affected males inherit the disorder from their mothers, who are carriers but are not normally affected by the disease.
- Haemophilia affects 1 in 5,000–10,000 live births.
- The condition is a disorder of the coagulation process, which means that the blood does not clot normally following an injury. In severe haemophilia even the most minor of injuries can cause severe blood loss.

Incidence and causes

- The clotting disorder is the result of a deficiency in specific blood clotting factors.
- Factor VIII deficiency (haemophilia A) accounts for 80% of all cases,
- Factor IX deficiency (haemophilia B) is less common.
- The severity of the haemophilia depends on the level of the blood-clotting factor in the plasma of the patient's blood and is classified as mild, moderate or severe.
- A child with mild haemophilia may only have a problem following surgery or major trauma, whereas a child with severe haemophilia may have a bleed without any apparent cause.

Signs and symptoms

- Haemophilia is not usually apparent at birth, unless abnormal bleeding occurs at the umbilicus or site of initial injections.
- The parents may only become aware that there is a problem when they are unable to stop their child from bleeding after a minor injury.
- Any child presenting to an Emergency Department who is not known to have haemophilia but who has excessive blood loss disproportionate to the injury should be investigated fully.
- Aside from the risk of excessive blood loss, a child affected by haemophilia who has an injured knee or elbow presents a more significant problem because of haemorrhage into the joint cavity (haemarthrosis).
- The affected joint is stiff, warm, red and swollen. Joint movement limitation occurs, and repeated haemorrhages may cause permanent deformities that could lead to long-term mobility problems.

Immediate management

- Children with haemophilia most commonly present to the Emergency Department following a minor injury when the parents have misplaced their factor injections or are unsure if the injury requires a factor injection.

In these cases:
- Carry out full ABC assessment
- Treat any problems that arise from the ABC assessment

- Assess injury and then seek advice from the paediatricians or the consultant whom the child is looked after in an outpatient capacity. Generally parents have telephone numbers of nurse specialists or specialist wards which can be contacted for advice.

History
- The treatment of each type of haemophilia consists of replacing the deficient factor to ensure clotting.
- Most children who are known to have haemophilia have the appropriate vials of factor at home and self-administer them should an injury occur. This minimizes attendances at the Emergency Department, and also enables the affected individuals to avoid frequent trips to hospital.

Examination
When a child with known haemophilia presents to the children's Emergency Department they should be assessed in the following way:
- The initial ABC assessment is carried out, but it is important to ensure that all those involved with the child are aware of the haemophilia status. Should these children require intubation and/or cannulation, only those with the appropriate level of experience should undertake the procedure to avoid any further blood loss or complications.
- If any major/minor injuries are present, ensure the department has access to the factor the child may require. This can take time to organize, so initiating this as soon as the child presents can help to minimize delays.

Investigations
- Only as required at the request of the consultant.

Treatment
- The treatment of haemophilia relies on injecting the required factor and then treating any secondary problems as they arise.
- There are two main types of factor injections available: recombinant and plasma products. Recombinant factors are regarded as free from any risk of blood infections as well as the theoretical risk of CJD.
- Other therapeutic agents include desmopressin and tranexamic acid.

Complications/prognosis
- Most common complication is arthritis or permanent joint damage due to repeated bleeding in the joint.
- The prognosis for children diagnosed with haemophilia is excellent, and recent advances suggest that gene therapy to treat haemophilia is a real possibility for the future.

Further reading
www.haemophilialife.co.uk/Haemophilia-Information/Home/tabid/194/default.aspx
Keeling D, Tait C, Makris M. (2008) United Kingdom Haemophilia Centre Doctors' Organisation. Guideline on the selection and use of therapeutic products to treat haemophilia and other hereditary bleeding disorders. *Haemophilia* 14:671–684.

① **Haemarthrosis**

Introduction

Haemarthrosis is bleeding (haem) into a joint space (arthrosis). This can occur apparently spontaneously, although more commonly it occurs following injury.

Incidence

- Rarely seen in children unless they are known to have a bleeding disorder (see Haemophilia, above)
- Sometimes seen in children with a history of significant trauma to the joint, particularly in 'knee twisting' ligament injury. Can occur up to 6 hours following sporting injury.
- May present following accidental ingestion or intentional overdose of anticoagulants such as warfarin or aspirin.

Signs and symptoms

- Acute onset of hot, painful swelling of a single joint, most commonly the knee which may have been preceded by trauma.
- The joint will be held in flexion, as this will be least painful for the child.
- There will be a limited range of movement.

Immediate management

- Analgesia: avoiding aspirin as this affects platelet function and worsens bleeding.
- PRICE physiotherapy guidelines should be followed to relieve joint symptoms:

Protection

- Use of splints, slings, crutches as applicable. Splints should be individually made, reflecting the degree of swelling and position of the affected joint. Children should be instructed in the use of crutches by an appropriately trained health care professional.

Rest

- Use of 'relative rest' or 'controlled activity'. Bed rest is virtually impossible in children with painful, swollen joints, 'sofa rest' whilst watching television should be encouraged. Controlled activity should be introduced once the joint has settled and normal mobility has been regained.

Ice

- Use of cold therapy, either through cold wraps (gel filled refrigerated bandages) or cold compresses where crushed ice can be applied to the affected area for short, timed, periods. The skin should be protected from contact with the ice by use of a towel or pillowcase.

Compression

- Use of supportive elastic wraps or bandage, applied loosely so as not to constrict the limb and cause more swelling and pain.

Elevation
- Supported elevation (sofa rest for legs, pillows supporting arms) for up to 72 hours following injury. Compression should not be used at same time as elevation.

History
- Some families may have a history of bruising/bleeding, but a negative family history will not necessarily mean that the child does not have a bleeding disorder.
- History of trauma.
- History of drug ingestion.

Examination
- A hot, swollen, tense joint will be apparent.
- The child will hold the joint in a position which provides maximum volume within the joint space (flexion) as this is least painful.
- The joint should NOT be manipulated into its normal position.

Investigations
Blood tests:
- Full blood count: as this will help in the elimination of the potential diagnoses of leukaemia, and infection. Additionally a low platelet count can be associated with a number of different aetiologies.
- Erythrocyte sedimentation rate: this will be raised if infection is a potential cause of the haemarthrosis.
- Clotting screen, including APTT, PT, fibrinogen: abnormalities in these will indicate inherited bleeding disorders as well as acquired coagulation disorders such as warfarin ingestion/overdose.
- X-ray: this will reveal soft tissue and/or bone injury such as fractures.

Nursing management
- Replacement of coagulation factor: in children with abnormal clotting for whatever reason.
- Physiotherapy: use of PRICE as outlined above and additional rehabilitative physiotherapy to regain normal joint function.
- Aspiration: if the joint is extremely tense, or if there are suggestions of sepsis, an unknown underlying diagnosis, or the swelling is not resolving with measures listed above.
- Joint aspiration will reduce pressure inside the joint and may in itself be diagnostic.
- Intravenous antibiotics: if the haemarthrosis is related to infection.

Complications/prognosis
- Risk of introducing infection into the joint with aspiration. This should only be undertaken when other diagnostic/therapeutic avenues have failed, and should only be performed by a health care professional who is experienced in this procedure.
- Restricted range of movement of joint, including contractures and muscle atrophy, leading to impairment of function if appropriate

emergency management procedures and/or rehabilitative physiotherapy are not undertaken.
• Arthritic damage with long term repeated bleeding.

Further reading

Guideline for the physiotherapy management of soft tissue injury with PRICE during the first 72 hours (ACSPM). June 1988. Available from National Library for Health www.library.nhs.uk

Nolan B, Vidler V, Vora A, Makris M (2003) Unsuspected haemophilia in children with a single swollen joint. *BMJ* 326:151–152

:⚙: Sickle cell crisis

Introduction
Sickle cell disease (SCD) is a genetically determined disorder of haemo-globin structure leading to severe haemolytic anaemia. In an acute sickle cell crisis, hypoxia, infections or other factors cause the red blood cells to change shape. This results in increased blood viscosity, obstructing blood flow and causing pain, tissue ischaemia, infarction, and cellular death.

Incidence
- Sickle cell disease affects approximately 170–180 children each year in the UK.
- Sickle cell disease is common in people of Afro-Caribbean descent, but also affects people from the Mediterranean, Middle East, Far East, and parts of India.
- A previous history and diagnosis of SCD and sickle cell crisis may be presented, and the child and family are generally aware of the condition.

Signs and symptoms
Painful vaso-occlusive crisis is the most common crisis in SCD.
- May affect all the organs of the body.
- The bones of the limbs and spine are commonly affected areas.
- In children less than 5 years of age this may present as hand–foot syndrome. Hands and feet will be tender and swollen (dactylitis). This is often the earliest presentation of SCD and is common in infants.
- The child may have their own treatment plan as the majority of painful crises tend to be managed at home.

NB: a vaso-occlusive crisis may not be the only reason why a child with SCD presents at the Emergency Department. It could be due to any other condition, so a definitive diagnosis must be made.

Immediate management
- Rapid clinical assessment.
- Administer high concentration oxygen via a nonrebreathing mask.
- Monitor cardiac activity via ECG.
- Secure intravenous access.
- Analgesia: if pain severe and not relieved by nonopioids, administer opioids, orally initially (morphine or diamorphine). Must be started within 30 minutes of arrival (http://www.ncepod.org.uk/2008sc.htm).
- If oral opioids are not effective administer parenteral opioids.
- Patient controlled analgesia may be considered.
- Nitrous oxide 50% and oxygen 50% (Entonox) can be used in hospital for the first 30–60 minutes only.
- Administer adjuvant nonopioid analgesia: paracetamol, NSAIDs.
- Monitor pain level, sedation level, respiratory rate, heart rate, oxygen saturation percentage, and respiratory depression every 20 minutes until pain is controlled and stable.
- Administer rescue doses of analgesia every 30 minutes for breakthrough pain.
- Assess level of dehydration.
- Assess neurological status using AVPU.

- Record temperature as infection can trigger a crisis.
- Once analgesia is effective a full assessment and examination can be undertaken as the child should be more co-operative.

Nursing management

- Position child to minimize their pain.
- Administer analgesic according to need; orally, subcutaneously or intravenously.
- Oxygen therapy (humidified): if oxygen saturations are less than 95% or blood gases are abnormal then admit the child.
- Increase oral fluid intake. IV fluids should not be used routinely. Nasogastric fluids should be considered if the child is reluctant to drink. Accurate fluid balance must be maintained.
- Sepsis screen if fever present.
- Chest X-ray if respiratory involvement is suspected.
- Antipyretics.
- Abdomen examined for tenderness, masses and swelling.
- Prescribe laxatives, antipyretics and antiemetics as required.
- Continuous vital sign monitoring may be indicated.
- Neurological status should be monitored. If altered, head imaging may be required.
- Routine blood test for full blood count, urea and electrolytes, liver function tests, and crossmatch for possible blood transfusion later.
- Psychological support for child and family.
- Reduce known triggers, e.g. cold, stress, where possible.
- Check prophylaxis status. All children should be immunized against pnuemococcus and take twice daily penicillin orally.
- Take daily folic acid.
- Refer to paediatrician; each hospital should have a named paediatrician with links to a designated sickle cell centre.
- Ensure shared care arrangements are in place for ongoing management of the child with SCD.

Complications

It is important to monitor for the following complications:
- Abdominal crisis
- Sequestration crises
- Stroke
- Acute chest syndrome
- Priapism

Advice

- Avoid known triggers.
- Continue with prophylactic medication.
- Provide parent and child education and support as identified.

Further reading

Aehlert B (2005) Mosby's Comprehensive Pediatric Emergency Care. Mosby. Philadelphia
Rees D (2003) Guideline for the management of the acute painful crisis in sickle cell disease. *British Journal of Haematology.* 120:744–752.
Meremicwu MM (2009) British medical evidence: http://clinicalevidence.bmj.com/ceweb/conditions/bly/2402/2402_background.jsp

Renal and reproductive problems

⚙ Renal colic in children

Presenting symptoms
- Characterized by acute onset severe pain, which is intermittent and radiates between the loin and the groin. In boys the pain can also radiate to the testicles. Pain due to renal colic is excruciating and is likened to the pain of childbirth or of broken bones.
- Nausea and vomiting.
- Haematuria (not normally visible, only detected on urinalysis).
- Fever (sometimes presenting as rigors).

Causes
- Ureteric calculi (renal stones); however, in children consider differential diagnoses including:
  - Severe urinary tract infection
  - Neoplasm
  - Congenital abnormalities such as pelviureteric junction obstruction and vesicoureteric junction obstruction.

Investigations
- Urinalysis for haematuria (pH > 7 indicates high levels of uric acid)
- Full blood count, U&Es, liver function tests, amylase
- CT scan (renal ultrasound and intravenous urography can detect the presence of renal calculi)

Management
Objectives of management should be to:
- Relieve pain.
- Diagnose cause of renal colic and treat accordingly.
- Prevent any further deterioration in renal function and return to normal homeostasis.

Pain management
Children should be assessed utilizing an age appropriate pain assessment tool. The following web link offers seminal advice regarding recognition and assessment of pain in children:

www.rcn.org.uk/_data/assets/pdf_file/0011/109829/002170.pdf

Once assessed appropriately, children should receive timely, appropriate and effective analgesia. Figure 11.1 is an algorithm for treatment of acute pain in children in emergency settings.

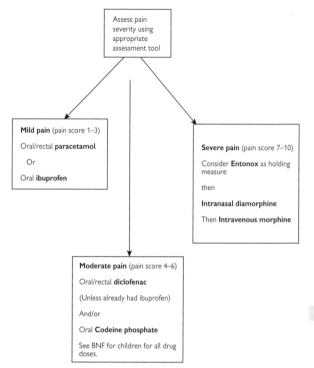

Fig. 11.1 An algorithm for treatment of acute pain in children in A & E (Adapted from Guideline for the Management of Pain in Children. British Association for Emergency Medicine; Royal College of Surgeons, 2004. Reproduced with permission by The College of Emergency Medicine)

Once pain is in under control, further treatment will depend on the cause of the renal colic.

Further reading

Edwards, JM et al (2004) Renal colic patient pain management in the emergency department. *Annals of Emergency Medicine* 44:58.

Royal College of Surgeons (2004) Guideline for the management of pain in children. British Association of Emergency Medicine.

ⓘ Urinary tract infection in children or young people

Introduction

This section covers inflammation of the bladder caused by either an infection or an irritation. Infections include urinary tract and sexually transmitted infections.

Cystitis is more common in girls than boys due to the close anatomical position of the urethra to the rectum.

Cystitis may be defined as complicated or uncomplicated. Complicated cystitis is defined by the presence of physiological or anatomical abnormalities of the urinary tract.

Presenting symptoms

- Acute pain on micturition.
- Need to pass urine frequently and urgently.
- May have blood in the urine.
- Abdominal pain.
- May be pyrexial.
- May cry/scream when passing urine.
- Pain or tenderness in the lower back or in the abdomen.
- Urine may be cloudy in appearance.
- Infant may present with poor feeding, lethargy and generally unwell.
- May vomit.

Immediate action

- Obtain a thorough history from the child/young person and their parents/carers. Is this the first episode of cystitis? Are there any pre-existing abnormalities of the genitourinary system that might increase the risk of cystitis occurring, e.g. bilateral urethral valves? Does the child have a Mitrofanoff appendicovesicostomy (urinary stoma)?
- Medically examine the child.
- Obtain a urine sample for microscopy, culture and sensitivity via MSU, clean catch, or suprapubic aspiration if other methods are not possible.
- Assess and manage pain.
- Commence oral antibiotics, or IV antibiotics if the child is acutely unwell, while awaiting laboratory results.
- Encourage good oral fluid intake and record balance.

Management

- Give advice regarding appropriate hygiene, e.g. for girls to wipe from the vagina backwards towards the anus to prevent the introduction of faecal bacteria into the vagina.
- Advise sexually active females to pass urine as soon as possible after sexual intercourse, and to observe good hygiene practices.
- If recurrent episodes of cystitis are occurring, consider further investigations, e.g. ultrasound.
- Treat the cause if a cause for the cystitis is established.

⑦ **Emergency contraception**

Introduction

Emergency contraception is a complex issue for a children's nurse. Our philosophy is that of family centred care, with the child or young adult as the primary focus. However, it is often the case that when seeking emergency contraception the young adult is either unwilling or unable to involve their family and will exclude parental involvement (see Fraser Guidelines, p.391).

The moral, ethical and legal issues surrounding contraception in this age group can cause much anxiety for nurses and medical staff. It is only by having a robust framework and intensive training that this service can be provided safely for both the young person and professionals involved.

Sexuality

- Part of the emergence of adulthood is the discovery of sexuality.
- 35% of girls and 46% of boys in the UK have their first sexual experience before the legal age of consent of 16 years.
- The rise in sexually transmitted diseases, particularly chlamydia, and the high teenage pregnancy rate are widely discussed in professional and popular media.

In relation to emergency contraception, one issue that staff may find difficult is discussing sexual intercourse with young women.

- Sexual intercourse needs to have taken place.
- Emergency contraception needs to be taken within 72 hours of sexual intercourse.
- If sexual intercourse took place over 72 hours earlier ask for medical advice. Refer to the gynaecology team on call who may opt to fit an intrauterine device.
- Remember that emergency contraception becomes less effective over time, and is only 20–30% effective in the last 12 hours of the 72 hours.

Confidentiality vs safeguarding children

Many young women seeking emergency contraception will be 'Gillick' competent. However, child protection issues have to be considered, and therefore it is important that the consultation can only be totally confidential if no other factors, such as abuse, emerge. This has to be explained at the start of the consultation.

The age of consent

- According to UK law the legal age at which a young person can consent to having sexual intercourse is 16.
- UK law also stipulates that sex with a child aged 12 or under is statutory rape.
- The law considers that a child under 13 years old is unable to understand the implications of their actions, and therefore needs to be protected.

Gillick competence

Often a teenager seeking emergency contraception is unaccompanied by her parents and may be accompanied by peers. In this instance the nurse is required to assess whether the young person is 'Gillick competent'. The General Medical Council's advice to doctors can be adapted for nurses too:

- The young person must understand the advice and any implications
- The healthcare professional should try to persuade her to tell her parents
- If the young person has had sexual intercourse and without intervention an unwanted pregnancy may occur
- It is in the best interests of the young person to receive advice and medication without parental consent or involvement
- Patients deemed to have learning difficulties may not have the mental capacity to give consent.

Age of partner

The age of the partner has implications for how the case should proceed. If the partner is older and the girl appears to be immature, take this into account, as a big difference in age or maturity may indicate an abusive relationship

Table 11.1 is a framework. Two 13 year olds might present on the same day. Chronological age is not a reliable indicator of maturity. This table is a guideline only and you can always seek advice from colleagues, the named nurse for safeguarding, and senior ED doctor or paediatric registrar.

Table 11.1 Framework for action depending on age of partner

Age of patient	Age of partner	Action
12 years	Immaterial	Refer to Children, Schools and Family/Emergency Duty Team (CSF/EDT)
13 years	13–15 years	Proceed if no other concerns
13 years	16–17 years	Proceed with caution
13 years	18+	Refer
14 years	13–15 years	Proceed if no other concerns
14 years	16–18 years	Proceed with caution
14 years	19+	Refer
15 years	14–16 years	Proceed
15 years	17–18 years	Proceed with caution
15 years	19+	Refer

Pregnancy test

A pregnancy test is required and consent is needed. If it is negative, proceed with emergency contraception. Remember to explain to the young person that a negative pregnancy test does not mean she is not pregnant from her recent sexual intercourse, and if her next period is late, she should seek medical help and have a pregnancy test at her GP, Family Planning or Genito-Urinary Medicine (GUM) Clinic.

If the pregnancy test is positive, give the young person time, and advise them of places to go for help including help lines.

Medication

When administering medication:

- Ask the patient if she is taking any other medication. Remember, if she is taking enzyme-inducing drugs (this includes St John's Wort) a higher dose of medication may be needed.
- Explain side effects.
- Always administer the medication in the department as this will prevent another girl receiving the medication.
- Advise that if vomiting occurs the drug may need to be repeated and that the patient should return to us, or another service if necessary.
- Remember, even if you have referred this child to the Children, Schools and Family team you should still dispense emergency contraception.
- Inform the young woman what to expect in relation to the effect of the medication.

Referring on

It is important to recognize the limitations of the emergency nurses/doctors, and referring the patient on is vital; however, the following issues must be dealt with:

- Does this young person mean to have sex with this partner again?
- Does she realise the risk of sexually transmitted infection?
- Refer to Family Planning or Genito-Urinary Medicine Clinic for contraception advice.
- Refer to GUM Clinic for screening for sexually transmitted diseases, but screening will not take place for 10 days.

Ethical/moral issues

Under the Abortion Act of 1967 (4), all nurses and doctors can refuse to dispense emergency contraception if they feel it is morally wrong to do so. Many faiths forbid the use of emergency contraception. However, remember that this may be a safeguarding issue, and it is expected that all staff would assess the patient and, if necessary, ask another practitioner to prescribe and dispense the medication.

It can be a challenging and divisive issue for a team if members of that team have moral objections to emergency contraception. It is important that this is discovered and addressed through training and mutual respect, before the situation arises where a young person is seeking advice.

Further reading

General Medical Council (2008) 0–18 years, guidance for all doctors. GMC. London.
Pocock M (2003) A critical analysis of legal and ethical issues regarding consent in childhood. *Nurse Prescribing* 1.

☠ Ectopic pregnancy (undiagnosed pregnancy)

Definition

Ectopic means 'out of place'.

The fertilized ovum implants at a site other than the endometrial lining of the uterus. Abnormal implantation sites include the fallopian tubes, interstitium, ovary, cervix, and peritoneum.

Causes

- Prior tubal infection
- Prior tubal surgery
- Prior genital infection or surgery
- Anatomical tubal abnormalities
- Anatomical endometrial defects
- Intrauterine contraceptive devices
- Contraceptive pill
- IVF treatment

Signs and symptoms

- Lower abdominal pain/cramps in supra-pubic or iliac fossa region
- Vaginal bleeding in 75% of cases (may be absent)
- Bleeding PV is brownish-red in colour
- Shoulder pain when patient lies down
- Fainting spells
- Painful fetal movements
- Gastrointestinal changes: diarrhoea, painful defecation, nausea and vomiting
- Lower back pain

Immediate management

- History of amenorrhoea and breast tenderness
- Assume the patient is pregnant until pregnancy tests and an ultrasound scan have ruled this out

Physical examination

- Temperature, pulse and respiratory rate may all be normal.
- If a ruptured tube has occurred then pulse will be fast. BP may be raised (initially) then become low due to shock.
- Vaginal bleeding may be mild or even absent.
- Abdominal palpation will elicit acute abdominal pain, mild to severe.
- Enlarged uterus.
- On vaginal examination, excrutiating pain if cervix is moved.
- Sloughing material visible in vaginal discharge.
- Shoulder pain is suggestive of peritoneal free fluid resulting from haemorrhage as a result of a ruptured fallopian tube.
- Clinical shock may result following rupture.
- No combination of clinical findings may reliably exclude ectopic pregnancy diagnosis.

Routine investigations

Group and hold two units of blood in case of surgical complications.

- Serum hCG levels (human chorionic gonadotrophin)
- Pregnancy test (urine)
- Serum progesterone to identify miscarriage
- Serum creatine kinase levels, marker of ectopic pregnancy
- Full blood picture to quantify blood loss and establish haemaglobin and packed cell volume (PCV)
- Clotting screen to establish risk of further clotting problems and potential disseminated intravascular coagulation (DIC)
- Rhesus factor to establish the need to administer Anti-D after the episode
- Urine culture (test initially)

Once IV access has been achieved for blood sampling, it might be wise to leave a cannula in situ for emergency IV fluids.

Diagnostic tests

Endovaginal ultrasound scan (particular care needs to be taken in gaining consent from the young patient)

- Identifies empty uterus
- Thick, brightly ectogenic structure
- Identifies pregnancy outside the uterus
- Adnexal mass indicating free, cul-de-sac fluid
- Intestinal ectopic pregnancy, where the fetus implants in a region of uterus closest to the fallopian tube, can be misdiagnosed as a uterine pregnancy due to the close proximity to the uterus.

Ultrasound scan

- May show haematosalpinx, where fallopian tube fills with blood or free fluid.
- Ruptured ectopic pregnancy, free of clotted blood in the intra-peitoneal gutter (Morison's pouch), may be visible.

Differential diagnosis

- Appendicitis
- Salpingitis
- Abortion/retained products of conception
- Ruptured uterine cyst
- Corneal myoma or abscess
- Ovarian cyst (benign)
- Ovarian tumour
- Cervical phase of uterine abortion
- Severe, chronic constipation
- Irritable bowel disease
- Pelvic inflammatory disease

Treatment

Medication

- Methotrexate ($50mg/m^2$) may be given IM.
- Stops the growth of the embryo.

- hCG levels should be checked day 4 and 7 after treatment.
- By day 7 the hCG levels should have fallen to <15% of initial levels, if not, a further dose may be given.
- <10% of women treated with methotrexate require surgical intervention.
- A transvaginal ultrasound scan should be performed following treatment.
- A surgical/gynaecological opinion is essential.

Exploratory/surgical intervention
- Laparotomy: pregnancy removed
- Salpingostomy: unruptured tubal pregnancy <4cm in diameter removed
- Salpingectomy: removal of ruptured tube

Nursing management
- Adolescents present differently to younger children: history-taking often requires excellent communication skills to overcome their shyness and self-consciousness regarding their sexuality.
- Be aware of genito-urinary problems in teenagers.
- Be aware of lifestyle changes and exposure to environmental precipitants.
- Anxiety can be secondary to symptoms, so the nurse needs to be empathetic in allaying the patient's fears.
- Monitor temperature, pulse and respiratory rate every 15 minutes.
- Continuous monitoring of blood pressure and mean arterial pressure (MAP) is important to detect early signs of deepening shock.
- Blood should be taken for group and crossmatch; hold 3 units.
- Observe the patient's level of pain or discomfort, as worsening pain or shoulder pain can indicate actual rupture of the fallopian tube and shock may follow.
- Analgesia is vital to alleviate pain and shock.
- Observe loss per vaginum and keep all pads to estimate blood loss.
- Urinary output should be recorded as an indicator of renal function, as a low BP will affect renal filtration and urine production.
- The nurse should ensure the patient is kept warm and nursed in a comfortable position. She should not be left unattended, particularly if she is a young person.
- Consent may be needed for a surgical procedure and so it is important to contact parents or family in the case of an underage patient.
- The patient should be kept fasting and a history obtained of any previous surgery, transfusions or anaesthetics in order to reduce the risk of allergic reactions to drugs or blood transfusions.
- Good documentation is essential in order to maintain a written record of all observations, procedures, drugs given and nursing care carried out.

Complications
- If tube ruptures and haemorrhage occurs: curettage and packing of uterine cavity may be necessary, as well as bilateral ligation of the internal iliac artery and possible hysterectomy.
- Abdominal pain is a common side-effect of methotrexate so the patient should have analgesia prescribed.

- Patient should be advised to drink lots of fluid, avoid sexual intercourse initially, and then to use a reliable method of contraception for at least 3 months due to the teratogenic risks of methotrexate.

Referral/counselling

- Follow-up by gynaecologist.
- Contraception advice.
- Counselling in regard to future risk.
- Counselling in relation to the lost pregnancy, particularly if it was planned.

Further reading

Ectopic Pregnancy Trust: Tel: 020 77332653 or e-mail: ept@ectopic.org.uk

The Miscarriage Association: http://www.miscarriageassociation.org.uk/ma2006/information/reading_list.htm

Stillbirth & Neonatal Deaths support group. http://www.uk-sands.org/

Royal College of Obstetricians & Gynaecologists (2004). http://www.rcog.org.uk/resources/Public/pdf/management_tubal_pregnancy21.pdf, accessed on 15 September 2008

Valley V (2006) Ectopic Pregnancy. Available at: www.eMedicine.com, accessed on 12 September 2008

Walker J (2002) Guidelines on Diagnosing Ectopic Pregnancy. E-mail: ept@ectopic.org.uk

Barr R (1983) Abdominal Pain in the Female Adolescent, Review. *American Academy of Pediatrics*, 4:281–289.

:✪: Concealed pregnancy

Introduction
- Pregnancy is sometimes hidden from family and friends.
- The UK has the highest teenage pregnancy rate in Europe; this currently stands at 32:1000 births.
- Half of all pregnant teenagers will not have had any antenatal care by 20 weeks gestation, putting them and their unborn babies at risk.

Social history/risk factors
Teenager/child may have:
- Mental health problems
- Learning difficulties
- Low self-esteem.

She may have a background of:
- Social deprivation
- Social care (fostering/residential homes)
- Physical abuse
- Sexual abuse
- Domestic abuse
- Involvement in crime
- Hesitancy in visiting GP or hospital
- Family may notice changes in personality, e.g. avoidance

These aspects of her history may only become apparent by liaising with Social Services, family members, or friends of the girl.

Immediate management
Look for signs that indicate possible concealment of pregnancy in the history
- Ambivalence
- Fearfulness
- Denial
- Sudden mood swings
- Loss of appetite, nausea and vomiting
- Pallor
- Dizzy spells
- Tightness of clothing around waist.

Examination for clinical signs of pregnancy
Enquire about the presumptive signs of pregnancy:
- Breast changes; tenderness, enlargement
- Nausea and vomiting
- Absence of periods
- Urinary frequency: some teenagers will complain of this normally
- Fatigue
- Uterine enlargement, swollen abdomen
- Quickening (fetal movement): a child/teenager will probably not recognize this sign as such but may describe it as 'wind'
- Skin changes, chloasma (pigmentation of face)

Probable signs of pregnancy
- Cervical softening (unlikely that a vaginal examination would be carried out due to the distress that this might cause to the girl).
- Braxton Hicks contractions, periodic uterine tightenings.
- Palpation of fetal outline through abdominal wall.

Examination
Positive signs of pregnancy
- Early pregnancy test, hCG levels high (98% accurate)
- Ultrasound scan with evidence of fetal outline
- Fetal heart audible by Doppler
- Palpation of fetal shape and movement through abdominal wall

Other clinical signs in later pregnancy
- Sugar and protein in urine: renal threshold lowered.
- Rise in BP, increase in blood volume increases cardiac workload.
- Breathing more difficult when abdomen enlarges.
- Anaemia from impaired iron absorption and demands of fetus.
- Reduced gastric motility and constipation.
- Backache/pelvic discomfort.
- Urinary symptoms:
  - bladder irritation
  - frequency
  - urgency of micturition
  - fluid retention/oedema of ankles and hands.

Differential diagnosis
- Hormonal changes due to contraceptives; discreet enquiry is needed.
- Gastric disorders.
- Amenorrhoea can be caused by anovulation, endocrine changes, illness, medication, metabolic changes and stress. Difficult to diagnose in an Emergency Department, but sensitive questioning or assistance from a relative might help here.
- Fatigue may result from anaemia, chronic illness, or depression.
- Abdominal enlargement can indicate ascites, obesity, and uterine or pelvic tumours.
- Quickening may be flatus, or increased peristalsis.
- Pigment changes are hormonal but can be due to contraception.
- Braxton Hicks contractions can resemble GI distress, or symptoms of a uterine tumour.
- 'Fetal' palpation could be a uterine tumour.

Treatment and nursing management
Once diagnosis is made
- Contact midwife or obstetrician at once
- Provide psychological care and counselling
- Enquire as to family support
- Social worker may be able to help with finance, housing, and legal issues

Assess wellbeing
- Make an appointment to see obstetrician/midwife at clinic or at home
- Record clinical observations to get a baseline of what is 'normal'
- Assess psychological state if possible, and provide resources and support contacts

Assess fetal wellbeing
- Abdominal palpation: it is important that someone the girl trusts is in the room when examinations are being performed

Ultrasound scan to assess:
- Fetal size: head size, length, abdominal girth, whether there has been growth restriction
- Placental size and location
- Amount of liquor surrounding fetus

Additional investigations
- Doppler scan to assess perfusion of placenta and cord
- Auscultate fetal heart rate

Nursing care
- Adolescent may be reluctant to give a full history. Skilled communication is needed to gain their trust and ascertain how at-risk they actually are.
- This is a potentially high-risk pregnancy, and so it is essential to contact a midwife so that she can liaise between the patient and the obstetrician and carry out the necessary care for mother and baby.
- Doctor/midwife should assess the risk of abuse/violence to this teenager and work closely with Social Services to ensure the safety of their patient. This requires astute observation of the interaction between the patient and the family members or friends who accompany her to the hospital.
- Always make sure the patient's body is covered with a warm blanket and never exposed; respect modesty.
- Always make sure that informed consent is given for all procedures.
- If the child/teenager is unable to fully understand what is being explained, engage the services of a paediatric social worker/counsellor, or appropriate interpreter if they do not speak English.
- Noninvasive forms of diagnosis should be used where possible, e.g. ultrasound scan rather than a vaginal examination.
- There should always be a nurse or midwife in the room when tests or procedures are being carried out; this is for the protection of the patient and the professional.

Psychological care
- A child under 13 years will feel very afraid and unsure about what happens next, and she will require psychological support.
- There are legal implications if the child is under 13 years of age as this situation is likely to mean that another person has had unlawful sex with a child, and this should be reported to the relevant authorities.
- If possible, the patient's parents should be informed with her consent, or another person whom she trusts should be called to be with her in the hospital.

- An older teenager may be more aware of the consequences and may handle the investigations and procedures in a more adult way, but she will still need support and reassurance in coping with this pregnancy.
- If the patient is sure she does want to keep the baby after birth, Social Services should be informed, but it is vital that she understands that there is no rush in making such decisions.

Further reading

Beuck L., Conerford K (eds) (2008) Maternal – Neonatal Nursing Made Incredibly Easy. London: Wolters Kluwer/Lippincott, Williams & Wilkins.
National Teenage Pregnancy Midwifery Network: www.rcm.org.uk/professional

☼ Torsion of testis

Introduction
- Torsion occurs when the testis rotates in the scrotum causing the spermatic cord to twist. This affects the blood supply to the testis initially causing venous engorgement followed by arterial ischaemia and eventually infarction.

Incidence
- Testicular torsion accounts for 80–90% of acute scrotal pain cases in adolescent males. The left side is twice as likely to be involved as the right due to the longer spermatic cord.

Cause
- May be precipitated by physical exertion or trauma.

History
- Sudden onset unilateral scrotal pain which gradually worsens and is more severe at the testis. In prepubertal males, the pain experienced may not be as severe.
- Right sided pain can radiate to the right iliac fossa, mimicking appendicitis.
- Nausea and vomiting have been noted in 30–40% of boys.
- Prior episodes of transient pain have been reported in 50% of boys.

Examination
- Unilateral redness, swelling and tenderness, but this may not be obvious in the first few hours of onset.
- Lack of or absent cremasteric reflex. The cremasteric reflex is noted when the inner thigh is stroked and the cremasteric muscle contracts causing the testis to elevate. This can be absent in a torsion.
- Testicular Doppler can show absent or poor perfusion to the testis, but is rarely indicated as this can cause a delay in treatment.

Treatment
- Urgent surgical exploration is required for any suspected torsion.
- Administer analgesia as prescribed.
- If the blood supply is restored promptly the testis should be salvageable.
- A viable testis is then surgically fixed in the scrotum to avoid reoccurrence (orchidopexy).
- Testicle is removal if unviable (orchidectomy). Fitting of a prosthesis may be undertaken.
- Attention must be paid to any potential body image issues.

Further reading
Matteson JR, Stock JA, Hanna MK, Arnold TV, Nagler HM (2001) Medicolegal aspects of testicular torsion. *Urology* 57:783–786.
Taskinen S, Taskinen M, Rintala R (2008) Testicular torsion: orchidectomy or orchidopexy? *Journal of Pediatric Urology* 4:210–213.

☼ Paraphimosis

Introduction

- Paraphimosis is a condition where the prepuce has been fully retracted to expose the glans of the penis and remains in this position. The trapped foreskin causes constriction, which interferes with circulation and nervous supply. This causes oedema which further increases constriction.

Incidence

- Paraphimosis is a rare condition.

Cause

- It may be spontaneous or iatrogenic such as when the prepuce is retracted for catheterization.

History

- Pain
- Oedema
- Sexual activity
- Catheterization

Examination

- Congestion of the prepuce and glans
- Difficult to return prepuce to normal position

Treatment

- Cooling techniques or a topical anaesthetic cream to allow manual compression, and then drawing the prepuce back over the glans.
- If all of these are unsuccessful then a reduction under general anaesthetic should be considered; a dorsal slit may be required to allow this. Only for the extremely rare recurrent episodes of paraphimosis should circumcision be considered.

Further reading

Mackay-Jones K, Teece S (2004). Ice, pins or sugar to reduce paraphimosis. *Emergency Medical Journal* 21:77–78.
Raman SR, Kate V, Ananthakristnan N (2008) Coital paraphimosis causing penile necrosis. *Emergency Medical Journal* 25:454.

⚙ Priapism

Introduction
- Priapism is a persistent erection not associated with sexual stimulation or desire.

Incidence
- It is very rare in children, but potentially serious when it occurs.

Cause
- Priapism occurs when there is a persistent engorgement of the corpora cavernosa of the penis, with preservation of blood flow to the glans and corpus spongiosum.
- High flow priapism usually results from trauma causing injury to the cavernosal arteries, with formation of an arteriovenous (AV) fistula causing increased flow through the corpora, and is noted to be painless.
- Low flow priapism is associated with conditions such as sickle cell disease and leukaemia; the ischaemic nature causes venous obstruction and is particularly painful.

History
- High flow priapism should include a history of penile or perineal trauma and a persistent painless erection. Straddle injuries are a particular common cause of this type of trauma. The priapism does not always occur immediately after the injury.
- Exclude underlying conditions such as leukaemia and sickle cell disease, especially when there is no clear history of trauma. Sickle cell disease produces a low flow priapism as the sickled cells increase the blood's viscosity and occlude the venous flow.

Examination
- A high flow priapism can be confirmed by immediate relief of the priapism upon perineal compression, with reoccurrence following removal of the compression (piesis sign).

Investigations
- Doppler and angiography aim to identify abnormal flow. Angiography is invasive, but is much more sensitive in identifying a fistula to allow for embolization.

Treatment
- There is no gold standard treatment for paediatric priapism.
- A watch and wait approach is considered to be acceptable and effective management in high flow priapism. This is because venous flow away from the penis is not compromised, and there should be no damage to the corporal bodies or risk of compartment syndrome.
- Embolization is the treatment of choice in adults as it will temporarily obstruct flow through the fistula to allow for it to heal. Embolization in children requires the skills of specialist radiology and anaesthetic staff.
- Pain should be assessed and managed appropriately.

- In low flow priapism the goal is to terminate the priapism without delay, to alleviate pain and to prevent any permanent damage to the corpora, which can cause fibrosis and potentially lead to impotence.
- Initially, treatment of the underlying cause of the priapism should be addressed, such as hydration in sickle cell anaemia.
- Specific treatment of the priapism involves aspiration of the corpora cavernosa, followed by intracavernous injection of an alpha-adrenergic agonist, which will constrict the arterial blood supply to the penis allowing venous drainage.
- Embarrassment and modesty issues must be taken seriously and addressed.

Further reading

Marotte JB, Brooks JD, Sze D, Kennedy WA (2005) Juvenile post traumatic high flow priapism: current management dilemmas. *Journal of Pediatric Surgery* 40:25–28.

Mockford K, Weston M, Subramaniam R (2007) Management of high flow priapism in paediatric patients: A case report and review of the literature. *Journal of Pediatric Urology* 3:404–412.

Endocrine and metabolic problems

ⓘ Diabetes mellitus

Introduction

Diabetes mellitus (DM) is a chronic, severe metabolic condition. It comprises a group of disorders with many different causes, all of which are characterized by a raised blood glucose level. This occurs because of a lack of the hormone insulin, or an inability to respond to insulin (Diabetes UK 2005).

Incidence

In England and Wales 17 children per 100,000 develop diabetes each year; in Scotland the number is 25 per 100,000.

There are a number of genetic variants of diabetes, but two main types are pertinent to children in contemporary society, type 1 and type 2.

Type 1 diabetes
- There is a cessation of insulin production in the pancreas.
- Aetiology is not completely understood.
- Thought to be the result of a cell-mediated autoimmune response to an infection.
- Some environmental factors may trigger type 1 diabetes in a child born with a genetic predisposition to this diabetic state.
- In childhood, the incidence of type 1 is greater than type 2, and the former is therefore more likely to be encountered in practice.

Type 2 diabetes
- The result of inadequate production of insulin, insufficient to meet the body's needs.
- The cells in the body may not be able to respond to the insulin that is produced.
- The incidence of type 2 is increasing at all ages and across races because of the increased levels of obesity.
- May account for as much as one fifth to one third of all new cases of DM. The increase in childhood obesity may also account for an earlier presentation of type 2 diabetes due to insulin resistance and beta cell exhaustion.

Signs and symptoms
- Polyuria
- Polyphagia
- Polydipsia
- Weight loss and lethargy
- Onset may be acute precipitated by the stress of an acute illness
- Onset can also be chronic and insidious over weeks or months
- On rare occasions, may be detected by the finding of glucosuria on routine urinalysis

Diagnosis is usually confirmed in a symptomatic child by finding:
- a markedly raised random plasma glucose (> 11.1mmol/l)
- glycosuria and ketonuria

- a fasting venous blood glucose level over 7mmol/l
- a raised glycosylated haemoglobin (HbA1c); this will help clarify the diagnosis.

Immediate management

The goals of treatment and nursing care are:

- to establish intravenous access for fluid management and insulin therapy
- to achieve glycaemic control, whereby an HbA1c level of less than 7.5% is maintained without frequent disabling hypoglycaemia
- to prevent diabetic ketoacidosis
- to prevent severe chronic complications associated with type 1 diabetes.

According to the National Institute for Clinical Excellence (2004), the fundamental aspects of treatment necessary to obtain safe and effective metabolic control are:

1. establishing the appropriate insulin dosages and regimes
2. establishing appropriate diet
3. exercise
4. stress/illness management
5. blood glucose and urine ketone monitoring.

Initial nursing care and management

Management from diagnosis of children and young people with type 1 diabetes mellitus requires:

- a multidisciplinary, family centred approach
- that children and young people should receive high-quality evidenced based specialist care
- a service that encourages partnership in decision making
- high quality information, education and support
- facilitation to be self managing, essential in achieving glycaemic control and reducing associated complications of hypoglycaemia, diabetic ketoacidosis, and the incidence of microvascular complications and delay in their progression (Diabetes UK 2005)
- initial and subsequent management will depend on the child's clinical condition, social and emotional difficulties and age.

Further reading

Couper, J (2008) Chapter 19.4. In: Roberton, D.M., South, M. Practical Paediatrics (6th edn). London: Churchill Livingstone.

Morrow, P (2008) Chapter 30. In: Kelsey, J, McEwing, G. Clinical skills in child health practice. London: Churchill Livingstone.

National Institute for Clinical Excellence (2004) Guidelines for the NHS on the management of type 1 diabetes in children and young people. RCOG Press, London.

Diabetes UK (2005) Resources to support the delivery of care for children and young people with diabetes. Diabetes UK, London.

☠ Diabetic ketoacidosis (DKA)

Introduction

Diabetic ketoacidosis is a state of metabolic decomposition due to a lack of insulin. It is a life threatening condition requiring emergency medical and nursing care (see Alert Box 1).

Incidence

- The condition occurs in children with type 1 diabetes.
- There may be an increased risk of ketoacidosis and ketonuria associated with type 2 diabetes.
- Incidence of diabetes in preschool-age children is increasing.
- Symptoms in younger age groups may be misinterpreted or their severity not appreciated.
- Children under 5 years may have a more severe biochemical derangement and clinical course than older children.
- Early identification is essential to reduce the morbidity and mortality associated with new-onset diabetes or known diabetics who have poor control, such as nonconcordant teenagers (Quinn et al 2006).

Box 1 Alert

Children and young people can die from DKA.
  They can die from:
- Cerebral oedema: this occurs more frequently in younger children and newly diagnosed diabetes and has a mortality rate of around 25%.
  Causes are unknown, but rapid reductions in blood glucose levels and/or a fall in serum sodium concentration can alter the plasma osmolality too quickly and may increase the risk.
  Guidelines aim to minimize this risk by producing a slow correction of the metabolic abnormalities.
- Hypokalaemia: this is preventable with careful monitoring and management.
- Aspiration pneumonia: nasogastric tube should be inserted in semi-conscious or unconscious children.
  British Society of Paediatric Endocrinology and Diabetes Recommended DKA Guidelines (2007)

Causes

- Previously undiagnosed diabetes mellitus
- Missed insulin injections, therefore giving rise to an increased blood glucose level
- Excessive glucagon
- Excessive glucocorticoids
- Infection or other illness
- Vomiting, trauma, burns, surgery
- Stress

Physiology

- A lack of insulin means that glucose in the blood cannot be taken up into the cells, giving rise to hyperglycaemia (>11mmol/L).
- Fat and proteins are broken down to provide energy.
- Fat is broken down rapidly and incompletely, producing ketone bodies in excess of the tissue cells' ability to metabolize them.
- Alterations in liver metabolism lead to further ketone production, which is accelerated when glucagon levels rise.
- Muscle tissues are unable to use ketones; this further contributes to an accumulation of these acids and acetone in the blood, which will eventually result in acidosis with low bicarbonate levels. Ketoacidosis is indicated by blood pH <7.3 and bicarbonate level <15mmol/L.
- Ketones have two other effects in addition to acidosis: they have a central action giving rise to nausea and vomiting, so increasing fluid loss and preventing oral replacement
- Ketone excretion in the urine gives rise to osmotic diuresis, resulting in further fluid loss and loss of Na^+, K^+, and Cl^-.
- High blood glucose gives rise to glycosuria and osmotic diuresis, increasing cellular dehydration, peripheral shut down and renal hypofusion.
- In addition, moderate or large amounts of ketones may be detected in the child's urine. Ketonuria if untreated may progress to ketoacidosis, which may be accompanied by deep breathing (Kussmaul respirations) and excessive weakness.

Characteristics

Has insidious onset over several days; presenting symptoms include:
- polyuria, thirst, glycosuria and general weakness
- anorexia, nausea, vomiting
- deep/rapid respirations (Kussmaul)
- ketone odour on breath, which is similar to the smell of 'pear drops'; however, some individuals congenitally cannot smell this.
- abdominal pain and muscle cramps
- dehydration
  - dry skin and mucous membranes
  - dark and sunken eyes
  - hypotension, tachycardia, weak pulse
- history of weight loss
- hypothermia due to peripheral vasodilation
- drowsiness and coma (these are late signs).

Immediate management and nursing care

Management and nursing care of children and young people with diabetic ketoacidosis should be performed according to the guidelines published by the British Society of Paediatric Endocrinology and Diabetes (2007).

Immediate emergency attention should consist of rapid assessment, and treatment is based on four physiological principles:
- restoration of fluid volume
- inhibition of lipolysis and return to glucose utilization
- replacement of body salts
- correction of acidosis.

Emergency management is aimed at stabilizing respiratory and cardiovascular status.

General resuscitation includes:

- **Airway:** assess airway patency. If comatose, or if the child has recurrent vomiting, secure the airway, insert nasogastric tube, aspirate, and leave on open drainage.
- **Breathing:** administer 100% oxygen by face mask.
- **Circulation:** assess for signs of shock indicated by poor peripheral pulses, poor capillary filling, tachycardia, and/or hypotension. A cardiac monitor should be used for continuous electrocardiographic monitoring, to assess T-waves for evidence of hyper- or hypokalaemia, and to monitor for arrhythmias.
- **Assess clinical severity of dehydration.** Accurate assessment may be difficult in DKA so the following guidelines proposed by Wolfsdorf et al (2006) may be helpful.
  - 5%—reduced skin turgor, dry mucous membranes, tachycardia.
  - 10%—capillary refill >3 seconds, sunken eyes.
  - >10%—weak or impalpable peripheral pulses, hypotension, shock, oliguria.
  - Note also the NICE guidelines (http://www.nice.org.uk/CG84).
- **Assess level of consciousness**: using the modified Glasgow Coma Scale.
- **Assess the weight of the child:** this is necessary to estimate fluid and insulin therapy.
- **Immediate insertion of cannula:**
  - to take blood samples
  - to replace fluids
  - to correct acidosis and electrolyte disturbances by administration of intravenous fluids and insulin therapy.
- Rapid correction should be avoided as it may result in untoward effects, including cerebral oedema, as previously indicated.
- Frequent monitoring of neurological status and metabolic parameters aids in the avoidance or early detection of complications.
- The child should receive care in a unit that has:
  - nursing staff experienced in monitoring and management
  - written guidelines for DKA management in children
  - access to laboratories for frequent and timely evaluation of biochemical variables.
- A child with severe DKA should be considered for:
  - immediate treatment in an intensive care unit
  - treatment in a unit that has equivalent resources and supervision, such as a children's ward specializing in diabetes care.

Nursing care, ongoing assessment, and monitoring are vital for the successful management of DKA, such that timely adjustments of the child's clinical and biochemical response to treatment are made.

- Documentation on an hourly basis must be strictly adhered to and should include:
  - clinical observations
  - intravenous fluids

- insulin therapy
- all fluid intake and output
- oral medications
- blood glucose monitoring
- urinalysis.

Nursing management–ongoing assessment and monitoring

- Assess neurological status frequently to observe for early signs of cerebral oedema (see Box 2).
- Respiratory function: record respiratory rate and depth and SaO_2 to identify need for O_2 administration.
- Assist in obtaining blood for blood gas analysis, blood sugar, urea and electrolyte estimation.
- Cardiovascular functioning: ECG monitoring; observe for flat T-wave, which may indicate hypokalaemia.
- Regular blood pressure and pulse monitoring.
- Gastrointestinal problems: if child is vomiting it may be necessary to pass a nasogastric tube to ensure safety and comfort; this also enables a more accurate record of total fluid output.
- Monitor the administration of insulin, IV fluids, and electrolyte supplements as prescribed.
- Maintain accurate records of fluid intake and output, and test urine for glycosuria and ketones.
- Regular monitoring of blood glucose to ensure that insulin requirements are adjusted accordingly.
- Continue to monitor child's condition until blood glucose returns to normal, the urine is free from ketones, and oral feeding is established
- Any concerns regarding the child's condition must be reported immediately to a senior doctor.
- All nursing interventions must be accurately reported and recorded.
- Throughout this period, attention to the hygiene and comfort needs of the child is required.
- Both the child and their parents require support and reassurance, and explanations for all interventions need to be provided.

Box 2 Signs and symptoms of cerebral oedema

- Headache
- Recurrance of vomiting
- Inappropriate slowing of the heart rate
- Rising blood pressure
- Decreased oxygen saturation
- Changes in neurological status: restlessness, irritability, increased drowsiness.
- Specific neurological signs: cranial nerve palsies, abnormal papillary responses.

Introduction to oral fluids and transition to subcutaneous insulin injections

Oral fluids should only be introduced when substantial clinical improvement has occurred and the child indicates a desire to eat. When oral fluids are tolerated, intravenous fluids should be reduced.

Subcutaneous insulin should commence when ketoacidosis has resolved.

- The most convenient time to change to subcutaneous insulin is just before a meal.
- The first subcutaneous insulin injection should be given before stopping the insulin infusion.
- Allow for sufficient time for the injected insulin to be absorbed.
- Children with established diabetes may resume their usual insulin regime.
- Newly diagnosed diabetics require titration of their insulin therapy according to their individual requirements.
- After transition to subcutaneous insulin, frequent blood glucose monitoring is required to avoid marked hyperglycaemia or hypoglycaemia.
- Management of DKA is not complete for a child until:
  - the cause has been identified and an attempt made to treat it
  - the five fundamental aspects of treatment as previously identified are implemented
  - the necessary educational and psychosocial support and follow-up care are co-ordinated by the multidisciplinary team in partnership with the child and their family
  - all care and collaboration is documented in the child's personal clinical record of care, treatment, and management.

Further reading

British Society of Paediatric Endocrinology and Diabetes (2007) Recommended DKA Guidelines Online. Available at: http://www.bsped.org.uk/dka.htm

Diabetes UK (2005) Resources to support the delivery of care for children and young people with diabetes. Diabetes UK, London

National Institute for Clinical Excellence (2004) Guidelines for the NHS on the management of type 1 diabetes in children and young people. RCOG Press, London

☼ Management of diabetes insipidus

Introduction
Diabetes insipidus (DI) is a relatively rare condition that arises from either an abnormality in the posterior pituitary gland (central DI), causing a lack of the hormone vasopressin, or a reduced sensitivity to vasopressin in the kidneys (nephrogenic DI). Vasopressin is also known as anti-diuretic hormone (ADH). This hormone is released when the body is dehydrated to conserve water through concentration of urine.

The lack of, or reduced sensitivity to, this hormone therefore results in hyperdiuresis, passing large volumes (diabetes) of dilute urine (insipidus) and excessive thirst.

Incidence
Very rare: 1 in 25,000 of the total population

Causes of central DI
- Head trauma
- Surgery
- Infection
- Brain tumour

Causes of nephrogenic DI
- Hypercalcaemia
- Chronic renal disease, or very rarely congenital abnormality of the kidney
- Nephrotoxic drugs

Signs and symptoms
- Excessive urination with very dilute urine.
- Bedwetting in previously dry child.
- Excessive thirst/desperate need for any fluid, e.g. the child will drink any fluid such as flower water or from the toilet.
- Signs of dehydration, such as a sunken fontanelle in babies.
- Fatigue/lethargy.
- History of recent head trauma or surgery.
- Loss of consciousness/fitting.

ALERT: control fitting and correct electrolyte imbalance.

Immediate management
- Dependent upon condition of child
- Protect airway if fitting

Investigations
- Urinalysis
- Urine osmolarity
- MRI brain
- Water deprivation test to confirm diagnosis

Nursing management
- IV access and infusion for fluid management
- Commence ADH replacement either IV or oral
- Monitor fluid balance
- Check bloods for electrolytes
- Will require further investigations into cause once stable

Ongoing treatment
- Replacement of vasopressin (ADH) with tablets or intranasal spray
- Review or stop nephrotoxic medication
- Patient will need to wear Medic Alert bracelet

Further reading
http://www.pituitary.org.uk/
http://www.nlm.nih.gov

☠ Management of cortisol failure

Introduction

Acute adrenal crisis is a life-threatening condition that occurs when there is not enough cortisol.

Cortisol is a glucocorticoid that:
- Helps regulate blood sugar (glucose)
- Holds back the immune response
- Is released as part of the body's response to stress

An adrenal crisis occurs when:
- The adrenal gland is damaged (primary adrenal insufficiency or Addison's disease)
- The pituitary gland is injured (secondary adrenal insufficiency)
- Adrenal insufficiency is not properly treated.

Addison's disease

Addison's disease results from damage to the adrenal cortex, which thus produces less cortisol.

This damage may be caused by the following:
- The immune system mistakenly attacking the gland (autoimmune disease)
- Infections such as tuberculosis, HIV, or fungal infections
- Haemorrhage
- Complication of meningococcal disease (possibly up to 52%)
- Tumours
- Use of blood-thinning drugs (anticoagulants)

Risk factors for the autoimmune type of Addison's disease include other autoimmune diseases.

Other causes include:
- Congenital adrenal hyperplasia and hypoplasia
- Radiotherapy
- Infection
- Cytotoxic therapy

Exogenous steroid therapy causing temporary cortisol failure

When inhaled, oral, or topical steroids have been taken for a prolonged period of time (usually several months or years) this leads to cortisol failure. This is usually temporary, but can become permanant. Steroids cause cortisol failure because they block the release of both CRH (corticotrophic releasing hormone) and ACTH (adrenocorticotropin) from the pituitary, thus reducing adrenal gland stimulation and leading to low levels of cortisol production. While the patient is receiving steroids they remain well, but if the steroids are stopped suddenly, or the individual is placed under stress, such as an operation, then they may have an adrenal crisis.

Incidence

Addison's disease, or adrenal insufficiency, affects between 1 and 4 in every 100,000 people across all age groups.

Signs and symptoms
- Abdominal pain/flank pain
- Lethargy/confusion/coma
- Dizziness
- Tachycardia/tachypnoea
- Hypotension
- Darkening of the skin

Immediate identification
- May be known to have underlying disease
- Wearing Medic Alert bracelet or similar
- History from family: check if taking steroids for asthma/eczema
- Signs of hypoglycaemia/hypotension
- Concurrent illness/accident
- Unconsciousness

ALERT: if known cortisol deficiency then IM/IV hydrocortisone should be administered immediately.

Immediate action
- Correct hypoglycaemia
- Correct dehydration and subsequent electrolyte imbalance

Management
- Referral to endocrine team for tests, such as the short synacthen test
- Treat underlying illness
- Commence regular hydrocortisone treatment
- Review asthma/eczema treatment if relevant

Nursing management
- Observations: frequent physical assessment for the first few hours of pulse, temperature, respiration rate, and blood pressure.
- Intravenous cannulation and infusion of isotonic solution of sodium chloride and glucose to help correct hypotension and hypoglycaemia.
- IV administration of glucocorticoids and mineralcorticoids.
- Vasopressor agents may be necessary to combat hypotension.
- A nasogastric tube may be inserted if the child is vomiting to prevent aspiration and relieve hyperemesis.
- Total bed rest; do not move child unless absolutely necessary.

Prognosis
- Good if identified and treated promptly.
- Discharge must include clear instructions to seek medical attention following any physically or psychologically stressful situation to prevent a recurrence of the crisis.

Further reading
http://www.pituitary.org
http://www.nlm.nih.gov
Bone M, Diver M, Selby A, Sharpless A, Addison M, Clayton P (2002) Assessment of adrenal function in initial phase of meningococcal disease. *Pediatrics* 110:563–569

☼ Hypoglycaemia

Introduction
Hypoglycaemia is the level of blood glucose at which physiological and neurological dysfunction begins.

Incidence/causes
Symptoms usually occur when:
- blood glucose level is less than 3.0–3.5mmol/l
- initially trying to stabilize diabetic state, if:
  - insulin dosage is excessive
  - insufficient food is eaten
  - extra exercise is undertaken.
- NB: children with inborn errors of metabolism may respond differently to hypoglycaemia.

Hypoglycaemia may be more common during the night when the glucose threshold for counter-regulatory hormonal responses is lower. Symptoms appear rapidly; this differentiates the hypoglycaemic coma from the coma of diabetic ketoacidosis.

Signs and symptoms
- Blood glucose <3.5mmol/l
- Hunger
- Weakness
- Shaking
- Sweating
- Drowsiness at unusual time
- Headache
- Behavioural changes

Immediate management
Requires immediate administration of fast-acting sugar to raise blood glucose. All children with type 1 diabetes should carry rapidly absorbed carbohydrates, e.g. GlucoGel®.

If a meal is not anticipated within the next hour a snack containing carbohydrate, fat, and protein is recommended. Check blood glucose level after 15 minutes.

Assess the need for additional carbohydrate or possibility of hyperglycaemia.

Loss of consciousness and convulsions
Treatment as for the unconscious patient
- Lie on side, check airway.
- Glucagon: administer by intramuscular or subcutaneous route. This may cause nausea and vomiting, so need to administer oral carbohydrate when child is awake. All families with a diabetic child should have glucagons at home and should be able to administer subcutaneously.
- Severe hypoglycaemia should be treated with 10% intravenous glucose.

Nursing management

When the child has recovered, check:
- consistency in routine
- that correct insulin dosage is being administered.

Encourage:
- regular blood glucose monitoring
- controlled snacking
- child/family compliance.

Ensure that any persons who are involved with the diabetic child on a daily basis are educated and trained in the recognition and treatment of hypoglycaemia.

Further reading

Diabetes UK (2005) Resources to support the delivery of care for children and young people with diabetes. Diabetes UK, London

National Institute for Clinical Excellence (2004) Guidelines for the NHS on the management of type 1 diabetes in children and young people. RCOG Press, London

Mental health problems

☼ Psychosis in childhood and adolescence

Defining psychosis

The word psychosis is used to describe conditions that affect the mind, where there has been some loss of contact with reality. When someone becomes ill in this way, it is known as a psychotic episode. This is serious, but uncommon in childhood, accounting for less that 1% of reported mental health problems.

Possible symptoms of a psychotic 'episode'

- *Confused thinking*
  Everyday thoughts are jumbled, sentences become unclear or nonsensical. A person might find it difficult to concentrate on conversations or remember things. Thoughts are perceived to speed up or slow down.

- *Delusions (false beliefs)*
  Young people can be convinced of their belief (e.g. working as a government spy), and will attempt to give plausible responses to any challenging argument.

- *Hallucinations*
  The person can see, hear, smell and taste things that are not actually there (e.g. 'voices' saying derogatory things).

- *Changed feelings*
  May feel cut off from the world, with everything moving in slow motion. Sometimes they may feel unusually excited or depressed. However, emotions are usually dampened.

- *Changed behaviour*
  May become either very active or lethargic. They may laugh inappropriately, or become angry and upset for no obvious reason. Behaviour is often in response to the above symptoms (e.g. someone may stop eating if a hallucination/delusion is that family members are trying to poison them).

Symptoms are often divided into **positive** and **negative** categories. Positive symptoms mean the addition of something that was not there prior to onset of illness (e.g. hallucinations/delusions). Negative symptoms mean the loss of previous character traits/behaviours/interests (e.g. isolation, lethargy, blunted affect).

A first episode of psychosis may be preceded by a prodromal phase (up to 3 years), which may contain subtle manifestations of the above symptoms (predominantly negative). These may or may not be noticeable to friends or family, and can often be hidden by the young person. The young person's family/friends may notice:

- Behaviour changes
- Deterioration in study or work
- The young person becoming more withdrawn and isolated
- The young person being less active than previously.

Types of psychosis

There are several types of psychosis in young people, including: drug-induced psychosis, bipolar (manic-depressive) disorder, organic psychosis, psychotic depression, brief-reactive psychosis, emerging schizophrenia, and schizophreniform disorder. Drug-induced psychosis is increasingly observed in adolescence, with the appearance of symptoms being associated with the use of or withdrawal from alcohol or drugs. In most cases, these effects will wear off as substance use decreases. However, with some the experience may last longer, as the substance use may have triggered an underlying vulnerability to psychosis that otherwise may have remained dormant.

Interventions in crisis situations

Medication

Young people will often be offered a low dose of atypical **anti-psychotic medication**. These drugs will often have fewer neurological side effects than older, traditional anti-psychotics, resulting in greater compliance and improved action on negative and positive symptoms. Young people may also be given **benzodiazepines** to prevent escalation of symptoms in the short term.

Communicate with the young person

For the majority of young people, their psychotic episode will be a very distressing and frightening experience, which may in a minority of cases manifest itself as aggression towards others. It is important to:

- Acknowledge and empathize with the young person's distress, and acknowledge their beliefs with regard to hallucinations/delusions. However, DO NOT collude with the hallucinations/delusions by saying that they are true.
- If possible assist the young person in activities that may provide a temporary alleviation/distraction from their distressing experience, e.g listening to music, watching television (though be aware that perceived messages through TV/music may form part of their hallucinations), talking about their interests, playing games, or writing letters.

Educate the family

Having to observe a child/sibling/friend experiencing a psychotic episode can be very distressing for those close to the young person. A phenomenon called **expressed emotion** (EE) can often be observed in such situations, manifesting as excessive criticism/anger towards the young person for their odd behaviour, or over-involvement in their daily lives, making the young person feel incompetent in their ability to undertake basic daily living tasks. It is important that families as well as young people are educated about the illness, and that coping strategies are explored. These all improve functioning levels and prognosis of the patient.

Referral to Child and Adolescent Mental Health Service (CAMHS)

The importance of early recognition and treatment of a psychotic illness cannot be overemphasized. This is especially the case for young people, who are vulnerable to disruption of their developmental pathways. The consequences of delayed treatment can be slower and less complete recovery and poorer long-term prognosis.

The management of a young person with psychosis as a paediatric inpatient can often be inappropriate for their needs (and disruptive to other children on the ward). Some paediatric units will have links to a hospital-based child mental health liaison team, who are available on a daily basis to advise and support the needs and management of these young people. They may then liaise with the local specialist community or inpatient CAMHS as appropriate. If such a team is not available, a direct referral to the local community CAMH team would be appropriate. These teams are staffed by a range of mental health professionals, and will be able to provide further specialist assessment and intervention.

In addition to local CAMHS there may be an Early Intervention in Psychosis service, who can offer intensive support for patients aged 14–35 for up to 3 years in the community.

Further reading

Birchwood MJ, Smith TP, Jackson C (1996). Early intervention in psychosis: the critical period hypothesis. *British Journal of Psychiatry* 172(suppl 33):53–59.
Kavannagh DJ (1992). Recent developments in expressed emotion and schizophrenia. *British Journal of Psychiatry*. 160:601–620.
www.sane.org.uk
www.youngminds.org.uk
www.rcpsych.ac.uk

☠ Self harm and parasuicide

Introduction

- Deliberate self harm (DSH) is self harm without suicidal intent, resulting in non-fatal injury; whereas parasuicide is self harm with the intent to take life, resulting in non-fatal injury.
- Both are behaviours, not illnesses, although two thirds of those presenting with DSH would be diagnosed as having depression.

Incidence

- There has been a dramatic rise in the last 20 years.
- 4.6–6.6% of people have self harmed, but this is likely to be an underestimate. Self report suggests that 13% 15–16 year olds have self harmed, with 7% in the last year.
- Half of those who attend emergency departments with DSH have also consumed alcohol.
- DSH is four times more common in girls under 16 years and twice as common in girls aged 18–19 years than in boys.
- 24% of young people who are in social care (foster care, care homes) have reported DSH/parasuicide.
- There are 24,000 attempted suicides by young people aged 10–19 years in England and Wales, one every 20 minutes.
- While suicide attempts are more common in girls, boys are more likely to be successful.
- 4–5% of all emergency department attendances are due to DSH, including more than 60,000 young people each year.

Reasons

- Young people often say that they do this in order to feel alive, release emotions, experience a sense of relief, express self hatred, or as a distraction from an intolerable reality. However, it may indicate deeper mental health issues.
- No single factor is shown to predict self harm, but a combination of external pressures from home/school life, emotions such as anger, guilt or frustration, and mental health or behavioural issues such as depression, conduct disorder, or impulsivity can lead to DSH.

Signs and symptoms

- Commonly involves self poisoning (overdoses including paracetamol, alcohol, and substance misuse) and self mutilation including cutting, burning, and scalding.
- Often accompanied by feelings of guilt and shame and a desire to keep the behaviour secret from others; hard to talk about the subject.

Immediate management

- Triage, assessment, and treatment should be undertaken by appropriately trained child health professionals in a separate children's area of the emergency department.

Treatment and nursing management

- Responsibility to facilitate disclosure of DSH falls to the healthcare professional, requiring a non-judgemental approach with care and respect for the young person behind the self harm behaviour, acknowledging their emotional distress.
- Issues of mental capacity, the young person's consent, parental consent and confidentiality should be taken into consideration. Encourage the young person to notify their parents, as the team should ideally gain parental consent for ongoing mental health assessment and treatment.
- Treatment for physical consequences of self harm should be offered regardless of willingness to accept psychosocial treatment.

Self poisoning

- Access TOXBASE.
- Activated charcoal should be available for immediate use; it can prevent or reduce absorption of the majority of drugs taken in overdoses, and is preferably given within 1 hour of ingestion, although up to 2 hours it is still effective for many drugs.
- Avoid multiple doses of activated charcoal.
- Emetics such as ipecacuanha should not be used.
- Gastric lavage and whole bowel irrigation should not be used unless specifically recommended by TOXBASE.
- Paracetamol levels should be measured for risk assessment 4–15 hours post ingestion.
- If paracetamol levels are raised treat with intravenous acetylcysteine.

Wounds

- Clean and check to ascertain depth.
- Tissue adhesive, or if requested skin closures, are the first line of treatment in wounds less than 5 cm.
- For wounds needing sutures, use local anaesthetic.
- Deeper wounds, with potential nerve involvement, need orthopaedic/ plastic surgical referral for repair in theatre.
- All children and young people should be admitted into a children's ward under overall care of a paediatrician; alternative placements may be needed depending upon age, circumstances of the child and family, time, child protection issues, physical and mental health of the child, and their preferences, and occasionally may involve admission to a mental health unit.
- The Child and Adolescent Mental Health (CAMH) team should conduct an assessment of needs and risks for the child including motivation for the DSH, suicidal intent, and hopelessness.
- Also need to assess the family, social situation and safeguarding issues and provide consultation for the young person, their family, the child health team, social services and education staff.
- Before discharge home, advise carers to remove all means of self harm, including medication.
- In cases of repeat DSH, consider offering developmental group psychotherapy with other young people (consists of at least 6 sessions).

Prognosis

- There are 600 successful suicides in young people aged 15–14 years each year in England and Wales, constituting the second highest cause of death in this age group. Of these, 44% have previously carried out DSH.
- One in ten people who self harm eventually kill themselves, with approximately 1% completing suicide in the year following presentation with a non-fatal act of self harm.
- Many who repeatedly self harm consider it a positive coping strategy, allowing them to have control, and as such it is a suicide prevention strategy.

Further reading

NICE (2004) Self harm: The short term physical and psychological management and secondary prevention of self-harm in primary and secondary care. NICE, London. http://www.nice.org.uk/Guidance/CG16

Mental Health Foundation and Camelot Foundation (2006) Truth Hurts: Report of the National Inquiry into Self-harm Among Young. http://www.camelotfoundation.org.uk/docs/self%20harm%20report%20lowres.pdf

TOXBASE: toxbase.org

:O: **Management of substance misuse**

Background

Alcohol misuse by children and young people is an increasing problem in the UK, with '77% of boys and 66% of girls drinking up to 10 and 6 units per week' (Rudolf and Levene 2006). It is part of the responsibility of children's nurses and all health care professionals to consider the long term health effects, both physical and emotional, to ensure that appropriate referral systems are in place, and to provide current information for young people and their families, to prevent long term problems.

Immediate identification of alcohol intoxication

- May have been witnessed, e.g. by friends.
- Blood alcohol concentration (BAC) will vary according to gender, size, how much food has been consumed, and how much alcohol has been ingested.
- Effects of 20mg of alcohol/100mL of blood may be a feeling of warmth and relaxation; at 50mg/100mL an individual will demonstrate less self control and will have impaired judgement.
- As BAC levels increase, the young person will become unsteady when attempting to walk, experience double vision, nausea, depression, and irritability.
- Gross intoxication will result in loss of vision, confusion, and loss of consciousness, and in some instances coma, paralysis of respiratory centre and death. (Adapted from Hughes et al in Bellis et al 2003)

ALERT: Other causes of symptoms such as confusion and decreasing consciousness should be ruled out before a definitive diagnosis of alcohol intoxication. For example:

- Significant brain injury (NICE 2007).
- Hypoglycaemia.
- Intracranial infection such as bacterial meningitis.
- Sepsis.
- Post convulsive state, effects of drugs (Paediatric Accident and Emergency Research Group 2008).

Immediate action

- Obtain as accurate a history of events as possible from witnesses and the transferring ambulance crew. Next of kin will be able to provide information about previous medical history.
- Follow the Resuscitation Council's Immediate Life Support algorithm:
  - Airway: check that airway is clear, as young people under the influence of alcohol can be nauseated and vomit; this increases the risk of aspiration with decreasing consciousness levels. Maintenance of a clear airway is essential and close observation should be continuous if consciousness level is impaired.
  - Breathing: observe for normal respiratory effort; oxygen will need to be administered to a young person with a decreased consciousness level in order to correct hypoxia.
  - Circulation: the young person may have lost fluid due to vomiting and may be cold from being outside. They will need to be kept

warm while being transferred to hospital, and intravascular access should be established as soon as possible.

- Disability: neurological assessment should be carried out using the Glasgow Coma Scale (GCS); a rapid assessment can also be obtained using the AVPU score.
- Exposure: conduct examination, requiring exposure of the young person's body, while ensuring dignity and respect. Determine the presence of any injuries, and look for puncture marks that might indicate intravenous drug use.

Management

- Young people who have been brought to hospital as a result of alcohol intoxication and a decreased consciousness level should be assessed according to the Resuscitation Council's Immediate Life Support guidelines (Cooper et al 2005), and if necessary given advanced life support. The guidelines on management of a child (aged 0–18) with decreased conscious level should also be followed (Paediatric Accident and Emergency Research Group 2008).
- Alcohol causes hypoglycaemia; therefore blood glucose levels should be monitored regularly, and intravenous dextrose solutions may need to be administered to counteract falling blood sugar.
- Young people are vulnerable under the influence of alcohol, and may sustain trauma injuries as a result of physical or sexual assault; these possibilities should be taken into consideration and managed in accordance with departmental guidelines.
- When recovered, a psychosocial assessment may be required to risk assess the needs of the young person; health promotion advice along with details of useful contact agencies should be provided.

Immediate identification of drug use

- Cannabis is an hallucinogenic drug causing relaxation, loss of inhibitions, paranoia, anxiety, and loss of coordination. Eyes appear red and tachycardia will be present.
- Ecstasy is a stimulant hallucinogen. It causes euphoria, increased energy, gregariousness, nausea, headache, reduced appetite, hypertension and tachycardia, and impairment of temperature control.
- Cocaine and the less refined 'crack' cocaine cause exhilaration, increased confidence, indifference to pain and hunger, and residual depression and fatigue.
- Amphetamines are a stimulant causing increased energy, stamina, confidence, headache, loss of appetite, dilated pupils, irritability, panic, and paranoia.
- Opiates, e.g. heroin, cause euphoria, sedation, respiratory depression, and bradycardia.

Adapted from Hughes (2001) and Rudolf (2006)

ALERT: It is possible that a combination of drugs may have been taken along with alcohol; an accurate history from any witnesses is essential for appropriate management, as well as past medical history from next of kin. As with alcohol intoxication, be aware of other disorders that may cause agitation or decreased consciousness.

Management

- Maintain a safe environment for both patient and staff.
- An immediate ABCDE approach should be taken, progressing to advanced life support if airway management requires intubation. Intravenous access will be required for reversing the effects of the drug and for fluid replacement.
- Advice should be taken from the local Poisons Unit by the accident and emergency team in the event of overdose of any drug, and acted upon accordingly.
- Monitoring should be according to the Paediatric Accident and Emergency Research Group (2008) guidelines. This would include cardiac monitoring, due to the effects of drugs on the cardiovascular system, and neurological assessment.

Further considerations

The effect of drugs on a young person leaves them vulnerable to assault, engagement in risky relationships, poor engagement with education, and can lead them to become involved in criminal activity.

Provision of access to specialist services such as CAMHS, drug advisory centres and information within the education, leisure, and health arenas will help to safeguard the young person, and support them to fulfil their full potential.

Further reading

Hughes K, Bellis MA, Kilfoyle-Carrington M (2001) Alcohol, Tobacco and Drugs in the North West of England: identifying a shared agenda. Public Health Sector, Liverpool John Moores University, Liverpool.

The Paediatric Accident and Emergency Research Group (2008) The management of a child (aged 0–18 years) with a decreased conscious level. An evidence-based guideline for health professionals based in the hospital setting. Nottingham: The Paediatric Accident and Emergency Research Group.

Resuscitation Council (UK): www.resus.org.uk

Cooper S, Johnston E, Priscott D (2005) Immediate Life Support (ILS) Training. Resuscitation Council (UK), London.

Rudolf M, Levene M (2006). *Paediatrics and child health*, Oxford. Blackwell Publishing.

National Institute for Health and Clinical Excellence (2007). *Head Injury. Triage, assessment, investigation and early management of head injury in infants, children and adults.* London, NHS.

☼ **Anxiety episodes/panic attacks in childhood and adolescence**

Defining anxiety (Thompson, 2005)

- A *normal emotional response*, which enables children and adolescents to cope with separation, competition, and threats/danger ('fight', 'flight' or 'freeze'). Objectively, normal and abnormal anxiety can be viewed as being on a continuum, the latter being characterized by:
  - *Physiological changes*: tachycardia, hyperventilation, sweating, tremor, jumpiness, sickness, abdominal pain, and headache.
  - *Changes in subjective awareness*: excessive worries/fears with regard to perceived threats to self or loved ones (including objectively 'normal' situations, such as meeting new people) and the perception that they will be unable to cope with any anxiety-provoking phenomena.
  - *Changes in behaviour* (Swadi, 2000): withdrawal, irritability and aggression. The young person may make subtle and overt attempts to avoid the anxiety-provoking scenario (i.e. avoiding school or social situations), which in severe cases disrupts normative social and academic development. In older adolescents the use of alcohol and/or substances may be used to cope with acute anxiety.

Disordered anxiety along the developmental pathway

Younger children: as described above, with fear of the dark and somatic complaints being potential features.

Middle childhood: separation anxiety (marked anxiety on separation beyond expectation for developmental stage), generalized anxiety disorder (not necessarily specific to a phobia), specific phobias (producing functional impairment or significant distress).

Adolescence: all of the above, with the possible addition of panic disorder, agoraphobia (fear of open environments), and social or school phobia (anxiety about performance in these situations and about meeting new people). Panic attacks (the severest attack of anxiety symptoms) are more apparent in this age group, but not necessarily indicative of a panic disorder (may be part of a phobic, generalized anxiety, or depressive disorder).

Issues/questions to consider in managing an acute anxiety episode/panic attack in a paediatric clinical environment

- The majority of children and young people are in this potentially unfamiliar environment because of a health problem, which may produce normal and appropriate feelings of anxiety. Anxiety responses are also influenced by temperament, genetics, family and social relationships, and traumatic events, which differ for different children/young people. What is a normal expression of anxiety for one may be deemed excessive when compared to another.

- It is very important to consider the child's stage of development: overt/high levels of distress on separation from caregivers in the first years of childhood is a healthy part of forming a bond with attachment figures (Bowlby, 1973), but perhaps can be viewed as problematic if a 15 year old responds to separation in the same way.
- Two useful questions in identifying abnormal anxiety are (Klein, 1995):
  - How well can the child recover from anxiety and remain anxiety free, when no longer exposed to the anxiety-provoking situation?
  - What is the degree of impairment to functioning, i.e. age appropriate social and academic activities?
- Acute episodes of anxiety or panic attacks may occur abruptly or unexpectedly in previously well-functioning children.

Interventions

Relaxation

When acutely anxious, children/young people may begin to hyperventilate, and this further exacerbates their anxiety symptoms. It is important to assist them to regulate their breathing, through the use of breathing and relaxation techniques.

- Square breathing involves getting the young person to focus on expelling all the air from their lungs, taking in a long slow breath, holding that breath, and finally slowly expelling the air from the lungs once more (all four stages should be equal in length). This may be difficult for younger children to follow.
- Appropriate use of physical touch, especially with younger children, can be helpful in regulating breathing, perhaps by placing the hand gently on the child's chest. It may be more appropriate to get a parent/carer to do this or give a hug to the child. This is not avoiding the anxiety, but can demonstrate support through the anxiety situation.
- Some children, with practice and guidance, may be able to visualize a place or situation in which they have felt calm and relaxed, which again will help them regulate their current anxiety symptoms.

Communicate with the child/young person

Reassure them that the panic/anxiety they are currently experiencing cannot physically escalate indefinitely, and that after a period it will plateau and subside. Avoid colluding with the child's attempts to avoid the anxious situation (possibly through the hyper arousal of a 'panic attack'), perhaps by omitting age appropriate information around a medical procedure. If attempts to minimize distress in this way are not perceived by the child as a true reflection of the actual procedure, this will reinforce their anxiety in the future. It is important to respectfully challenge such colluding behaviour in parents/carers.

Medication

Medications considered for use with older children and adolescents experiencing acute anxiety/panic attacks include selective serotonin reuptake inhibitors (SSRIs) and benzodiazepines. For short-term intervention benzodiazepines can be effective in reducing distress, clarifying the clinical presentation, and enabling the young person to communicate their difficulties.

Referral to Child and Adolescent Mental Health Service (CAMHS)

If the presentation of anxiety is severe and persists beyond the stressful situation, it may be appropriate to refer on to the hospital child mental health liaison team (if available as a resource) or local community CAMHS team for further assessment and support.

Further reading

Department of Health (2004). *National Service Framework for Children, Young People and Maternity Services*. London. Department of Health.

Klein, R.G., Pine. D.S. (2006). 'Anxiety disorders'. In Rutter, M., Taylor, E. (eds). Child and Adolescent Psychiatry, 4th Edn. Oxford: Blackwell Publishing. Pp 486–509.

Swadi, H (2000) Substance misuse in adolescents. *Advances in Psychiatric Treatment* 6 pp. 201–10.

The Royal College of Nursing (2004). *Children and Young People's Mental Health Every Nurse's Business*, London Royal College of Nursing.

Thompson, M. (2005). 'Problems in older children: anxiety'. In M. Cooper, C. Hooper, M. Thompson, (eds), Child and Adolescent Mental Health: Theory and Practice. London: Hodder Arnold.

www.childanxiety.net
www.rcpsych.ac.uk
www.youngminds.org.uk

ⓘ Depression in children and young people

Age definitions
In accordance with the National Institute for Health and Clinical Excellence guidelines on the identification and management of depression in children and young people, a child is aged between 5 and 11 years and a young person from 12 years up to their 18th birthday (NICE 2005).
Response to current trends:
- The Royal College of Nursing (2004:1) suggests that there is 'increasing evidence that mental ill-health in childhood and adolescence is becoming very common'. It may be, of course, that it is being recognized and diagnosed more often today.
- It is essential that nurses are equipped with the correct knowledge and understanding of conditions such as depression, so that they can make appropriate risk assessments and care provisions for children and young people.
- Standard 9 of the National Service Framework for Children, Young People and Maternity Services states the requirement that 'all staff working directly with children and young people have sufficient knowledge, training and support to promote the psychological well being of children, young people and their families and to identify early indicators of difficulty' (Department of Health 2004).

Emergency presentation
Children and young people may present to a range of agencies in need of urgent mental health assessment; these may include primary health care services such as GP surgeries, or walk in centres, social workers, police and emergency departments. Therefore, professionals must be able to make an initial assessment, and should have referral access to a 24 hour Child and Adolescent Mental Health Service (CAMHS) (Department of Health 2004).

Identification of symptoms of depression in primary care, schools and community settings: psycho-social risk factors
- Age.
- Gender.
- Family discord.
- School relationships/academic stressors.
- Peer relationships.
- Bullying.
- Physical, sexual or emotional abuse.
- Comorbid disorders, including drug and alcohol use.
- History of parental depression.
- History of single loss events.
- Multiple risk factors, including ethnic and cultural factors.
- Homelessness.
- Refugee status.
- Living in institutional settings.
(NICE 2005)

Management of young people with a depressive disorder presenting in an emergency department

- Young people may present in an emergency setting as a result of deliberate self harm, trauma injury secondary to risk taking activity, or alcohol or substance abuse. There may be an associated depressive disorder in these young people, but assessment, treatment and stabilization of their physical condition will be the priority. In some conditions this may include advanced life support interventions.
- Taking a detailed history of medical, mental health, and psychosocial events prior to admission to the emergency department will establish any pre-existing depressive disorders already being treated, or any significant risk factors leading to admission.
- When it is medically appropriate, a mental health assessment should be carried out by the CAMHS.
- A young person should be interviewed alone as well as with a parent or carer, as the latter may not have been aware of how their child has been feeling (Fairclough in Glasper, McEwing and Richardson 2006).

Treatment and management

- According to the NICE guidelines (2005), treatment of depression is deter-mined by classification defined by the World Health Organization ICD-10:
  - Mild depression.
  - Moderate and severe depression.
  - Severe depression and psychotic symptoms.
- The level of severity will also determine the degree of supervision the child or young person will require.
- It is important to consider the individual child or young person's 'functioning in a number of settings, for example, school, with peers and with family' (NICE 2005:9) rather than focusing totally on presenting symptoms.
- The NICE guidelines also provide a list of key symptoms for consideration in diagnosing depression, and should be used as a point of reference.
- The use of assessment tools such as KIDDIE–SADS (K-SADS) and Child and Adolescent Psychiatric Assessment (CAPA) assist with accurate diagnosis of depression by CAMHS professionals.
- The five question PATHOS screening questionnaire may be used by practitioners treating adolescents in emergency departments as a result of intentional drug overdose.

The building of a supportive and collaborative working relationship with the child or young person and their family is essential in the effective assessment and treatment of depression (NICE 2005). This must be ac-companied by access to specialist services as required, and provision of up-to-date information on the condition and services available.

Further reading

Department of Health (2004). *National Service Framework for Children, Young People and Maternity Services.* London.

Fairclough A (2007). *Depression.* In Glasper EA, McEwing G, Richardson J (eds). *Oxford Handbook of Children's & Young People's Nursing.* Oxford, Oxford University Press.

Kingsbury S (1996) PATHOS: a screening instrument for adolescent overdose: a research note. *Journal of Child Psychology and Psychiatry* 37:609–611

National Institute for Health and Clinical Excellence (2005). Depression in Children and Young People – Identification and management in primary, community and secondary care. London: NICE.

ⓘ Fabricated or induced illness

Paediatric nurses must always remain vigilant to the possibility that carers can and do cause harm to children through fabricated or induced illness. Terminology to describe the fabrication or induction of illness in a child has changed over time, and includes Munchausen's syndrome by proxy and factitious illness.

The focus should always remain upon the impact of fabrication or induction of symptoms and signs on a child's health and development and how best to safeguard their welfare.

The mother's and/or other carer's possible actions may consist of:
- Fabrication: false reporting of signs and symptoms, which may include fabrication of past medical history.
- Interference: e.g. with specimens of bodily fluids and with IV lines.
- Falsification: of hospital charts and records, and of letters and documents.
- Direct interference with the child (induction).

Incidence/causes

The presentation of fabricated/induced illness is very variable.
- Age: most common with younger children.
- Range of presenting symptoms.
- Varying severity of initial illness.
- Differing lengths of time of falsification or illness induction before identification and action.
- Fabrication may escalate to illness induction.
- Child may collude and self perpetuate.

NB: children subject to fabricated or induced illness may also suffer from a genuine medical condition.

Effects on the child

- Repeated investigations, procedures and treatments
- Health and life are threatened if illness is induced
- Deprived of full education
- Socially isolated
- Anxiety and confusion about health

Signs and symptoms

- Reported symptoms and signs found on examination not explained by medical condition.
- Investigations do not explain reported symptoms.
- Signs are reported or symptoms observed only by a parent (or particular adult), or when a parent (or particular adult) is present.
- Inexplicably poor response to prescribed treatment.
- New symptoms are reported on resolution of previous ones.
- Repeated presentations to a variety of health professionals with a variety of problems.

- Child's normal daily activities are being curtailed beyond that which might be expected for any medical disorder from which the child is known to suffer.
- Parent disputes negative findings and requests further investigations. Parental behaviour:
- Unusually detailed knowledge and interest in child's condition
- Predicts when further episode of illness will occur
- Not easily reassured or questions negative findings
- Unusually involved in details of child's treatment
- Constantly by inpatient child's side
- Not distressed or unusually calm in face of a seriously ill child
- Observed tampering with specimens or equipment (rare)

Action

- Ascertain whether a child's symptoms and signs have an explanation as a verified illness.

NB: in all situations it is good practice when making records to attribute observations to the reporter or observer, e.g. 'mother said', 'nurse saw', but in fabricated/induced illness situations this is of vital importance.

- Consider discrepancies between reported symptoms and independent observations.
- Once concerns have been raised, all observations and samples must be tactfully taken by nursing staff without parent participation. How samples were obtained should be recorded.
- If there are still discrepancies and professional concerns, an internal professionals meeting should be called by the lead paediatrician/ professional or Named Professional to clarify suspicions, to consider observation, to suggest further investigations required to identify or exclude a medical cause for the child's reported symptoms, and to agree a management plan. Attendance needs to include not only internal health professionals, but also invited external professionals who can provide a fuller picture, e.g. social care colleagues, health visitors, a GP, school nurse, etc. A child protection referral will be made when judged necessary.

Observations

The purpose of observation is to gain a complete and detailed picture of the child's state of health and an understanding about the child's reported symptoms and signs. It is important that:

- Observation is constant and everything is documented.
- All care and treatment is carried out by hospital staff.
- All input and output is documented.
- All interactions with parents and carers and other interactions are documented.
- Any concerns are immediately reported.
- Parents are informed that there is no clear diagnosis, and to help clarify the diagnosis it is important that clinical staff are able to more closely and constantly observe their child's reactions.

- If there are any safety concerns, e.g. concerns regarding illness induction, the parent(s)/carer must never be allowed unsupervised access to the child or anything that will be administered to the child (e.g. access to the ward kitchen, etc.).
- Named Professionals will provide constant support and ensure constant review of action required including liaison with and referral to social care.

Further reading

The Royal College of Paediatrics and Child Health (2002) Fabricated or Induced Illness by Carers. London: RCPCH

Department of Health (2002) Safeguarding Children in Whom Illness is Fabricated or Induced. London: DH

Unscheduled care management

⑦ Legal framework in emergency care and accountability of the practitioner

Practitioners must have a working knowledge of legal and ethical issues relating to autonomy and consent to treatment. The Department of Health (2004) defines consent as a patient's agreement for a health professional to provide care. For consent to be valid the patient must:

- Be competent to take a particular decision
- Have received sufficient information to take it
- Not be acting under duress.

Obtaining consent from patients is essential prior to the provision of treatment or care. While mentally competent adults can make informed choices regarding their health, achieving autonomy is a gradual developmental process. Children and young people require legal protection until they are mature enough to make informed choices about their health. The law recognizes that children and young people under 18 years of age are significantly different to adults in their decision making abilities, and need legal protection and provision until they are mature enough to make their own informed choices. Legislation also enables them to give their own consent to treatment as they develop and mature.

The child under 16 years old

Where a child lacks capacity to consent, then a person with 'parental responsibility' or the court can give that consent by proxy (on behalf of the child). Parental responsibility is defined as:

All the rights, duties, powers, responsibility, and authority which by law a parent of a child has in relation to the child and his property.

(Children Act 1989 Section 3 (1))

- Parental responsibility is automatically conferred upon the mother, and pertains to the father if he was married to the mother when the child was born or shortly after.
- Single fathers did not have parental responsibility as an automatic right until the implementation of the Adoption and Children Act 2002 in December 2003 (England and Wales), which states that the unmarried father, if he jointly registers the birth with the mother, also has parental responsibility.
- The change in parental responsibility is not retrospective, and so does not apply to unmarried fathers of children born before December 2003.
- Other people such as legal guardians, person/s with a residence order, or adoptive parents may also have parental responsibility.
- Parental responsibility is not lost when parents divorce, and most parents retain this when a child is accommodated by the local authority or police.
- Parental responsibility is only valid if the parent is acting in the best interests of the child (known as the welfare principle).
- Parental responsibility diminishes as children mature and ceases when a child reaches 18 years of age in England, Wales and Northern Ireland.
- In Scotland parental responsibility ceases when a child reaches 16.

Children develop at varying rates and, as Gillick v West Norfolk and Wisbech Area Health Authority (1986) established, competent minors can consent to their own treatment or care. The standard principles used with regard to contraceptive treatment are known as the Fraser guidelines, which include a set of criteria that must apply when health professionals are offering treatment or care to those less than 16 years of age.

Mature minors cannot refuse treatment that may be needed in life saving situations.

The Fraser Guidelines

1. The young person understands the health professional's advice.
2. The health professional cannot persuade the young person to inform his or her parents or allow the doctor to inform the parents that he or she is seeking contraceptive advice.
3. The young person is very likely to begin or continue having intercourse with or without contraceptive treatment.
4. Unless he or she receives contraceptive advice or treatment, the young person's physical or mental health (or both) is likely to suffer.
5. The young person's best interests require the health professional to give contraceptive advice, treatment or both without parental consent. (Department of Health 2004)

A mature minor is also entitled to an obligation of confidentiality, unless the health professional believes that maintaining confidentiality may be harmful for that child or others, e.g. in a child protection situation.

16- and 17-year-olds

Sixteen and 17-year-olds are deemed mature enough to give their own consent for medical, surgical and dental treatment and investigations (Family Law Reform Act 1969 Section 8(1) and 8(2).

- This principle is also included in the Mental Health Act 1983.
- An unconscious 16- or 17-year-old can still be given life saving treatment in an emergency.
- Parents of an incapacitated young person under 18 years are still able to give consent by proxy.
- Where a 16- or 17-year-old refuses to give consent for treatment or care their autonomy may be challenged by practitioners or in law, e.g. in Re W (a minor: medical treatment) (1992) the Court of Appeal overruled W's refusal to receive life saving treatment.
- From October 2008 parents can no longer give consent for their 16- or 17-year-old to be admitted to a psychiatric unit for treatment (Mental Health Act 2007)

Further reading

Adoption and Children Act 2002

Children Act 1989 Section 3 (1)

Department of Health (2004) Best practice guidance for doctors and other health professionals on the provision of advice and treatment to young people under 16 on contraception, sexual health and reproduction. Gateway reference 3382

Family Law Reform Act 1969 Section 8(1) and 8(2). http://www.legislation.gov.uk/ukpga/1969/46

Gillick v West Norfolk and Wisbech Area Health Authority (1986) AC 112, (1985) 3 All ER 402, (1985) 2BMLR 11 HL

Mental health act (1983) http://www.dh.gov.uk/en/PublicationsandStatistics/Legislation/Actsandbills/dh4002034

Mental health act 1983 and 2007 http://www.dh.gov.uk

Re W (A Minor) medical treatment (1992) *All Eng law rep* 4 pp. 627–49.

ⓘ Trephining subungual haematomas

Definintion

A subungual haematoma is a collection of blood beneath a nail, often caused by a crush injury or repetitive trauma to the nail bed through an activity such as running. As the fingertips and toes are sensitive areas, a subungual haematoma can be extremely painful, and it is the level of pain, along with the cosmetic appearance of the nail, that brings people to the Emergency Department. The treatment of a subungual haematoma depends on three main factors:

- Whether a fracture of the terminal phalynx has occurred through the crush injury (if there is a fracture present then trephining the nail will turn the fracture into an open or compound fracture)
- The size of the haematoma (if the haematoma is small and causing a low level of pain then the nail can be managed conservatively with elevation and ice)
- If the nail is disrupted or the nail margin not visible then expert advice should be sought from an orthopaedic/plastic surgeon depending on the hospital policy.

The trephining procedure involves making a hole in the nail directly above the haematoma to release it.

- Prior to the trephining, the nail and finger should be cleaned thoroughly and placed in a sterile field.
- The treatment should be carried out aseptically and universal precautions should be followed as the haematoma may spurt if there is pressure involved.
- The hole itself can be made by hot cautery or 'drilling technique'.

Hot cautery

- Performed either using a trephining machine or a paper clip straightened and heated, with the hot end placed on the nail until the nail is burned through and the haematoma is expressed. NB: distraction strategies should be considered.
- This method can be unpleasant due to the smell of burning nail, and also because the use of a heated paper clip appears antiquated.

Drilling

- Using a blue (22 gauge) needle held vertically to the nail bed and rolled between the practitioner's thumb and index finger creating a drilling action to make a hole in the nail.
- The hole made by this method is smaller than one made by hot cautery and because of this the procedure may need to be repeated if the hole seals over.

Both methods are effective and local policy should be checked by the practitioner to decide which method is to be used. Once the haematoma has been drained the nail should be covered with a dry dressing and the appropriate follow-up arranged in either hand clinic or Emergency Department review clinic. In all cases the patient should be advised to keep the finger dry and clean and take regular analgesia.

Whichever method of trephining is selected the procedure itself is relatively straight forward and gratifying for the practitioner as the relief is immediate. However, with all treatments in the children's Emergency Department the main skill is to adequately explain to the child and the parent that trephining the nail is less painful than leaving the subungual haematoma in place. The child must give their consent so that they keep still for the trephining. This is vital to ensure that the practitioner is not at risk of a sharps injury or a burn. In these cases the use of a play therapist cannot be underestimated (See Communicating through Play, p. 14). If the child is uncooperative despite the use of a play therapist and adequate discussion it may be more appropriate to manage the child conservatively, but this decision should be made following discussion with the parents and doctors involved.

Further reading

Richardson M (2004) Selecting a treatment option in subungual haematoma management. *Nursing Times* 100:59.

⑦ Bandaging and securing dressings

Introduction

Whenever a child in the Emergency Department requires a dressing or bandage, the first consideration for the practitioner when selecting the appropriate dressing is the compliance of the child. Although you may have the perfect dressing in your trolley for the injury you are faced with, if the child will not allow you to apply and secure the dressing then you may need to be creative! Negotiation skills and communication form a crucial part of nursing children in any department, and these negotiation skills are often tested fully when faced with wound dressings in the children's Emergency Department.

The key principles of bandaging and securing any dressing are always to:
- optimize conditions for healing
- ensure the bandage does not cause any further harm
- ensure that it will cause minimal distress when it needs to be removed; again this often means that creativity is needed with children.

In the children's Emergency Department the most common use of bandages is to secure dressings such as burn dressings or wound coverings, as there is little research which supports the use of limb bandages with sprains and soft tissue injuries in children.

When dressing a burn or other wound in the Emergency Department, advice from colleagues and local policy should be sought as most departments have specific guidelines for the primary dressings of these specific injuries. Once this advice has been sought and the primary covering has been selected, consideration should be given to the best way to ensure this primary dressing is held securely in place in a way that ensures that healing takes place and is acceptable to the child and the parent. Consideration should also be given to changing of this dressing, e.g. a burn dressing may be held in place very securely with Elastoplast when first applied, but when the dressing requires changing its removal may cause excessive pain, which will distress the child and almost certainly make it more difficult to redress. In this situation a larger nonadhesive dressing may look disproportionate compared to the size of the burn, but may cause the least amount of distress to all those involved and may ensure the child complies with the dressing to maximize healing.

General method for applying dressings

- Ensure analgesia is given approximately 30 minutes prior to the dressing application or change.
- Prepare the dressing trolley; first clean it thoroughly and then ensure you have everything needed for the dressing. Wash hands and follow universal precautions.
- Explain the procedure to the child in an age appropriate manner; parents should also be fully aware of the process. Involve a play specialist if available.
- Position the child so that they are safe and comfortable and the wound is easily accessible.

- Keep the child warm: this is especially important with burn dressings, as the child may have been treated with cold water to cool the burn initially.
- Perform the dressing using aseptic non-touch technique. Explain what is happening to the child the entire time, as this will help to reassure them.
- Dispose of old/unused dressings appropriately and wash hands.
- Explain to parents how to look after the dressing at home, giving advice leaflets if available. Ensure the parents are aware of when to return for dressing changes or of how to remove the dressing at home.
- Document the procedure in the notes.

Further reading

NHS Choices (2008) How do I apply a bandage? http://www.nhs.uk/chq/Pages/1052.aspx? CategoryID=72&SubCategoryID=721

NMC (2010) Record keeping for nurses and midwives. http://www.nmc-uk.org/Documents/ Guidance/nmcGuidanceRecordKeepingGuidanceforNursesandMidwives.pdf

⑦ **Replacing gastrostomy devices**

Introduction

- Children who cannot independently maintain adequate nutritional, fluid or pharmaceutical input via the oral route may have a gastrostomy device inserted.
- The gastrostomy is a tube that provides direct access to the stomach via the abdominal wall, through which nutritional/fluid/pharmaceutical intake can be maintained and supplemented.
- Gastrostomy devices can also be inserted solely for means of stomach decompression and venting purposes.

Background information

- Gastrostomy devices are available in different formats and from various manufacturers. Practitioners are advised to refer to manufacturers' advice and local policies and guidelines pertinent to devices used. With regards to paediatrics, the most popular devices seem to be PEG (percutaneous endoscopic gastrostomy) tubes and low profile skin level gastrostomy devices.
- The bulleted lists below recognize some basic differences between these two types of gastrostomy tube.
- **PEG gastrostomy**
  - Freka Tube (Fresenius Kabi), CorFlo PEG Tube (Merck).
  - Surgical or endoscopic insertion.
  - Tube external to abdomen.
  - Usually secured via internal disc and external fixator plate, stitches or cage design.
  - Generally inserted as the initial/primary gastrostomy.
  - Surgical replacement required approximately every 2 years.
- **Low profile gastrostomy**
  - Mic-key Button (Vygon), Corflo Cubby Button (Merck), Mini Button (AMT Inc).
  - Insertion by trained parent, carer or health professional.
  - Skin level device, cosmetically preferred to PEG.
  - Secured via inflatable balloon.
  - Usually inserted minimal 6 weeks post stoma tract formation and primary PEG insertion.
  - Replaced every 3–12 months (dependent on life of individual device and local health policy).
- This section is focused on the replacement of low profile gastrostomy devices. These are also referred to as skin level, button or balloon button devices.

Incidence and causes

- As a planned procedure, low profile gastrostomy devices are commonly replaced at between 3 and 9 monthly intervals, dependent on local policy.
- In some regions it is known for low profile gastrostomy devices to be used until they are no longer viable, and are then replaced.

- Low profile gastrostomy devices can become unexpectedly removed from the stoma tract or develop faults. This will result in the device needing to be replaced immediately.
- Incidence for emergency gastrostomy device replacement may include the device being pulled out or physically damaged, device not been used in accordance with manufacturer's instructions, incorrect size/ measured gastrostomy device in place, stoma site trauma and infection.

Signs and symptoms

The following may cause the gastrostomy device to come out of the stoma tract and/or be unusable:

- Stoma tract/gastrostomy tube infection: redness around the stoma site, inflammation, discharge, pain, bleeding and foul odour.
- Trauma: pain and bleeding from the stoma site. The stoma tract is unintentionally dilated/damaged from a traumatic event resulting in the device becoming unstable, loose, or removed from the stoma tract, e.g. the device being forcibly pulled while in situ with the balloon inflated.
- Device misuse: non- or incorrect inflation of balloon, inaccurate measurement of tract leading to wrong size device being inserted, incorrect equipment attached to access port of device, and contraindicated fluid, nutrition and/or medication being administered via the device.

Immediate management

- Typically the most important aspect of gastrostomy/stoma tract care is to ensure that the tract does not close. The stoma site may begin to close within 1 hour after a device has been removed (www. appliedmedical.net/BalloonButtonGuide.pdf).
- If there is no spare replacement gastrostomy device available to you and you cannot reinsert the current device (due to its physical state, for hygienic reasons, or as per local policy), then place a dressing over the stoma entrance and seek medical advice immediately (www. corecharity.org.uk/Peg-Feeding.html).
- If possible, you should always consult the manufacturer's guidance for the specific low profile balloon gastrostomy device you are using.
- Do not replace a device if the stoma tract is infected, traumatized, or not fully formed (i.e. recent post operative insertion).
- If you have an appropriate replacement low profile balloon gastrostomy device available, the stoma tract is viable and you are qualified to do so, then you can go ahead and replace the device.
- Wash and dry hands thoroughly (http://www.hpa.org.uk/web/ HPAwebFile/HPAweb_C/1194947384669).
- Put on gloves.
- Remove the new low profile gastrostomy from the packaging and, using the balloon valve, inflate the balloon with 5 mL of sterile water or saline. Observe the balloon; it should look symmetrical with no signs of leakage or damage. Deflate the balloon.
- To remove the old device, attach a 5 mL syringe to the balloon valve of the low profile gastrostomy in situ in the patient. Holding the gastrostomy device securely, withdraw the syringe plunger until all of the water is removed from the balloon.

- Gently remove the device from the stomach using slow and steady pressure; you can use a small amount of water-soluble lubricant to help ease it out if required.
- Lubricate the tip of the new low profile gastrostomy device with some water-soluble lubricant and gently insert into the stoma, until the external base of the device is flat against the skin.
- Whilst holding the gastrostomy device in place in the stoma, inflate the balloon via the balloon port/valve with 5 mL (or prescribed volume) of cool boiled water or saline.
- Gently pull the gastrostomy away from the skin until it stops; this checks that the balloon is secure, ensures that the balloon is positioned against the stomach wall, and helps pull the stomach wall and abdomen together to maintain the stoma tract.
- Check that the low profile gastrostomy is in the correct position (within the stomach). Dependent on local health policy, this may require aspirating gastric contents and checking that the aspirate result corresponds to the recommended result for gastric acid.
- If the appropriate result is obtained and low profile gastrostomy placement is confirmed in the stomach, then the procedure is complete. If not, X-ray verification could be required.

Additional information

- This is generic advice. Refer to individual manufacturer guidelines.
- The guidance described does not apply to the insertion of G-tubes or similar balloon gastrostomy feeding tubes.
- Please always be mindful of the child's privacy, dignity and psychological welfare when using or handling a gastrostomy device.
- Changing a low profile balloon gastrostomy can potentially cause anxiety, pain and discomfort. Administration of appropriate analgesia, if possible prior to the procedure, is advisable.
- If the gastrostomy has needed to be replaced due to a physical or material defect, then it is possible for the faulty device to be examined and tested to establish the cause of the event. Investigation can determine whether the event was due to bacterial/fungal colonization or infection, manufacturer defect, client misuse, etc.

Further reading

NHS (2007) Best Practice Statement. Caring for children and young people in the community receiving enteral tube feeding. Edinburgh: NHS Quality Improvement Scotland.
Draper R (2009) PEG Feeding Tubes – Indications and Management. www.patient.co.uk/showdoc/40024638.

⑦ Management and placement of nasogastric tubes in children (troubleshooting)

Introduction
Nasogastric (NG) tube placement in children is a common procedure, often used as a short term method of enteral nutrition or administration of medicine for children who are unable to take food/medicine orally. See Table 14.1 for how to insert an NG tube.

Indication of need for nasogastric tube insertion
- Need for enteral nutrition
- Administration of medicines
- Aspiration of stomach contents

ALERT: Contraindications
- Anatomical deformity
- Trauma (i.e. nasal injuries or skull fractures)
- Recent oral, nasal or oesophageal surgery
- Severe gastro-oesophageal reflux
- Upper gastrointestinal stricture

Table 14.1 Inserting a nasogastric tube
ALERT: Always make an initial risk assessment for each patient prior to feeding and administering medication via a nasogastric tube.

	Action
1.	Prepare equipment: Appropriate nasogastric tube Water or water based lubricant Gallipot 50 mL enteral feeding syringe pH indication paper Hydrocolloid dressing Tape Scissors Disposable gloves and apron
2.	Explain and discuss procedure with child and family and obtain consent.
3.	Wash and dry hands, put on plastic apron and clean work surface.
4.	Prepare hydrocolloid dressing and tape for securing the nasogastric tube.
5.	Put on disposable gloves and remove nasogastric tube from packaging, ensuring that the packaging and nasogastric tube are not damaged in any way.

Table 14.1 Inserting a nasogastric tube (*Continued*)

Action
6.   To determine the length of tube to be inserted: measure from the nostril to the ear, and then from the ear to the stomach, just pass the xiphoid process.
7.   Record the reading, and mark or hold the point on the tube in your less dominant hand. **NB:** supportively holding the child or infant can provide comfort and support for the child and aid in passing the nasogastric tube. Wrap infants in a blanket and sit older children up with their head supported.
8.   Select a clear nostril and lubricate the tip of the nasogastric tube using water or a water based solution.
9.   Pass tube into nostril, angling slightly upwards and slide backwards along the floor of the nasopharynx. Gently feed the tube downwards; you may need to stop to allow the tube to pass through the cardiac sphincter into the stomach. Getting an infant to suck on a pacifier or an older child to take sips of water will assist in passing the tube. **ALERT:** Never force the tube. If the child becomes distressed, starts gasping or coughing and becomes cyanosed, stop the procedure immediately and withdraw the tube.
10.   Insert the tube until the mark or point on the tube reaches the child's nostril and check the tube is in the correct position by obtaining aspirate and following the flow chart shown in Fig. 14.1.
11.   Secure the tube by putting hydrocolloid dressing onto the child's cheek and then secure the tube on top with tape.
12.   Ensure adequate documentation takes place recording the size of the nasogastric tube, date and time of insertion and nostril it is inserted into.

Management and confirming correct placement

Checking the position of a nasogastric tube should take place:
- Following insertion
- Before commencement of feeds
- Before administration of medicines via the nasogastric tube
- At least once a day during continuous feeds
- Following any episodes of vomiting, retching or coughing
- Following indication of tube displacement (e.g. loose tape or visible tube appears longer)
  (National Patient Safety Agency, 2005)

Troubleshooting

A child appears to have a blockage in their nasogastric tube. No aspirate can be obtained.

- Attempt to inject 1–5mL of air down the tube with a 20mL or 50mL syringe.
  - If successful wait 15–30 minutes and try aspirating again.
- Consider the material and how long the nasogastric tube has been in place. Follow manufacturer's guidelines on how frequently nasogastric tubes should be changed, as some can deteriorate and lose flexibility when in contact with gastric secretions for a length of time.
- If unsuccessful in passing air down the nasogastric tube, then remove tube and replace with a new one following appropriate guidelines.

Testing nasogastric feeding tubes

The National Patient Safety Agency (NPSA) (2005) recommends, following a number of reported incidents and deaths, that the methods that should be used to test the position of a nasogastric tube are:

- Measuring pH of aspirate, using pH indicator strips/paper to confirm the appropriate acidity of the aspirate.
- Radiography.

THE FOLLOWING ARE UNSAFE METHODS AND SHOULD NOT BE USED:

- 'Woosh test' (auscultation of air through the feeding tube).
- The use of blue litmus paper to test the acidity and alkalinity of the stomach aspirate.
- The absence of respiratory distress as an indicator of correct position.
- Observing bubbling at the end of the tube at expiration when the proximal end of the tube is under water.
- Observing the appearance of aspirate as a single testing method.

Troubleshoot

A mother arrives in a GP surgery with her 4 month old child. She is concerned as she has trouble obtaining aspirate prior to each feed, which in turn delays the times of feeds and distresses the child if she has to reinsert the tube.

- Is the child on any medication? For example, domperidone is a gastric emptier so would affect the amount of gastric contents.
- Follow flow chart (Fig. 14.1) for confirming nasogastric tube placement, advance tube 1–2 cm and try aspirating again.
- Remove nasogastric tube and reinsert, ensuring that a new measurement is taken for the length of the tube.

Troubleshoot

A child is admitted into a walk-in centre with a localized skin reac-tion/redness around the side of the face and nostril in which a nasogastric tube is inserted, with no history of trauma.

- Consider sensitivity/allergy to dressings.
- Remove tube and consider the need for replacement of tube and use of nasogastric tube in an alternative material.
- If reinserting nasogastric tube, insert into opposite nostril and secure on opposite side of face.
- Possible latex allergy. Insert using latex free gloves and refer to dermatologist to determine allergy source.

Troubleshoot

You are teaching parents in the emergency department about aspirating to test the position of a nasogastric tube.

Remember:

- 0.5–1mL of aspirate is considered a sufficient amount to test on pH indicator paper/strips.
- Aspirate of pH 5.5 or below allows you to commence feeding, as it is unlikely that the aspirate is from the lungs. However, if there is any doubt of the tube position, and especially if the pH is between 5 and 6, then feeding must not commence (NPSA 2005).
- If the aspirate is of pH 6 or above you must not feed, as it is possible that the aspirate is that of pulmonary secretions. If the patient's clinical needs allow, leave for up to 1 hour and retest the tube. If not, gain advice and consider re-placing the tube or checking position by X-ray.

Confirming correct placement
See Fig. 14.1 below.

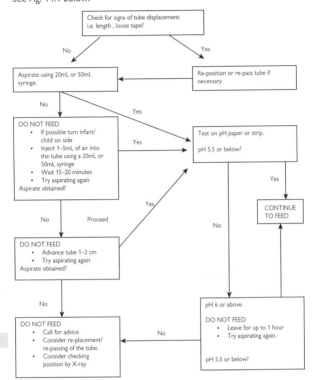

Fig. 14.1 Confirming the correct placement of nasogastric feeding tubes.
Adapted from NPSA (2005) guidelines for infants and children.

Further reading

National Patient Safety Agency (2007) Nasogastric Tube Incidents: Summary Update. http://www. npsa.nhs.uk/nrls/alerts-and-directives/alerts/nasogastric-feeding-tubes/

National Patient Safety Agency (2005) Reducing the harm caused by misplaced nasogastric feeding tubes. Interim advice for health care staff. February 2005. NHS

http://www.rcn.org.uk/newsevents/news/article/uk/new_publication_on_restraining_children_available

http://www.ich.ucl.ac.uk/clinical_information/clinical_guidelines/copy%20of%20copy2%20of%20cpg_guideline_00109

http://www.patient.co.uk/showdoc/40000186/

⑦ The role of the Paediatric Assessment Unit

The changes in the General Practitioner contract came into effect on 1 April 2004. Of profound interest to nurses working in paediatric emergency care was the ability of GPs to opt out of traditional out-of-hours services. This has fuelled a shift in the management of sick children from general practice to hospital, through attendance at either an emergency department or a paediatric emergency assessment unit (PEAU).

Short Stay Paediatric Assessment Units (SSPAU) and Paediatric Assessment Units (PAU) are an integral component within the paediatric emergency care setting, and are designed to meet the needs of children and young people.

The Royal College of Paediatrics and Child Health suggests that SSPAUs and PAUs can improve the provision of safe emergency services for children, and that these units should be developed more widely.

The units cater for children with acute illnesses, acute illnesses within a chronic condition, and other urgent referrals from the community. SSPAUs also receive referred children. They facilitate the prompt assessment, observation, investigation, and treatment of children in a safe and dedicated child-focused environment, staffed by senior paediatric nursing staff and experienced children's and emergency doctors, without resorting to inpatient areas.

The units are particularly effective when catering for specific conditions, including breathing difficulties, fever, vomiting and diarrhoea, abdominal pains, rashes, and skin problems, as well as most viral infections. These conditions have been noted as the most common reasons for attendances in an emergency department.

The length of stay within the PAU setting can be tailored to the specific condition, observational period and treatment line (i.e. 4, 6 or 8 hours).

Current evidence supports a view that acute paediatric assessment services are a safe, efficient, and acceptable alternative to inpatient admission.

The main purpose of the units is to prevent inappropriate hospitalization and reduce the number of children being admitted for inpatient care. Patients who need to be admitted for further observation or treatment have been assessed, initially treated, stabilized, and given a prescribed care plan before leaving the PAU environment. The solution to providing high quality emergency and urgent care for young people and children is highly trained, skilled staff, with clear patient pathways and the ability to use best practice supported by a network.

The majority of children in the hospital setting can be managed without any investigations if they are assessed early by appropriately trained paediatric staff. SSPAUs and PAUs along with accident and emergency settings utilize the PEWS (Paediatric Early Warning Score) tool to promptly identify and initiate emergency treatment. Being able to identify children at risk of clinical deterioration and to facilitate timely emergency care is clearly important. These tools have the potential to optimize patient outcomes, improve quality of care and reduce the length of stay within the hospital setting.

Further reading

Tume L, Bullock I (2004) Early warning tools to identify children at risk of deterioration: a discussion. *Paediatric Nursing* 16.

Aitken P, Birch S, Cogman G, Glasper EA, Wiltshire M (2003) Quadrennial review of a paediatric emergency assessment unit. *British Journal of Nursing* 12:234–241

Index